'The Battle for Health'

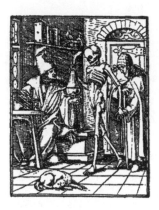

The History of Medicine in Context

Series Editors: Andrew Cunningham and Ole Peter Grell,
Department of History and Philosophy of Science,
University of Cambridge

Titles in this series will include:

Medicine from the Black Death to the French Disease
edited by Roger French, Jon Arrizabalaga,
Andrew Cunningham and Luis García-Ballester

*Faith, Medical Alchemy and Natural Philosophy:
Johann Moriaen, Reformed Intelligencer, and the Hartlib Circle*
J. T. Young

The Making of the Dentiste, *c. 1650–1760*
Roger King

'The Battle for Health'

A Political History of the Socialist Medical Association, 1930–51

JOHN STEWART

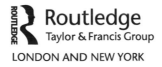

Routledge
Taylor & Francis Group

LONDON AND NEW YORK

First published 1999 by Ashgate Publishing

Reissued 2018 by Routledge
2 Park Square, Milton Park, Abingdon, Oxon, OX14 4RN
52 Vanderbilt Avenue, New York, NY 10017

Routledge is an imprint of the Taylor & Francis Group, an informa business

A Library of Congress record exists under LC control number: 98034699

Typeset in Sabon by Manton Typesetters, 5-7 Eastfield Road, Louth, Lincolnshire, LN11 7AJ

ISBN 13: 978-1-138-35041-0 (hbk)
ISBN 13: 978-1-138-35042-7 (pbk)
ISBN 13: 978-0-429-43590-4 (ebk)

Contents

Acknowledgements

I wish to thank the Wellcome Trust for supporting my research into the Socialist Medical Association. This has taken the form of research and travel expenses; and, in the academic year 1997–98, a Research Leave Fellowship. Part of that year was spent at the Wellcome Unit for the History of Medicine, University of Oxford, where much of this book was written. I am grateful to the Unit's former Director, Jane Lewis, for providing me with this facility. The archivists and staff of the British Medical Association; the British Library of Economic and Political Science; the Bodleian Library, Oxford; Churchill College Archives, Cambridge; the Public Record Office, Kew; and the Museum of Labour History are to be commended for their patience and their knowledge of the sources for which they are responsible. Particular thanks are due to Brian Dyson and his colleagues at the Brynmor Jones Library, University of Hull, which holds the archives of the Socialist Medical Association and of Somerville Hastings. Stephen Brooke, Harry Hendrick, John Macnicol, David Nash, and Charles Webster were kind enough to constructively criticise various chapters, as were the editors of the series in which this volume appears, Andrew Cunningham and Ole Grell. Errors of fact and interpretation are, of course, entirely my own responsibility. Finally, two colleagues at Oxford Brookes University, Anne Digby and Harry Hendrick, have over the years been unfailing sources of support, personal and intellectual; I am deeply indebted to them.

Abbreviations

AGM	Annual General Meeting
BMA	British Medical Association
BMJ	British Medical Journal
EC	Executive Committee (usually of the Socialist Medical Association)
EMS	Emergency Medical Service
GMC	General Medical Council
GP	General Practitioner
ILP	Independent Labour Party
LCC	London County Council
MP	Member of Parliament
MPC	Medical Planning Commission (of the British Medical Association)
MPU	Medical Practitioners' Union
MTT	Medicine Today and Tomorrow
NALT	National Association of Labour Teachers
NEC	National Executive Committee (of the Labour Party)
NHS	National Health Service
PEP	Political and Economic Planning
PHAC	Public Health Advisory Committee (of the Labour Party)
SJCIWO	Standing Joint Committee of Industrial Women's Organisations (of the Labour Party)
SMA	Socialist Medical Association
SMSA	State Medical Service Association
SPSL	Society for the Protection of Science and Learning
TUC	Trades Union Congress

CHAPTER ONE

Introduction

The National Health Service (NHS), often portrayed as the crowning achievement of the post-war Labour governments' 'welfare state', celebrated its fiftieth anniversary in 1998. One organisation which, at least by its own account, played an important role in the service's creation was the Socialist Medical Association (SMA), founded in 1930 and affiliated to the Labour Party the following year. The SMA campaigned for a unified state medical service universal in scope and free to all; served by full-time salaried staff, including medical practitioners; organised around the key institution of the health centre; emphasising preventive rather than curative medicine; and under democratic control, primarily at local level. Association members also held that medical practice, when allowed to work cooperatively and without economic barriers to the care of all patients, in itself provided a model for socialism. The way in which a socialised service was set up was therefore of equal importance with the care being delivered. These radical and innovative ideas together constituted the Association's vision of a socialised medical service, such a service being significant both in its own right and as part of the wider transition to a socialist society. In the course of its early history the SMA was able to attract, as members or supporters, prominent individuals such as the first Minister of Health, Christopher Addison; the propagandist for science, Ritchie Calder; and the medical scientists and practitioners Major Greenwood, Aleck Bourne, Richard Doll, David Stark Murray, and Somerville Hastings.

The Association has received a mixed press in scholarly studies of the political origins of the NHS. Some historians and social scientists have ignored it entirely, or suggested socialist ideology was unimportant in the formation of the new service. Others have highlighted, with varying degrees of emphasis, the SMA's participation in the debate over medical reconstruction, especially within the Labour Party. Of particular note here are the studies by Frank Honigsbaum and Charles Webster, both of whom place the Association's activities in their broader medico-political context. Ray Earwicker's unpublished doctoral thesis on the labour movement and the origins of the NHS situates the SMA in the wider field of left-wing proposals for health care reform, and is thus a vital source of information. Stephen Brooke's research on the Labour Party during the Second World War provides crucial insights into the political and policy context in which the Association operated, as well as giving credit to its role on party committees. Important as these secondary works are, none is concerned, nor claims to be concerned, solely or even primarily with the SMA. Two histories of the organisation have appeared, both by founder members and leading activists in the period under consideration. The first, by Charles Brook, came out in 1946, the year of the National Health Service Act; the second, by David Stark Murray, in 1971. Invaluable as primary sources, these nonetheless have the weaknesses as well as the strengths of books written by participants in the historical events they describe. There is thus no modern, scholarly study devoted exclusively to the SMA, a gap the present text seeks to fill.[1]

The Association was strongly of the opinion that it had played a positive and influential part in the creation of the National Health Service. Writing on the eve of the 'Appointed Day' in 1948, the day when the service actually came into operation, Murray agreed that the labour movement had long understood the need for improved health. But, he continued, it was the work of the 'small group of pioneers' who founded the SMA which had made these desires 'clear and practical' and which had 'culminated in their fruition in the national health service tomorrow'.[2] This study offers support, albeit qualified support, for this view. It argues that up until the end of World War II the Association had a central role in the formulation of Labour Party health policy, was actively involved in the wider medico-political arena, and that it hence made a significant contribution to the debates and discussions which resulted in the formation of the NHS. After the war, and with the coming of a Labour government, matters became more problematical. The SMA had deep reservations about aspects of the plan put forward, and subsequently implemented, by Labour's Minister of Health, Aneurin Bevan. In turn, Bevan was clearly sceptical about Association members, whom he privately described as 'pure but impotent'.[3]

The Labour Party as a whole had mixed feelings about its affiliate medical organisation. On the one hand, it had cause to welcome the SMA's activities, for two reasons. First, the Association put forward relatively coherent blueprints for a socialised medical service, a far from straightforward task in the 1930s and 1940s given the complexities and anomalies of both pre-war and wartime health care provision. In advancing these plans the SMA was able to employ both professional expertise and political vision. This gave its proposals credibility, even if they were not always fully agreed to by others in the labour movement or others in the medical profession.

Second, the SMA contributed directly to Labour thinking on health care in two specific ways. It was instrumental in placing the question of health service reform before Labour Party conference in the first half of the 1930s, and the consequent official commitment to a state medical service. The Association's status was then recognised and enhanced by its strong presence on the party's Public Health Advisory Committee, a body charged in the 1940s with devising a scheme for a national health service. Up until 1945, therefore, the SMA was at the heart of Labour's health policy formation. Furthermore, the organisation gained vital administrative experience through its role in running the medical services of the London County Council (LCC) after its capture by Labour in 1934. In the inter-war period an important strand in Labour thought continued to see 'municipal socialism' as a plausible social democratic strategy and the capturing of local institutions as one way of undermining the hegemony of the National Government. The Association held strongly to this view, and used its LCC achievements to further the case for a devolved and directly accountable health service.

However, despite the SMA's importance in laying the groundwork for the NHS some of its key, if radical, aspirations remained unfulfilled. Ultimately Bevan was able to convince his Cabinet colleagues, the wider Labour Party, the medical profession, and indeed the British people that his was the best plan for the reconstruction of health care provision. He agreed that compromises and concessions had, of necessity, been made to the doctors. Nonetheless Bevan could reasonably point out that in the face of political and professional objections, and serious structural constraints, a universal, comprehensive, and free service had been introduced. The Association was, as suggested, to claim credit for its role in the formation of the NHS, and that all that was best in the new service derived from its ideas. It also recognised, however, that Bevan had got his own way over what it considered vital issues. The Association was especially critical of the service's tripartite structure, the failure to introduce a salaried service, the lack of democratic control, and the effective abandonment of plans for health centres. One implication of these compromises and concessions was that a truly socialised health service had not been achieved, and some leading Association members clearly never forgave Bevan for what they saw as a betrayal.[4] These differences also highlight the important point that the Association was not alone in having views on medical reconstruction, either within the labour movement or more generally. Its plans had to compete with other proposals, on occasion put forward by those with more political influence than it could usually exert.

There is a further dimension to this 'failure' on the SMA's part to have its version of a socialised service fully realised. Although primarily concerned with medical issues, the SMA was not a narrowly-focused organisation. Its members were socialists as well as health workers, and it therefore engaged with wider political matters. In so doing the

Association invariably tended to the left of the labour and socialist movement, and this did not always endear it to the party leadership, nor to other important parts of the movement such as the Trades Union Congress (TUC). In itself this might not have mattered too much. However in the mid-1930s the Association agreed to admit members of the Communist Party. On a number of occasions this left-wing bias, particularly when it involved communist agitation, led to actual or potential areas of embarrassment and friction between the Association and the Labour Party. This tension was further exacerbated by the nature of the party itself and the political and bureaucratic system within which it operated once in government.

The differences between the Labour leadership in general, and Bevan in particular, and the Socialist Medical Association are of historical interest and significance. But they are also more than that. The Association's critique of the NHS raised important and as yet not entirely resolved questions, for example on the nature of the relationship between the medical practitioner and the state. At a time when the future of the NHS is being constantly debated, these issues take on a stark contemporary relevance. The present work critically analyses the Association's history and development from its foundation in 1930 down to the fall of the Labour government in 1951. This was the period when the SMA had the greatest opportunity to influence the debate over health service provision, and the emphasis is therefore very much on its *political* activities. The text is organised as follows.

Chapter Two examines left-wing medical politics prior to 1930, focusing especially on the activities of those individuals, organisations, and ideas which influenced the Association. Attention is paid to Sidney and Beatrice Webb, who in large part set the progressive agenda for health care reform; to the Labour Party's ideas on health care post-1918; and to the State Medical Service Association (SMSA), a body which, as its name suggests, sought the restructuring of the medical services under state supervision. Significantly, some of the founding and leading members of the SMA were involved in medical politics during this period. A key figure here was Somerville Hastings, a prominent doctor in his own right; a leading member of the SMSA; on a number of occasions an important spokesman on health matters for the Labour Party; sometime member of parliament and latterly member of the LCC; and first President of the SMA.[5]

By 1930 Hastings, along with other leading left-wing medical practitioners such as the London general practitioner (GP) Charles Brook and the Scottish pathologist David Stark Murray, had decided that the SMSA had run its course. These socialist medical activists were critical of the SMSA's lack of political clarity and its organisational isolation, and thus felt that what was now required was a medical body specifically committed to socialist politics. Chapter Three examines the setting up of the SMA and its subsequent organisational development; the principles on which it was based; and its ideas on medical reorganisation. Affiliation to the Labour Party was of crucial importance, and a key moment in the Association's history. It was through the Labour Party, therefore, that the SMA's socialist and health care aims were to be realised. However, the seeds of a long-term problem were also sown with the admission of Communist Party members from 1936.

Although still a numerically small body, the SMA began to exert a certain amount of influence during the first decade of its existence. Chapter Four places the organisation in the context of the health concerns of the broader labour movement; and in the wider medico-political sphere. Of particular significance was the Association's success in initiating debates on the future of the health services at Labour Party conferences in 1932 and (especially) 1934. In retrospect, the SMA saw this as the first real step on the road to the National Health Service. Further progress came with the reconstitution of the party's Public Health Advisory Committee, on which there was a strong Association presence. Significantly, however, the SMA did not have the medical reform field to itself, even on the political left. Part of its energies were devoted to arguing against rival schemes for health service reconstruction, socialist or otherwise. Chapter Five discusses a further important aspect of the SMA's work in the 1930s, and one of its undoubted major achievements, its participation on the LCC. The largest single provider of health care services in the country, and probably the world, the council after 1934 was an Association stronghold and this experience helped convince the SMA that local control was crucial to a socialised medical system. The LCC's health policies were also of wider significance, for example in influencing Ministry of Health civil servants as they began to examine reform of the medical services.

However, the SMA was not solely concerned with domestic issues, and Chapter Six discusses its approach to international affairs, this being underpinned by its argument that both socialism and medicine at its best were not confined by national boundaries. We therefore examine the Association's practical aid to medical refugees from Nazi and fascist persecution; its involvement with the Republican side in the Spanish Civil War; its critique of official plans for civilian protection in the event of war; and its belief that, despite the horrors of modern warfare, medicine could make both technical and organisational advances in time of war. The lessons it drew from these events confirmed its commitment to a socialist health strategy. This chapter also discusses a rather more problematic issue for the Association, its internal divisions in the early years of the war over what political position to adopt towards the conflict.

The Second World War opened up important opportunities for the Association, and was a period when its membership began to rise rapidly, in itself a sign of contemporary optimism about social reconstruction. Chapter Seven analyses in particular the SMA's involvement with the Medical Planning Commission set up by the British Medical Association (BMA); and its response to one of the founding documents of the post-war 'welfare state', the Beveridge Report. The nature of 'total war', and the accompanying problems of medical organisation, further vindicated for the SMA its views on the need for socialised health services. These themes are again evident in Chapter Eight, which examines the Association's continuing role on Labour's Public Health Advisory Committee, and its reaction to the Coalition Government's White Paper on the future of the health services. It was at this point that the organisation was at the peak of its influence within the Labour Party and clearly felt that it stood a strong chance of having its vision of a socialised medical service realised. The Association was also, however, highly conscious of both alternative plans on the political left; and the need to combat what it saw as 'medical reaction', especially as embodied in the principal professional organisation, the BMA.

As Chapter Nine illustrates, these concerns were to a significant extent justified. The NHS certainly satisfied many SMA demands, but it also ignored or played down others. The Association was especially concerned about the lack of democratic control; the tripartite system of administration; the method of remunerating medical practitioners; and the failure to introduce health centres on any significant scale. At first it was prepared to support Bevan, believing him to be a politician who would resist medical reaction and introduce a truly socialised health service. But disappointment over Bevan and his compromises and concessions soon surfaced, and the Association's critique of the NHS forms a central part of this chapter. This found little support in the broader labour movement, however, and from its position of relative strength at the end of the war the SMA became increasingly marginalised.

The final chapter therefore examines the Association's standing by the fall of the second Attlee administration in 1951. By this time the financial restraints under which the Labour governments operated had resulted, as far as the SMA was concerned, in further erosion of the principles on which a socialised medical service should be based. The Association certainly acknowledged the achievements of the NHS, but was increasingly anxious as to when the next steps towards a socialised – as distinct from national – health service would take place. The repeated references to a national 'sickness' service was one, rather cynical, manifestation of this anxiety. To these concerns were added the Association's own problems of recruitment and level of membership participation. As will become apparent throughout this work, although the SMA at its peak could claim several thousand members, much of the policy making and administration was nonetheless carried out by a handful of individuals. It was, furthermore, an organisation based principally in London. These structural problems further eroded the Association's effectiveness. We conclude, therefore, with an overall assessment of the SMA's significance, focusing especially on its role in the creation of the NHS. But it is also suggested that a number of the issues it raised, wittingly or otherwise, have contemporary validity for those concerned with the nature and organisation of social welfare and with the means and ends of socialism.

Notes

1. Frank Honigsbaum, *The Division in British Medicine*, Kogan Page, 1979; Charles Webster, 'Labour and the Origins of the National Health Service', in Rupke, Nicolaas (ed.), *Science, Politics and the Public Good*, Macmillan, 1988; Ray Earwicker, 'The Labour Movement and the Creation of the National Health Service', unpublished PhD thesis, University of Birmingham, 1982; Stephen Brooke, *Labour's War*, Oxford, Oxford University Press, 1992; David Stark Murray, *Why a National Health Service?*, Pemberton Books, 1971; and Charles Brook, *Making Medical History*, Percy B. Buxton, 1946. Others who note, albeit with considerable differences in emphasis, the role and interventions of the SMA and/or the part played by 'socialism' in the creation of the National Health Service, include Harry Eckstein, *The English Health Service*, Cambridge, Mass., Harvard University Press, 1958; Daniel Fox, 'The National Health Service and the Second World War: the Elaboration of Consensus', in Smith, H.L. (ed.), *War and Social Change*, Manchester, Manchester University Press, 1986; Daniel Fox, *Health Policies, Health Politics: the British and American Experience, 1911–1965*, Princeton, New Jersey, Princeton University Press, 1986; Martin Francis, *Ideas and Policies under Labour, 1945–1951*, Manchester, Manchester University Press, 1997; Rudolf Klein, *The New Politics of the NHS*, 3rd edn, Longman, 1995; Almont Lindsey, *Socialized Medicine in England and Wales*, Chapel Hill, University of North Carolina Press, 1962; Arthur Marwick, 'The Labour Party and the Welfare State in Britain, 1900–1948', *American Historical Review*, December 1967; Vicente Navarro, *Class Struggle, the State and Medicine*, Oxford, Martin Robertson, 1978; John Pater, *The Making of the National Health Service*, King Edward's Hospital Fund, 1981; Steve Watkins, *Medicine and Labour: the Politics of a Profession*, Lawrence and Wishart, 1987; Charles Webster, *The Health Services since the War: vol. 1, Problems of Health Care – The National Health Service before 1957*, HMSO, 1988; and *idem*, 'Conflict and Consensus: Explaining the British Health Service', *Twentieth Century British History*, 1990, 1, 2 – this is an important review of the historiography of the National Health Service.

2.   Irwin Brown (David Stark Murray), *Back-Room Boys of State Medicine*, Socialist Medical Association, 1948, p. 1.
3.   Jennie Lee, *My Life with Nye*, Jonathan Cape, 1980, p. 177.
4.   See, for example, John Stewart, 'The "Back-Room Boys of State Medicine": David Stark Murray and Bevan's National Health Service', *Journal of Medical Biography*, November 1996.
5.   On Hastings's career down to the 1940s see John Stewart, 'Socialist Proposals for Health Reform in Inter-War Britain: the Case of Somerville Hastings', *Medical History*, 39, July 1995. For his life as a whole see *idem*, 'Somerville Hastings', in the forthcoming *New Dictionary of National Biography*, London and Oxford, British Academy/Oxford University Press, 2004, and the entry in Honigsbaum, *The Division in British Medicine*, pp. 327–8.

CHAPTER TWO

The Genesis of the SMA, 1900–1930

The physical condition of the working class had long been a labour movement concern. As leading SMA member David Stark Murray put it, rather melodramatically, during the passage of the National Health Service Bill in 1946, when it came to such a service 'Keir Hardie (and he wasn't the first) thought of it in 1868 when he first went down a pit'.[1] Early socialist analyses tended to see in the abolition of capitalism the solution to all problems, including those related to health. This attitude persisted well into the twentieth century, and one of the principal arguments of the SMA was to be that capitalism per se *and* the capitalistic organisation of medical care both contributed to individual and national ill health. One of the central problems of social democracy is highlighted by such analysis: that is, which is to be prioritised: economic reform which ultimately will be to the material benefit of the whole population, including the working class; or social reform to ameliorate, in the relatively short term, the conditions under which working class people are currently disadvantaged?

Nonetheless, by the beginning of the twentieth century it was increasingly acknowledged that reform of existing medical provision was an urgent necessity, and that such reconstruction could in itself contribute to the transition to a socialist society. As Webster points out, the Labour Party was, from its foundation in 1900, committed to the abolition of the Poor Law, which in itself implied the creation of medical services free from the stigma of pauperism. The early 1900s also saw the formation of several left-wing medical pressure groups, and Murray further claimed in 1946 that the original 'pioneers' of state medicine were to be found in the Edwardian period. He gave particular credit to the SMSA, discussed further below, and to individuals such as Dr George Geddis of the Independent Labour Party (ILP), who had attacked private practice and proposed in its place a state salaried system. As Murray put it, Geddis 'visualised the profession as a disciplined army waging war against the forces that threaten the national health', a telling metaphor given the SMA's identification of the 'battle for health'.[2]

However, as Murray argued on yet another occasion, it was 'the early Fabians who first made health a truly political subject'. Dr F. Lawson Dodd, for example, later to become a member of the SMSA and treasurer to the Fabian Society, as well as being the originator of the famous Fabian summer schools, told a Society audience in 1907 that long

before 'industry as a whole is taken over by the State ... the medical
service will be nationalized'. Competition within the medical profession, as currently existed, was harmful in that it reduced fees, destroyed
'fraternal cooperation', and hindered scientific progress. Hospital services too were inadequate, and overall a 'co-ordinated State medical
service' was required. Interestingly, for as we shall see this was to be an
SMA concern, Dodd emphasised the benefits of such a scheme for the
middle class, and his speech was one of a series on 'Socialism and the
Middle Classes'.[3]

The Webbs and the medical services

But the first really important left-wing articulation of the need for the
reform of health care provision came from that quintessentially Fabian
partnership, Sidney and Beatrice Webb, initially through the Minority
Report of the Royal Commission on the Poor Law. Beatrice presented
her memorandum on the medical services of the Poor Law and Local
Government Public Health Departments to the Royal Commission in
September 1907. This was, typically, both highly detailed and historically informed. The dual nature of the existing system – that is the
division of responsibilities between the Poor Law and local government
– resulted in the two different parts working to different principles and
aims, the outcome being 'chaos, almost ludicrous in its paradoxes'.[4]
This notion of anarchy in the health services – manifested by overlaps,
omissions, and lack of any coordination or planning – was to be central
to left-wing critiques over the next thirty years. Webb's solution, con-
forming to her more general aim of breaking up the Poor Law, was a
unified, preventive service, although at this stage she saw no need for an
end to private practice or the voluntary hospitals.

The Webb memorandum was published in 1910 as *The State and the
Doctor*. Here the point was made that despite untold millions being
expended on health, the end result was two separate and ill-coordinated
services, one consequence of which was a huge, undiscovered, volume
of disease, particularly among the young. Even where help was given,
this was not always to best effect. From the 'standpoint of national
health' medical relief might be seen as 'worse than useless'. It encouraged individual patients to have 'faith in the taking of medicine instead
of reliance on hygienic regimen', and thereby counteracted the 'efforts
of the Public Health medical service in the promotion of personal
hygiene'.[5]

Once again, the stress on preventive medicine was to be a central
theme of left-wing medicine in the coming years, if generally without

the moralising so typical of the Webbs. The problems of housing and employment conditions were also to be highlighted more than the personal shortcomings the Webbs clearly found so distasteful, although their emphasis on individual responsibility could have the effect of showing up blatant anomalies in the system. They pointed out, for example, that those who had 'neglected the elementary duties of personal cleanliness' by becoming infested with lice could receive free treatment and, in some cases, replacement clothes, all without the stigma of pauperism. By contrast, the individual who contracted an occupational disease 'in the earning of his daily bread' had no rights to medical treatment unless he or she became destitute. Apart from any other reason, therefore, health reform was needed to 'curb physical self-indulgence … and positively heighten the desire and capacity of all persons to maintain themselves'.[6] As we shall see, SMA members were to argue that, when a fully socialised health service was in place, individuals would have significant responsibility for the maintenance of their own bodies. Duties as well as rights were to be emphasised in the Association's vision of health care in a socialist society.

The Webbs thus argued the pressing need for a unified service, 'based on Public Health rather than upon Poor Law principles'. In terms of organisation, they assumed the continuance of local authority control, albeit supervised by 'a single Central Department' which would bring under one roof all the currently scattered health responsibilities of the various branches of national government. The role of this body was, however, 'not to centralise administration, but, on the contrary, to set local life in motion', and these local bodies would be under democratic control.[7] Local control of health services was to be another key aspect of the SMA's proposals for a socialised service. This emphasis on localism was a characteristic not only of Association thinking, but also formed an important strand in Labour Party attitudes towards social welfare.

Of course there were areas of health policy where the Webbs were either ambiguous, or sought to maintain or reinforce the existing system. On the question of voluntary hospitals – institutions maintained by private donations or subscriptions – they noted inadequacies in the current level of provision and serious gaps in coverage of places and social groups, and felt it unlikely that this would change. On the other hand, there was no suggestion of voluntary hospitals being abolished, and it was even felt that certain types of case might be beneficially transferred to these from public institutions.[8] Similarly, the Webbs did not think that medical treatment should necessarily be free. In 'the public interest' neither the speed with which a patient received treatment, nor its efficiency, should be hampered by money. Nonetheless, there was no reason why costs should not be recovered from those able to pay. This would also help resolve another potential problem, that any unified service would be 'detrimental to the interests of the private practitioner, if not the medical profession as a whole'. This was a belief which was, for the Webbs, based on a misapprehension. The main aim of fees and charges was to

> confine the medical services of the Health Department to that section of the population which must, in the interests of the community as a whole, be provided with medical attendance at the public expense.

For all others, the 'prosperous workman, or the stingy person of the lower middle class', there would be no incentive to use public services, since they would be charged as in private medical practice. Hence those who could afford it would exercise their right to free choice of doctor, and this would ensure – indeed enhance – the private practitioner's prosperity. Furthermore, this 'free choice' of doctor should be confined to the private sector. This did not mean, though, that there was no place for state salaried practitioners. Each public health department was to have available 'the necessary staff of whole-time salaried officers, including clinicians as well as sanitarians, institution superintendents as well as domiciliary practitioners'.[9]

Sidney and Beatrice Webb proposed significant and far-reaching changes in health care provision while suggesting that some existing features remain in place. Subsequent reformers, including the SMA, were to be deeply influenced by their ideas. In particular, the importance of preventive medicine, a unified service, and local authority control were to be central to the Association's plans for a socialised health service. Other aspects of the Webbs' thinking, however, were to be rejected, especially the continuance of voluntary hospitals and of private practice.

The contemporary response to the Webbs of one individual, Somerville Hastings, is particularly noteworthy in the context of this study. Hastings, the single most important figure in the SMA's early history, was later to recall the role of both his medical training and his religious background in shaping his political beliefs. In the local village chapel, for example, he found 'the cradle of democracy', and Hastings was to remain committed to the view that true democracy and socialism were mutually reinforcing. It is highly possible that these retrospective remarks were filtered through the philosophy of R.H. Tawney, whom Hastings knew and with whom he clearly shared a number of preoccupations. Prior to 1914 Hastings was politically active in both the ILP and the Fabian Society (not being a trade unionist, he was ineligible at this stage for Labour Party membership); attended Fabian summer schools at Harlech, and was friendly with prominent Society figures such as Dodd and George Bernard Shaw (the latter speaking on Hastings's behalf during his various attempts to be elected to the Commons in the 1920s and 1930s); and participated in meetings at the Webbs' house.[10]

Hastings was clearly deeply impressed by the Minority Report. His own copy is copiously underlined, and the passages highlighted are interesting in view of the development of his own ideas. As part of their discussion of the Poor Law Medical Services, the Webbs argued that 'its lack of coordination between domiciliary inspection and institutional treatment' was one reason why it was 'practically useless'. Similarly, the Minority Report's authors stressed the need for a State Medical service concerned with 'searching out disease' and 'aiming always at preventing either recurrence or spread of disease'. These phrases and sentences, specifically picked out by Hastings, were to become central to his own critique of existing health care provision.[11]

Hastings also responded publicly to the Minority Report, in a pamphlet written with two colleagues. He and his fellow authors argued that the Poor Law had to be finally broken up, a process already well under way. Similarly, the current dual system of health was inefficient, and no doctor who had worked in impoverished areas could fail to see the need for change in 'the present confused methods of looking after the health of the poor'. As the Webbs suggested, unification would be cheaper and administratively simpler. At this point, Hastings and his colleagues were prepared to go along with the idea of private practice being effectively protected and enhanced by a unified public service. Should a reformed service become 'Socialistic', then doctors should have nothing to do with it, since they would both lose income from patients and be forced to pay for the state service by way of taxes and rates. Rather curiously, for there was no significant ambiguity about the Minority proposals, the authors sought clarification from the Webbs on this issue. However they also saw a role for a greatly expanded, and salaried, public medical service. They suggested that a large proportion of doctors, possibly one third, were already state employees, and that 'it may reasonably be anticipated that the proportion will be greater under the Minority scheme'. Again to reassure those who would remain outside the public sector, the authors claimed that this expansion of state practitioners would benefit those in private practice by relieving pressure on an overcrowded profession. The Report's implementation would thus involve more work for doctors in both the public and the private sectors.[12]

Nonetheless, and here again there is something of a difference from the Webbs, it was stressed that public service doctoring was good in itself. It would bring security in the form of salary and pensions, and the idea that the publicly employed doctor would experience a 'crushing of his individuality' was rejected. On the contrary, freedom from financial worries would open up whole new areas of medical experience for the individual practitioner. This notion of the benefits doctors would enjoy, both intellectual and economic, in a state service, was something the SMA was to emphasise in the 1930s and 1940s as it sought to win over the hostile mass of general practitioners to its version of a state medical system. In 1910, however, Hastings and his colleagues had more modest aims. Raising, like the Webbs, the importance of preventive medicine, they concluded that the Minority proposals were of significance not just for doctors, but for society as a whole. The combination of a well-organised public sector working in cooperation with a skilled, if private, medical profession would do much to enhance the 'health and with it the self-respect of our people'. Underlying the proposals was an 'intense desire to prevent what evil can be prevented'.[13]

The State Medical Service Association

The Webbs provided an important schema for socialist medical reformers, one which would continue to be influential into the 1940s. However, theirs was not the only model. In 1911 Benjamin Moore, Professor of Biochemistry at Liverpool University, who in the following year was going to be instrumental in founding the State Medical Service Association, published his proposals for medical reform. Moore suggested that a 'National Health Service' would both strengthen the 'physique of the race' and save national resources. Realistically, however, the creation of such a system would take a whole generation, partly because of the anticipated hostility of the medical profession. Moore felt that without this 'vested interest' – a phrase which recurs throughout left-wing critiques of health care provision – his new service would be staffed from the start by full-time, salaried doctors. Although this would not happen immediately, it should remain the ultimate aim. Similarly, Moore saw the need for a unified hospital service. As will become apparent as this book progresses, these were to be two of the main SMA preoccupations. Significantly, however, Moore at this stage sought to appeal not just to the medical left, but across the political spectrum, despite his own socialist beliefs.[14]

The SMSA held its inaugural meeting in July 1912, and by the end of the year had organised itself into various committees. Among these was the propaganda committee, which Somerville Hastings joined in late 1912 and of which he was, by early the next year, secretary. The organisation was primarily concerned (unsurprisingly given Moore's role in its foundation) with a salaried service and a unified hospital system. Its eight founding principles were as follows. First, a state medical service to be administered by a Board of Health under the supervision of a Cabinet-rank minister, the Minister of Public Health. The need for a separate Health Ministry was prominent among reformers' demands in the Edwardian era. Second, one of the service's 'primary objects' should be the unification of preventive and curative medicine. Third, entry to the medical profession should be by one state examination only. So far, this was not dissimilar to the plan put forward by the Webbs and by Hastings and his colleagues, especially with respect to the first two points.[15]

However, the other five founding principles of the SMSA began to move off in a potentially different direction. First, the *whole* (my emphasis) profession was to be organised along the lines of other existing state services. Second, medical salaries should be increased gradually according to length of service and position, and should attract pension rights. This was not necessarily different from what reformers such as the Webbs had proposed, but the stress on the salaried principle is important. Third, and again in theory compatible with previous reformers' aims, the public ought to have a choice of doctor, while no practitioner should be required to take on more than a certain number of patients. Important, though, is the notion that this is predicated on a salaried, and full time, service. Fourth, and here there is a much more obvious break with, for example, the Minority Report, all hospitals should be nationalised, and used for the various types of medical care and treatment in conjunction with the patient's own doctor. Finally, the services of all state doctors should be available to everyone, irrespective of income. This is in obvious contrast to the Webbs' idea of encouraging those who could to consult private practitioners.[16]

There were possible ambiguities here: for one thing it is not made entirely clear whether private practice was to be totally abolished. Furthermore, important issues were not, as yet, addressed: there was no obvious equivalent, for instance, of the Webbs' emphasis on the role of democratically elected local authorities. Honigsbaum therefore rather overstates the initial similarities between the Webbs and the SMSA: the former were not entirely averse to private practice, the latter did not look clearly at the question of administration and control.[17] However it is evident that the Socialist Medical Association was to owe a huge intellectual debt to both the SMSA and the Webbs. Hastings was later to claim, for example, that the SMSA was among the first to recognise the necessity of preventive medicine, a principle central to SMA thinking.[18]

Moore's own ideas were further clarified in 1913. In line with contemporary social thought, the gains in 'national efficiency' which a state medical service would bring were highlighted. These would be not only financial but also through, for instance, the saving of between 80–100 000 child lives per year. Moore again emphasised matters such as the creation of a salaried medical profession. This was, he suggested, the only way in which doctors would escape from 'drudgery ... to a land of devoted service' wherein they would be able to pursue their altruistic desire to bring health to their fellow human beings. Moore also argued for an expansion of health insurance and gave more specific details than previously as to how a state service might be administered. He was convinced that central control under a Minister of Health was vital, not least in preventing overlap of function. But Moore also recognized the role of – albeit reorganised – local authorities. He shared the Webbs' contempt for the Poor Law Medical Services, and suggested the creation of an intermediary layer between centre and locality. The aim here was to avoid over-bureaucratic, centralised control.[19]

Once again, such proposals were to be key aspects of the SMA programme for socialised health care, and it is apparent that Moore's arguments here were in a number of respects close to those of the Webbs. Indeed, despite the differences stressed above between the SMSA and the Webbs, Sidney was an Association vice-president, a platform from which he could expand on his plans for medical reform. In November 1912, for example, he addressed the Service Organisation Committee, set up to examine the possible construction of a state service. Webb pointed out that at present health services were 'controlled locally and that many Local Authorities took great pride in their work'. It would thus be difficult to take such functions away from them and place them under 'central management' which, furthermore, involved 'rigidity and fixity of methods of administration'. He therefore recommended a devolved system based on existing local authorities, 'stimulated towards efficiency by substantial "Grants in Aid" from the Board of Health'.[20]

A further instance of the attempt to work out a blueprint for all aspects of a socialised medical service can be found in an SMSA meeting in early 1914. At this the customary resolution demanding a state medical service was passed. Among those who spoke was the Bermondsey GP, and later MP, councillor, and SMA founder member, Alfred Salter. As well as describing the health problems of working-class districts, to one of which he devoted his entire medical and political career, Salter also suggested a 'democratisation' of the medical profession. By this he appears to have meant a much more broadly-based entry into the profession, and he suggested that medical education might be altered to take this into account. Apart from anything else, this would ensure a 'necessary increase' in the supply of doctors. The demand that doctors more accurately reflect the composition of society was later taken up by the SMA. Similarly, the question of control of the health services continued to be raised in SMSA meetings. Sidney Webb, for example, told one gathering that 'doctors should not be members of governing committees but should work through advisory committees'. In true Webb style, he then appears to have argued for the importance of medical administrators. As Murray points out, the issue of administrative control being debated here was to recur right down to, and beyond, the founding of the NHS.[21]

By the outbreak of the First World War the need for, and the nature of, a socialised medical service was being debated by 'progressive' social reformers and doctors. There were differences of emphasis between them, not surprisingly given their attempts to build a new health care system from first principles. The significance of this left-wing intervention should not be exaggerated. The SMSA, for instance, was a small organisation, with fewer than 150 members in 1912, and was well aware of the obstacles confronting its tentative proposals. An Executive Committee meeting in December 1913, at which Hastings was present, discussed the 'panel' system set up by the 1911 National Insurance Act and noted the bitter opposition of the 'great majority' of panel doctors 'to the ideals of the SMS Association'. The SMSA also had problems in broadcasting its message. It had initially hoped for support for its policies from the journal *Medical World*, but this failed to materialise. Similarly, a decision on whether to broaden the scope of the organisation 'to appeal more directly to the public' was deferred in 1914. It was felt that a 'definite scheme' for a state service should first be drawn up, and a sub-committee of eight, including Hastings and Salter, was formed for this purpose.[22]

In the wider context the labour movement, the most apparently sympathetic constituency for those seeking a socialised medical service, had shown itself divided over the extremely modest health provisions of the 1911 Act. Many in the political wing of the movement were sceptical about the insurance principle, expressing concern about both the limited coverage provided by the Act and how it was financed. By contrast the trades unions and leading political figures such as Ramsay MacDonald and Beatrice Webb were broadly in favour of insurance, although it is notable that the Webbs had, by 1914, recognised the system's limitations. This was particularly so, as both they and other reformers pointed out, in respect of working class women.[23]

Nonetheless in the pre-First World War discussions over the nature and aims of medical care it is possible to find, as Murray on more than one occasion suggested, in the 'writings of a handful of men around 1910–14 ... the real origin of all that is important in health services'. More specifically, and implying an important shift of perspective in the period, Murray also claimed that from the time of the Minority Report 'the call of earlier political reformers for improved health conditions became a call for an organized medical service'. The period saw too the emergence of a number of individuals who were to have an important role in left-wing medical politics after World War I. As we have seen, Salter and Hastings were already active and, according to Murray, Moore was a significant influence on H.H. MacWilliam, later author of the important 'Walton Plan', discussed further in Chapter Four.[24]

Moreover, within the broader labour movement, calls were being made prior to 1914 for a more comprehensive state medical service. Labour MPs such as George Lansbury sought, unsuccessfully, to expand the terms of the health part of the 1911 Act. Marwick contrasts contemporary Labour demands for hospital nationalisation and a state medical service with the 'Webb idea of a service for the very poor only' – although as noted this is something of an exaggeration – suggesting that from now onwards Labour would insist on a 'comprehensive, classless ... service'.[25] This is an important point, one which in the long term has significant validity. It is also evident that a sense of the origins and development of the health services was important to Murray and his SMA colleagues, for they stressed the part played by left-wing medical activists campaigning over a long period for what appeared to be achieved after 1945. In turn, historical evidence could be used to counter the claims of bodies such as the BMA that it was they who were responsible for the NHS. But although the SMA was able to draw on historical traditions and precedents in its arguments for a national health service, it was also conscious, as subsequent chapters will illustrate, of the need to adapt to changing circumstances. More problematical was its ability to persuade, in the last resort, the rest of the labour movement of the historical and contemporary validity of its case.

The decline of the SMSA, and the development of Labour's health policies

The SMSA kept up its activities during the First World War, albeit under difficult conditions, with Hastings continuing to play a leading role. The war itself raised the question of the shape of the health services once hostilities ceased, part of the wider debate within the British left over what form post-war society should take. Various attempts were made to draft parliamentary Bills, and discussions held with government ministers. As the Executive Committee noted in the autumn of 1917, the 'great social upheaval' of the war had led to 'changes in public opinion'. This in turn indicated the 'advisability of instituting an Association for propaganda on a wider basis than hitherto', with the aim of advancing the cause of national health and physical welfare.[26]

The meaning of this can only be fully understood in the light of the subsequent General Meeting of the Association, where it was announced that a 'Welfare Group' had been formed whose specific aim was to work for the SMSA's objectives 'through and with the Labour Party'. This was to be independent of the Association, 'as it was important that the SMSA should remain a non-Party organisation'.[27] What this effectively meant was that Moore and Hastings became members of the Labour Party's Public Health Advisory Committee (PHAC), and indeed were largely responsible for the creation of this body, discussed further below. Importantly for the future development of socialist medical politics, certain key SMSA activists – notably Hastings – were clearly beginning to doubt the efficacy of the Association's 'non-party' stance, and were prepared for both ideological and practical reasons to concentrate their energies on the Labour Party.

Another important SMSA response to the war and its implications for the medical services came in a *Lancet* article by Moore and Charles Parker in the summer of 1918, copies of which were distributed to all Association members. Restating the case for a 'State Medical Service', the authors first identified 'Five Essentials': a Ministry of Health, headed by a minister of Cabinet rank; a Medical Research Service; an expanded Public Health Service; cooperation between preventive and curative services; and a Public Clinical Service. Elaborating, Moore and Parker argued for medical services to be comprehensive and free; for there to be a full-time salaried service; and for an administrative structure with central control but local administration. Voluntary hospitals were to be allowed to remain, but the public hospital system considerably expanded.[28] The rather more conciliatory approach to the voluntary hospitals notwithstanding, this was not dissimilar to earlier SMSA pronouncements on medical reorganisation.

However, two further points should be noted. First, Moore and Parker's article was part of a wider contemporary debate over the future of the health services. Not only did they contribute to the *Lancet*'s series of articles on the subject, so too did Sir Bernard (later Lord) Dawson. Dawson subsequently chaired the committee which in 1920 produced a report – the Dawson Report – which sought to protect the general practitioner and the panel system while recognising the need for medical reorganisation through, for example, the institution of 'health centres'.

As Webster puts it, the participants in this debate were seeking to gain 'the high ground of medical planning'. Second, Moore and Parker likewise pressed strongly for 'health centres', an idea embryonically present in pre-1914 SMSA writings. This was to involve locating all primary health functions in such institutions, which were also to be closely linked with local hospitals. They were, in addition, to be used to change the role of the general practitioner, who was to be integrated with other medical services and work as part of a team. This would give GPs the opportunity for further medical training through specialisation. Further, they would become salaried employees of the state, rather than independent contractors, and patients would have the right to a free choice of doctor.[29]

As Murray rightly points out, the Dawson Report is 'often spoken of as if it invented Health Centres', but this was not the case, for two reasons. First, the proposals of Moore, Parker, and the SMSA pre-dated those of Dawson. In 1946 Murray claimed that Parker was advocating health centres in 1912, and even this was not when they were first conceptualised. And while he did not 'visualise the Health Centre as we do today', Parker was nonetheless more advanced in his thinking on the subject than the 'official medical spokesmen' of the mid-1940s. Second, what Dawson envisaged did not approximate to what a *real* health centre should involve: for example his report showed 'no inkling of group practice'. This view has been largely substantiated by Webster and others, who see in Dawson's scheme a reaction and antidote to left-wing medical thought. Interestingly, although with a frustrating lack of chronological clarity, Brook later recalled that '(L)ong before the National Health Service' Alfred Salter had founded the Bermondsey Public Health Centre, where a range of medical and allied services were apparently available.[30]

If the Dawson Report was intended to forestall left-wing medical agitation, then it appears to have been successful, at least as far as the SMSA was concerned. According to Murray, the organisation met only once in 1919; then not until 1921; and then not until 1928, when it was partially revived and renamed the National Medical Service Association. During 1928 and 1929, by which time Hastings was its chairman and effectively its leader, various attempts were made to renew activities despite Moore's view that it ought to be wound up. A grant of £50 was given to the PHAC for the publication of a book on public health. The organisation's aims were restated, including its determination to remain non-political. This in turn caused it to decline the offer, in early 1931, of amalgamation with the Socialist Medical Association. However, despite the presence of medical activists such as Hastings, Salter, Hector Munro and Ethel Bentham – all of whom were also involved with the SMA – the 1931 meeting was the last recorded.[31]

A number of reasons can be put forward for the SMSA's decline. First, Murray suggests that the Dawson Report, and its apparent advocacy of health centres, led some members to believe that 'the job was finished', while 'failing to realize just how long a battle still had to be fought'. Second, the political climate of the 1920s was different from that of Edwardian progressivism and of wartime and immediate post-war hopes of social reconstruction, as exemplified by reformers' expectations of the newly created Ministry of Health. Economic depression, the return of a Conservative administration, and the hostility of the medical profession meant that the radical restructuring of the health services was not high on the list of governmental priorities. As Honigsbaum points out, this was a time when even routine checks of panel records were denounced as 'medical socialism'.[32] On the other hand, the post-war period saw Labour's emergence as the main opposition party, and many of the medical left's more committed socialists began to devote their energies to Labour politics. As a non-aligned organisation, the SMSA was going to be squeezed in such circumstances. The SMSA clearly served an important function in the development of socialist medical thought, but by the 1920s was effectively marginalised.

At the same time a number of left-wing medical activists had, by the 1920s, become involved in the Medical Practitioners' Union (MPU), founded in 1914. Although an organisation with which the SMA was going to have troubled relations – for example over medical refugees – and which remained determinedly 'non-political', the MPU had an important role in mobilising general practitioners on, in principle at least, a trade union basis. This was acknowledged by its affiliation to the TUC in 1934. By the late 1920s individuals who were to be important in the SMA had gained leading MPU positions. Charles Brook was elected to its executive in July 1929, while its general secretary, Alfred Welply, became the Association's first treasurer.[33] The SMA did not, therefore, come from nowhere. Its leading members had considerable experience of medical politics by 1930, the lessons of which they sought to bring to the new organisation. They also, of course, operated in the context of the Labour Party, whose post-war health policies we now examine.

Webster argues that during the 1920s 'there was a notable decline in Labour central leadership on the health front', with health matters usually subsumed under housing and social security proposals. Arthur Marwick, on the other hand, finds a 'flurry of special conferences and policy documents in the 1920s', surprisingly ignored by historians of both the welfare state and the Labour Party, although he also notes that at least in the short term this had little impact on overall policy.

Paradoxically, both of these positions are largely correct, and this relates to the point made earlier, namely the social democratic dilemma of whether to prioritise economic reconstruction or social welfare. It was possible for the labour movement to emphasise economic and industrial matters while on occasions – although not to the extent Marwick suggests – producing important statements on the future of the medical services. As Earwicker points out, social improvement was only of 'secondary concern' in the Party's policy discussions in the immediate post-war period, with even here health taking a low priority. On the other hand, a document such as that on the curative and preventive medical services could be full of 'positive and detailed proposals' which 'firmly established the guidelines for medical debate within the movement up until the NHS Act of 1946'.[34]

Two further points must be borne in mind. First, politics takes place not only at the centre, in parliament or on national executive committees. Local activity remained extremely important in this period, and many labour and socialist activists saw their main political commitments as being with Boards of Guardians or local authorities. This had particular implications for social policy, including health, since such bodies continued to be important providers of welfare. They were also seen as more accountable, and thereby 'democratic', than the Commons in London, especially in an era when Labour had only limited success at national level. Local control of medical services was to be central to the SMA's proposals for a democratic health service, and in line with an existing tradition in left-wing thinking on social welfare.[35] Second, like all political parties, the Labour Party was not homogeneous. If it tended to prioritise economic and industrial matters, this was because of the importance within it of male, manual worker, trades unionists. Other groups and individuals, however, paid rather more attention to welfare matters. These included women's organisations and professionals such as doctors. It is in these circumstances that the party's health policy proposals and, in particular, the activities of future SMA members, are examined.

At Labour Party conference in 1918, a motion on health was proposed – by Dr Marion Phillips of the Women's Labour League – and unanimously carried.[36] One of its principal features was the centralising of all health services under a Ministry of Health, but with local authorities having responsibility for policy implementation. This should be placed in the broader framework of Labour's plans for 'reconstruction' and, in a famous phrase, a 'new social order'. One outcome of these concerns was the Public Health Advisory Committee, one of a number of such bodies created in the post-war period, in this particular case as a result, as we have seen, of pressure by Moore and the SMSA. Among its members were Moore and Parker; Beatrice Webb; and future SMA activists G.P. Blizard (committee secretary until 1920), Alfred Salter, Ethel Bentham and, most importantly of all, Somerville Hastings. The setting up of the committee was the subject of typically cautious correspondence from Sidney Webb to the *British Medical Journal (BMJ)*, in which he denied that Labour was interested in a state medical service, or that it was committed to any particular plan. Nonetheless he did press the need for some extension of municipal services and their unification under a single authority, very much standard Webb ideas.[37] His caution was, however, an early indication of some of the institutional constraints the committee was to face.

Its most important publication, which came out in various versions from 1918 onwards, was a collection of memoranda dealing in a highly detailed way with a broad range of medical topics. This was the document so highly praised by Earwicker.[38] Worth noting are its suggestions that medical practice had failed to keep pace with medical science, and that greater emphasis should be placed on preventive medicine; that a remodelled health service should be under democratic control, nationally and locally; and that health centres, based on local hospitals and with doctors working cooperatively rather than independently, should be the norm. Furthermore, a state medical service should be 'free and open to all', and financed by a 'charge upon communal funds' rather than by insurance. Realising, perhaps, both the radicalism of their proposals and the administrative problems associated with the replacement of one system, highly disorganised and overlapping as it was, with another, the committee also proposed a 'transition stage' between the two. This clearly derived from Moore and Parker's *Lancet* scheme of 1918. It was also notable, in light of the later SMA position on the subject, that in 1919 the committee agreed to delete from the earlier version the demand for 'whole-time' salaried service. This followed shortly after a letter from the Labour Party suggesting that the current version not be published in view of its 'conflicting findings'.[39]

The debt this important document owes to the Webbs and the SMSA is evident. Of particular interest is the adoption of the idea of health centres, an issue which was to become central to SMA plans for a socialised medical service. We have already noted how Moore and Parker's proposals in this respect had affected more 'conservative' thinking, and in particular the Dawson Report. To this should now be added the impact of the PHAC's work. As Webster puts it, one further way of looking at the Dawson Report is as a 'counterblast to Labour proposals, written from the perspective of a medical élite desperately searching for a means to salvage the general practitioner from impending redundancy'.[40]

However, reservations have to be made about the activities of the PHAC. First, the committee as a whole rejected the proposals of a sub-committee looking into the role of general practitioners in a socialised medical service. While appearing not to rule out entirely the future of private practice, the sub-committee nonetheless went a long way towards a salaried state service. According to Marwick, the 'influential minority' behind this rejected proposal had Hastings as a leading figure. Hastings, both in his own right in the 1920s and as founding president of the SMA thereafter, was to continually press the need for an end to private practice. This contextualises the earlier point concerning the deletion of a full-time salaried service from the original document.[41] It was almost certainly episodes such as this which caused Hastings and Moore to report to the SMSA Executive in September 1918 that 'schemes for a State Medical Service were not receiving due attention' on the PHAC. Consequently the committee chairman, W.R. Anderson, was to be asked to press this issue and to put aside time for discussion of Parker and Moore's *Lancet* article.[42]

Second, the place of all the advisory committees set up after 1918 was highly ambiguous, not least because some of their 'expert' members came from outside the ranks of the labour movement, and this was as true of the PHAC as any other. The autonomy and initiative in policy making that might have resulted was, however, not acceptable to the unions, and by 1924 the committees were effectively brought to heel by the TUC. This meant that those with radical proposals for social reform found it difficult to put these forward inside the party itself. This was despite the efforts of individuals such as Hastings, who was clearly anxious to maintain as close a relationship as possible between the committee and the Labour Party.[43]

All this contributed to what Duncan Tanner describes as a 'general climate of anti-intellectualism' which did little to encourage new policy initiatives. Little wonder, then, that the PHAC became, in Webster's expression, 'relatively inert', even after reorganisation in the late 1920s, by which time Hastings was its chairman. In the early 1930s it produced, jointly with the Standing Joint Committee of Industrial Women's Organisations (SJCIWO), a report on *Hospitals and the Patient*. The Joint Committee, chaired by Hastings and also including SMA members Esther Rickards and Amy Sayle, concluded that for hospitals 'only a coordinated system can give full service'; and that for a long time voluntary hospitals had been run for the convenience of honorary staff and doctors rather than patient comfort. Such points were to be part of a wider criticism of the voluntary hospital system put forward by the SMA. However, by this stage the PHAC did not have any properly defined function. It was suspended in 1932, and only became of significance again in the late 1930s, when revived by Hastings.[44]

The Health Committee's problems notwithstanding, two other Labour Party interventions on health matters in the 1920s are worth noting. The first concerned what was described as the hospital 'crisis'. In 1922 a joint Labour Party/TUC publication called for a radical reorganisation of hospital provision, very much along the lines advocated by Moore and Parker in 1918. This was followed in April 1924 by a conference organised by Labour's National Executive Committee (NEC) and attended by interested parties such as the BMA and the MPU. In a letter to the conference the first Labour Prime Minister, Ramsay MacDonald, urged that what was now required in hospital provision, as in other areas of national life, was 'the application of the scientific spirit, the coordination of effort, and the elimination of waste', themes taken up at the meeting itself by Hastings. The only way out of the 'present impasse', he argued, was for the state to take responsibility for 'providing hospital treatment for all who needed it'. Labour viewed health as a 'national concern', and believed it positively dangerous to have hospitals reliant on charity or private enterprise. As Marwick suggests, no significant consensus was reached because of the diverse interests represented, and in particular because of Labour's arguments for the integration of voluntary hospitals into a public system, a point not lost on the supporters of these institutions.[45] Nonetheless the conference was important in articulating a particular view of hospital reorganisation; in demonstrating Labour's willingness to participate in health debates; and in providing Hastings with another public platform.

The other major Labour health initiative of the period concerned nursing. The PHAC and a sub-committee of the SJCIWO prepared a report for consideration at a conference in January 1927. In the first instance this dealt with nurses' training and conditions of employment. The relatively low level of pay of nursing staff was noted, and among the report's recommendations was that the profession should more vigorously pursue trade union organisation. It was also observed that

> owing to the tradition of the profession, the average nurse thinks of a Trade Union as a body of manual workers continually taking part in strikes. She does not realise that every profession has found organisation necessary. Thus, doctors and lawyers have formed their own professional associations, and Civil Servants, teachers, and health visitors have also their own Trade Union associations.[46]

As we shall see, the need for professionals to organise and to rally to socialism was to be consistently emphasised by the SMA, which was also eventually to allow nurses to become full members. Such points were made at the conference itself, notably in the opening speech by, once again, Hastings.[47]

In the aftermath of the First World War, therefore, the Labour Party did concern itself with health issues, although it did not pursue the early promise of a plan for comprehensive reorganisation, and latterly responded to what were perceived as two particular crises – hospitals and nursing – rather than continuing to address more general issues of reform and restructuring. As suggested earlier, however, this does not mean that particular groups within the labour movement did not address health matters in a more systematic way. Women and local activists (and these were overlapping categories[48]) were concerned with health and medical issues, and the local model of welfare provision remained influential in the labour movement until the 1940s.

Somerville Hastings in the 1920s

Another such group was, of course, health care professionals. The SMA was founded by doctors in the Labour Party, and it is therefore appropriate to examine what some of these were saying in the decade prior to 1930. Murray, for example, wrote a series of articles for *The Scottish Co-Operator* dealing not only with health and the medical services, but also with some of the reasons for their importance to modern society. It was, he argued, possible to assess a nation's level of political development by the measures it employed for health promotion, and on such criteria Britain was, along with the rest of the world, 'extremely backward'. Furthermore, in the healthy human body itself, and especially in blood circulation, could be found 'a perfect system of distribution, transportation, and co-ordination'. This was, in other words, a model for socialism and socialised medicine, and in contrast to the 'foolish, selfish, competitive methods' on which the contemporary state was organised. Hastings too used such organic metaphors. In a talk to new students at the Middlesex Hospital in 1923 entitled 'Team Work in Nature', he suggested that Darwin had shown that the natural world was characterised not only by competition, but also by cooperation. The latter was also to be found in medicine, where staff of all types 'are united in the single purpose of healing the sick'.[49]

Hastings is a particularly useful individual on whom to focus for this period, for the following reasons. First, he was a prolific writer, publishing a wide range of material in various formats. Second, Hastings was already well established in left-wing medical politics, by the 1920s being effectively the leader of the SMSA, a member of the PHAC, and on a number of important occasions the health spokesman of the

Labour Party. Also, as shall be shown, he was going to have a controversial role in the labour movement investigation into family allowances. Third, Hastings was becoming involved in Labour politics at national level. After unsuccessfully contesting the parliamentary seat of Epsom in 1922, he was twice elected MP for Reading, first in 1923 – when he was appointed a parliamentary private secretary at the Board of Education – and again in 1929. This prefigured his political role on the LCC, of which he became a co-opted member in 1929 and elected member in 1932, and his career as MP for Barking after 1945. Finally, Hastings was to be a key founder member of the SMA, playing a leadership role in the Association throughout the period of this study.[50]

For Hastings, ill health was part of a wider structural problem of capitalism. Poverty, he explained in 1926, included not only 'poverty of this world's goods'. It also encompassed 'poverty of education, ... of leisure, ... of ideas, ... of opportunity, and poverty of health'. Poverty was 'body- and soul-destroying' as was attested by data on, for example, infant mortality and the rejection of potential army recruits as a result of poor physique. Socialism alone was the answer.[51] What was required in health care provision, therefore, was what was required in society as a whole: a fundamental restructuring.

As far as medical practice was concerned, at its heart lay teamwork which, alongside the associated ideas of planning and coordination should be expanded in health care

> first, because it is part of the spirit of the age to provide for its needs by collective action; and secondly, because ... the public provision for sickness already instituted has undoubtedly made for the general good.

Coordination was important at the centre, by way of the Ministry of Health, but was also needed 'at the peripheries'. Here the role of the general practitioner was crucial although, it was emphasised, not in the traditional role of isolated and independent medical entrepreneur. Rather, the GP should be part of the health team, hence the significance of health centres, associated and integrated with local hospitals. While Hastings was prepared to concede that the voluntary hospital system had some significant achievements, nonetheless public health was suffering because hospitals worked as isolated units, and had little real contact with general practitioners. Overall, therefore, what was required was a comprehensive, national scheme with, in each locality, the hospital at its centre and with the aim of providing 'the best possible service free to everyone who wished it'. Prophetically, Hastings was suggesting in the mid-1920s that a nationalised hospital system was 'inevitable within 10 or 20 years'.[52]

Here, then, was a large element of Hastings's vision of a socialised medical service. It had to be under public control, unified, and properly planned, coordinated, and integrated. Such a system would benefit the whole of society. In an article in 1922, he explained how the middle class would gain. That an article of this type was thought appropriate for publication in a socialist newspaper was significant in itself. First, it showed the desire of the Labour Party to win over middle class, professional voters. This can be seen as part of the more general transformation of inter-war social democracy from an ideology based on the working class to one emphasising the 'people' or the 'nation'.[53]

Second, Hastings's piece demonstrated his concern to alleviate the fears of a particular middle class professional group – medical practitioners – about the possibilities of state medicine. As will become evident, the dichotomy between democratic control and professional rights was one which the SMA tried hard, but probably unsuccessfully, to resolve in the coming years. This was to lead to a number of apparently contradictory statements by individuals such as Hastings over the proper place of the professions in a democratised health service. In 1928, for example, he lamented the fact that since the setting up of the Ministry of Health ten years previously, there had only been one Minister (Christopher Addison, later an SMA member) with knowledge or experience of medical matters. Ten years later, however, Hastings expressed the view that not 'a few people are of the opinion that Mr Neville Chamberlain was the best Minister of Health this country has ever had' because of his passing of the 1929 Local Government Act, which gave local authorities the right to appropriate Poor Law hospitals.[54]

In 1922, however, Hastings was trying to keep matters as straightforward as possible for his intended middle-class readers. He suggested that the existing health system favoured only two groups: the very rich, who could afford expensive treatment; and the very poor, who could receive free services in hospital. In between, there was no doubt that 'the middle class man or woman with a family may be very hard hit in the case of a long illness or severe operation'. Even those in the employed working class were better off, since they benefited from health insurance. All this would change under a Labour administration which would 'provide the best that medical science can give, free of all cost to all who need it'. This would mean an end to 'almoners with their inquiries' and 'long hospital waiting lists'. Furthermore, Labour would 'provide not only the service of a general practitioner, *working under much better conditions than under the present panel*' (my emphasis), but also 'the services of consultants, specialists and dentists when required, together with those special methods such as vaccines, X rays, electricity, etc., which are so costly at present'.[55]

Hastings was thus pitching his appeal to the middle classes at both a personal and a national level, and made sure that he emphasised the professional rights of the GP. Rational self-interest, which could be advanced under this Labourist version of socialism, was counterposed to the anarchy, injustices, and waste of capitalism, in health as elsewhere. Waste and inefficiency were important political issues in the post-First World War era – we have already seen MacDonald's comments on this – and Hastings further showed how these took a particularly pernicious form in sickness and disease through an examination of child health. The labour movement as a whole had an ongoing interest in child health, partly out of simple humanitarianism, but also because healthy children were required for an efficient economy and, ultimately, the transition to a socialist society.[56]

Hastings himself had retained an interest in child welfare throughout his life, and this was recognized by his membership of the Curtis Committee which looked into the matter in the late 1940s. For present purposes, his views on child welfare also help to further illuminate his approach to health and health service organisation. From the 1920s Hastings served on a number of committees concerned with the physical well-being of the young. Drawing on his own experience as a school medical officer, he produced memoranda for the Labour Party and for the TUC on matters such as rheumatism in children. In one of these, and using an analogy which he employed on numerous occasions, he argued that just as education was free, so too should be child health provision. 'Indeed from the national point of view', he continued, 'it is much more necessary to attend to the health of children than to educate them'. The PHAC also considered the issue of child health in the early 1920s. In particular, the relationship between unemployment and its physical and mental effects on children was examined. Although no definite link could be established, it was nonetheless felt that 'the cumulative effects of ... poverty are incalculable'. This in turn damaged 'physique, nerves, temper, and morals', matters in which unemployed parents were powerless to act.[57]

Hastings expanded on this in 1923 in his significantly titled *Labour, the Children's Champion*. Everything should be available for the full development of all children, for the only way in which the country's resources could be completely utilised was 'by giving to every child the opportunity of reaching the position for which he or she is best suited'. In his maiden Commons speech he further argued that children were 'the most important capital we can possess', and should so be protected at all costs. All this, of course, had health implications. But the Labour Party stood for 'free doctoring for all', and hence demanded that

> the State should provide everything necessary to cure your children
> when they are ill, that there should be no difficulty in getting a
> first-class doctor to come and see them at home when this is
> necessary, and that the doctor should be able to arrange for their
> admission as in-patients to hospital, or send them to a convalescent
> home, and to order nourishment as well as medicine when this is
> required.[58]

The comprehensiveness of this vision is striking, with health services
collectively provided and with doctors empowered, in the case of children at least, to demand the provision of food. Further illustration of
this approach to health care is to be found in Hastings's role in the
labour movement debate over family allowances.

   The poverty which could accompany the birth of children had long
been understood among the working class and its political representatives, and more widely since around the beginning of the twentieth
century. More problematic was what action to advocate. One possible
solution – which appealed to certain sections of the labour movement,
including the ILP and some feminists – was family allowances, whereby
cash payments would be made to mothers to help in the raising of their
children. Such proposals were, however, controversial, and the trade
union movement was for the most part hostile to cash allowances
because of the feared impact on wages and wage bargaining. In an
attempt to resolve the issue, a joint committee of the Labour Party and
the TUC was set up in the late 1920s.[59] Among the witnesses to this
committee were Alfred Salter and, as one of the two representatives
from the PHAC, Hastings. As the Interim Report of the joint committee
records, both pointed out that as far as the health dimension of family
allowances was concerned, mothers could not be expected to have
'expert knowledge' since, although acting with the 'best intentions',
they might nonetheless provide unsuitable food for their children. Hastings and Salter felt that such 'ignorance' was certainly disappearing, but
that as matters currently stood it was crucial that

> the best possible expenditure of the available money should be
> studied, and this is most easily done by the provision of social
> services, etc., through the public authorities.

Both emphasised the need for the expansion of the public health services, and the report's proposals in this respect were close to the kind of
service for which Hastings had previously pressed.[60]

   Hastings reiterated these arguments in a debate, in the pages of *The
Labour Woman*, with the ILP's Jennie Lee (later Bevan's partner). Hastings had no doubt of the need to spend 'vast sums of money' on the
nation's 'most valuable asset', its children. But although commending
the skills of the working class mother, he nonetheless doubted whether

they had the 'requisite knowledge' to buy the nutritionally best food. All the evidence suggested, therefore, the need for collective public services and a state medical service. The latter would 'provide the child with all he needs ... when he is ill, without any cost to the parents'. Such arguments clearly influenced the decision of the TUC (and thereby the Labour Party) to reject cash family allowances.[61]

There are obviously a number of factors at play here. While no doubt well-intentioned, Hastings's and Salter's scepticism about the abilities of working-class mothers comes across as biased by both class and gender. As one (female) participant in the TUC debate put it, there was a clear difference between the 'professional classes in the Labour Movement today' and 'organised working mothers'.[62] But there was more to it than this. The analysis of Hastings and colleagues such as Salter encompassed two important themes. First, medical science was becoming increasingly complex, and even doctors could not be expected to embrace all its aspects. In such circumstances, professional – 'scientific' – advice became of greater and greater significance, even if at the apparent expense of mothers' autonomy. This was another variant on a theme already identified, and which was to cause the SMA endless problems, the nature and limits of professional power. Second, welfare services were best provided, for economic reasons if no other, on a collective rather than an individual basis. As Hastings put it, 'by cooperative effort we can provide for our needs not only much better, but also much more cheaply'.[63] Once again, such collectivism was to be crucial to the SMA, not least in the creation of a socialised medical service, a key component of the transition to socialism.

The need for a Socialist Medical Association

It was suggested above that it is, paradoxically, possible to argue that both Webster and Marwick make important points about the attitude of the labour movement to health matters in the 1920s. On the one hand, it is clear that conferences, debates, and various publications addressed issues of health and health care organisation, and that embryonically there existed proposals for some form of socialised medical system. There is also evidence that a reorganisation of medical services, as part of the broader project of breaking up the Poor Law, was considered by the Labour government in 1924.[64] At an individual level, Hastings in particular was publicly developing his ideas on socialised health care and was increasingly influential on the PHAC. He also had gained a certain amount of success at national political level; taken, in 1929, the first step on his way to becoming a leading member of the

Labour LCC; and acted on a number of occasions as a health spokesman for the Labour Party.

On the other hand, an examination of the most public declarations of
Labour's policy proposals, general election manifestos, reveals a range
of remedies for social problems such as unemployment, pension rights,
education, and housing, but almost nothing specifically on health services. This situation was not helped by the constraints under which the
PHAC operated, and its clearly limited impact at this stage on party
policy making. Furthermore, socialist medical activists were by this
time aware that the SMSA was effectively defunct, despite the prominent part played in it by overtly left-wing doctors such as Hastings, and
that its position of non-alignment was increasingly anachronistic. The
situation therefore appeared to require the creation of an explicitly
socialist medical organisation, clearly linked to the Labour Party and
campaigning within it, and within the medical profession, for a fully
socialised health service. It was in this context that the Socialist Medical
Association was founded.

Notes

1. Irwin Brown (David Stark Murray), 'We Thought of it First', *MTT*, vol. 5,
   no. 6, June Quarter 1946, p. 10.
2. Webster, 'Labour and the Origins of the National Health Service', p. 185;
   Honigsbaum, *Division in British Medicine*, pp. 54, 106–7; Irwin Brown
   (David Stark Murray), 'Hats Off to the Pioneers', *MTT*, vol. 5, no. 5,
   March Quarter 1946, pp. 11, 10.
3. Murray, *Why a National Health Service?*, p. 4; *Fabian News*, vol. XVII,
   no. 7, June 1907, p. 46; on Dodd see Honigsbaum, *Division in British
   Medicine*, p. 82; and Norman and Jeanne Mackenzie, *The First Fabians*,
   Weidenfeld and Nicolson, 1977, p. 347.
4. Quoted in A.M. McBriar, *An Edwardian Mixed Doubles*, Oxford, Oxford University Press, 1987, p. 232. This part of the chapter owes much
   to McBriar's analysis, pp. 231–6. For labour movement reaction to the
   Minority Report, see also Earwicker, thesis, p. 69ff.
5. Sidney and Beatrice Webb, *The State and the Doctor*, Longmans, Green,
   1910, pp. 212, 214.
6. Ibid., pp. 215–16, 260.
7. Ibid., pp. 218, 222, 224, 250.
8. Ibid., pp. 230–31.
9. Ibid., pp. 233, 256–8, 250.
10. DSH, File 1, 'Articles', typescript 'Founders of the Labour Movement I
    have Known', n.d. but mid-1960s; DSH, File 25, 'Religion and Social-
    ism', typescript 'The Origin and Dangers of the Welfare State', n.d. but
    late 1940s; Stewart, 'Socialist Proposals', p. 339.
11. DSH, File 68 'Publications', Hastings's own signed copy of *Break up the
    Poor Law and Abolish the Workhouse: Being Part I of the Minority*

Report of the Poor Law Commission, Fabian Society, 1909. The passages quoted are at pp. 287, 293.

12. H. Beckett-Overy, Somerville Hastings, and Arnold Freeman, *The Medical Proposals of the Minority Report: an Appeal to the Medical Profession*, H. and W. Brown, 1910, pp. 3, 9, 8.
13. Ibid., pp. 7, 8, 15–16.
14. Benjamin Moore, *The Dawn of the Health Age*, J. and A. Churchill, 1911, pp. 180, 187–8, 190, v; Honigsbaum, *Division in British Medicine*, p. 55.
15. DSM (2) 1, Executive Committee meetings 13 November 1912 and 2 April 1913; *Lancet*, 1912, II, p. 342. The point about the importance of a separate Ministry of Health is made in Frank Honigsbaum, *The Struggle for the Ministry of Health*, Occasional Papers in Social Administration no. 37, 1970, p. 32.
16. *Lancet*, 1912, II, p. 342.
17. Honigsbaum, *Division in British Medicine*, p. 54.
18. Somerville Hastings, 'Public Health', in Herbert Tracey (ed.), *The British Labour Party*, Caxton Publishing, 1948, vol. II, p. 134.
19. Benjamin Moore, *First Steps Towards a State Medical Service*, State Medical Service Association, 1913, pp. 3, 14, 15ff., 19, 28, 21ff.
20. Honigsbaum, *Division in British Medicine*, p. 54; DSM (2) 1, Service Organisation Committee, 28 November 1912.
21. On Salter's life and career see Fenner Brockway, *Bermondsey Story*, George Allen and Unwin, 1949; *Lancet*, 1914, I, p. 1154; Murray, *Why a National Health Service?*, p. 12.
22. DSM (2) 1, General Meeting, 25 October 1912; Executive Committee, 23 December 1913; Special General Meeting, 9 June 1913; Executive Committee, 21 May 1914; Special General Meeting, 6 August 1914; and Executive Committee, 2 July 1914.
23. Marwick, 'The Labour Party and the Welfare State in Britain, 1900–1948', pp. 385–6; Bentley B. Gilbert, *The Evolution of National Insurance in Britain*, Michael Joseph, 1966, pp. 435–7; Earwicker, thesis, p. 76ff.
24. Murray, *Why a National Health Service?*, pp. 8, 6, 7; *idem*, 'The National Health Service in Britain', in Evang, Karl, Murray, David Stark and Lear, Walter J., *Medical Care and Family Security*, New Jersey, Prentice-Hall, 1963, p. 91.
25. Pat Thane, 'The Labour Party and State "Welfare"', in Brown, K.D. (ed.), *The First Labour Party*, Croom Helm, 1985, pp. 206–7; Marwick, 'The Labour Party and the Welfare State in Britain, 1900–1948', pp. 386–7.
26. Murray, *Why a National Health Service?*, p. 12; DSH microfilm, Bundle 2, Biographical Information; John N. Horne, *Labour at War: France and Britain 1914–1918*, Oxford, Oxford University Press, 1991, Chs 6 and 7; DSM (2) 1, Executive Committee, 30 October 1917.
27. DSM (2) 1, General Meeting, 6 February 1918.
28. Benjamin Moore and Charles Parker, 'The Case for a State Medical Service Re-Stated', *Lancet*, 1918, II, pp. 85–7; DSM (2) 1, Executive Committee, 13 September 1918.
29. Charles Webster, 'The Metamorphosis of Dawson of Penn', in Porter, Dorothy and Porter, Roy (eds), *Doctors, Politics and Society: Historical Essays*, Amsterdam, Rodopi, 1993, p. 215; Moore and Parker, 'The Case for a State Medical Service Re-Stated', p. 86.

30. Murray, *Why a National Health Service?*, p. 14; Irwin Brown (David Stark Murray), 'We Thought of it First', p. 9; Webster, 'Conflict and Consensus', pp. 136–8; *MTT*, vol. 11, no. 11, September/October 1958, p. 5.

31. David Stark Murray, 'Before Our Time: The Real Pioneers of the NHS', *MTT*, vol. 12, no. 5, 1959, p. 6; DSM (2) 1, General Meeting, 18 April 1928; General Meeting, 6 July 1928; Meeting, 12 December 1929; Provisional Executive Committee, 19 December 1929; and Provisional Executive Committee, 27 February 1931.

32. Murray, *Why a National Health Service?*, p. 14; Honigsbaum, *The Struggle for the Ministry of Health*, p. 59.

33. Honigsbaum, *Division in British Medicine*, pp. 54ff, 182; MSS.79/MPU/1/2/1, Minutes of Council, 18 July 1929; Murray, *Why a National Health Service?*, p. 22.

34. Webster, 'Labour and the Origins of the National Health Service', p. 187; Marwick, 'The Labour Party and the Welfare State in Britain, 1900–1948', pp. 389, 391; Ray Earwicker, 'The Emergence of a Medical Strategy in the Labour Movement 1906–1919', *Bulletin of the Society for the Social History of Medicine*, no. 29, December 1981, p. 6.

35. See also Earwicker, thesis, Ch. 6.

36. The full text of this is contained in Marwick, 'The Labour Party and the Welfare State in Britain, 1900–1948', p. 388ff, to which this section of the discussion is much indebted.

37. Honigsbaum, *Division in British Medicine*, p. 55; *BMJ*, 1918, II, pp. 175–6; and 1918, II, pp. 301–2.

38. Labour Party, *Memoranda Prepared by the Advisory Committee on Public Health: The Organisation of the Preventative and Curative Medical Services and Hospital and Laboratory Systems Under a Ministry of Health; The Position of the General Medical Practitioners in a Reorganised System of Public Health; The Ministry of Health*, Labour Party, 1921. Earwicker, 'The Emergence of a Medical Strategy in the Labour Movement 1906–1919', p. 6, refers to the 1919 version; Webster, 'Labour and the Origins of the National Health Service', p. 186, to the 1918 and 1922 versions; and Marwick, 'The Labour Party and the Welfare State in Britain, 1900–1948', pp. 389–40, to undated versions.

39. Labour Party, *Memoranda Prepared by the Advisory Committee on Public Health*, pp. 2, 5, 6, 10; see also Marwick, 'The Labour Party and the Welfare State in Britain, 1900–1948', p. 390; LP/JSM/PH/2, Minutes of the Advisory Committee on Public Health, 3 June 1919; LP/JSM/PH/1, Minutes of the Advisory Committee on Public Health, 20 May 1919.

40. Webster, 'Labour and the Origins of the National Health Service', p. 186. Marwick is particularly dismissive of the Dawson Report as compared with what the political left was producing at the time: 'The Labour Party and the Welfare State in Britain, 1900–1948', p. 389.

41. Labour Party, *Memoranda Prepared by the Advisory Committee on Public Health*, p. 11 – some extant versions of this document have an insert at this point which reads: 'Part II of the Memoranda here printed, "The Position of the General Medical Practitioners in a Reorganised System of Public Health", drafted by a Sub-Committee, was ultimately rejected by a majority of the full Advisory Committee on Public Health, which then adopted Part I unanimously'; Marwick, 'The Labour Party and the Welfare State in Britain, 1900–1948', p. 389.

42. DSM (2) 1, Executive Committee, 13 September 1918.
43. Honigsbaum, *Division in British Medicine*, p. 87; Ross McKibbin, *The Evolution of the Labour Party 1910–1924*, Oxford, Oxford University Press, 1974, pp. 214–21, 234–5; on Hastings's efforts in this direction, see LP/JSM/PH/20, Minutes of the Public Health Advisory Committee, 19 October 1920.
44. Duncan Tanner, *Political Change and the Labour Party, 1900–1918*, Cambridge, Cambridge University Press, 1990, p. 436; Webster, 'Labour and the Origins of the National Health Service', pp. 187, 190; Labour Party Research Department, *Reports on Hospitals and the Patient; and a Domestic Workers Charter*, Labour Party, 1931, p. 15; Labour Party, *Report of the Thirtieth Annual Conference of the Labour Party*, Labour Party, 1930, p. 44; Honigsbaum, *Division in British Medicine*, p. 255.
45. Trades Union Congress and the Labour Party, *The Labour Movement and the Hospital Crisis*, Trades Union Congress and the Labour Party, 1922, p. 1; Labour Party, *The Hospital Problem: The Report of a Special Conference of Labour, Hospital, Medical and Kindred Societies, held in the Caxton Hall, Westminster, on April 28th and 29th, 1924*, Labour Party, 1924, pp. 2, 3; Marwick, 'The Labour Party and the Welfare State in Britain, 1900–1948', pp. 390–91; Brian Abel-Smith, *The Hospitals 1800–1948*, Heinemann, 1964, p. 320.
46. Labour Party, *Draft Report on the Nursing Profession*, Labour Party 1927, p. 23.
47. *BMJ*, 1927, I, p. 253.
48. See, *inter alia*, Pamela Graves, *Labour Women*, Cambridge, Cambridge University Press, 1994, especially Chapter 5; and Pat Thane, 'Women in the British Labour Party and the Construction of State Welfare, 1906–1939', in Koven, Seth and Michel, Sonya (eds), *Mothers of a New World*, Routledge, 1993.
49. DSM (2) 4, *Scottish Co-Operator*, 3 January 1925, p. 7; and 23 May 1925, p. 485; *Lancet*, 1923, II, pp. 774–6.
50. Stewart, 'Socialist Proposals', *passim*.
51. Somerville Hastings, *Why this Poverty?*, Reading, Reading Labour Party, 1926(?), pp. 1–3.
52. *Lancet*, 1928, I, pp. 67–9; 1922, I, p. 703; 1926, I, p. 180.
53. Gosta Esping-Andersen, 'Citizenship and Socialism: De-Commodification and Solidarity in the Welfare State', in Rein, Martin, Esping-Andersen, Gosta and Rainwater, Lee (eds), *Stagnation and Renewal in Social Policy*, Armonk, New York, M.E. Sharpe Inc., 1987, p. 84.
54. Somerville Hastings, 'Labour and the Middle Class – II', *London Labour Chronicle*, September, 1922, p. 7; *idem*, 'The Future of Medical Practice in England', *Lancet*, 1928, I, p. 69; DSM 4/1, Somerville Hastings, 'Some Notes on the BMA Scheme For a General Medical Service For the Nation', 18 October 1938.
55. *London Labour Chronicle*, September 1922, p. 7.
56. On this see John Stewart, 'Ramsay MacDonald, the Labour Party, and Child Welfare, 1900–1914', *Twentieth Century British History*, 4, 2, 1993; and *idem*, '"The Children's Party, therefore the Women's Party": the Labour Party and Child Welfare in Inter-War Britain', in Digby, Anne and Stewart, John (eds), *Gender, Health, and Welfare*, Routledge, 1996.
57. DSH, File 9, 'School Medical Service', *passim* and *Recovery of Cost and*

the School Medical Service, by Dr Somerville Hastings, February 1925; Advisory Committee on Public Health, 'Notes on the Effect of Unemployment on the Health of Children', May 1922, in *Labour Party Executive Committee Minutes and Associated Papers*. This particular paper can be consulted either at the Labour Party archive in Manchester, or on the microfilm/microfiche edition published by Research Publications.

58. Somerville Hastings, *Labour, the Children's Champion*, TUC/Labour Party, 1923, pp. 3, 11; Parliamentary Debates, 5th series, vol. 169, col. 1907.

59. This episode is covered in more detail in Stewart, '"The Children's Party, therefore the Women's Party"', pp. 170–73.

60. TUC/Labour Party, *Joint Committee on the Living Wage, etc: Interim Report on Family Allowances and Child Welfare*, TUC/Labour Party, 1928, pp. 5, 23, 31–2.

61. *The Labour Woman*, 1 August 1930, pp. 121–2; TUC, *Family Allowances: Text of the Minority and Majority Reports issued by the TUC and Labour Party Joint Committee: Verbatim Report of the Debate at the Nottingham Conference*, TUC, 1930, pp. 4–5, 16.

62. Ibid., p. 23.

63. *The Labour Woman*, 1 August 1930, p. 121.

64. See, for example, *Poor Law Reform: Memorandum by the Minister of Health, 1st August 1924, to the Cabinet*, Arthur Greenwood Papers, Bodleian Library, University of Oxford.

CHAPTER THREE

'The People's Health'

This chapter examines the founding of the Socialist Medical Association and its consequent organisational development in the 1930s, including affiliation to the Labour Party in 1931. It further analyses the principles on which the Association argued for a socialised medical service. Unsurprisingly, these built on the ideas put forward by medical reformers since the turn of the century. The great change in the 1930s, however, was that now an explicitly socialist medical organisation – the SMA – was in existence, and affiliated to the main opposition political party. The Association could anticipate, at some future point, a Labour administration in which its own ideas on health and health care might be highly influential. A sense of optimism and of urgency informed the SMA's arguments in this period although it was, as shall become apparent, fully aware that its scheme was not the only proposed solution to the reconstruction of the health care system.

The founding of the Socialist Medical Association

Both Murray and Brook give accounts of the circumstances surrounding the SMA's formation. In addition to the general context described in the last chapter, at least three immediate factors seem to have been involved. First, the question of a state medical service had again been under discussion by left-wing medical activists, both in the National Medical Service Association (successor to the SMSA) and, more specifically, as a result of an article by Hastings on the future of medical practice which appeared in the *Lancet* in 1928. Second, Brook, following a speech to an LCC meeting, had been contacted and visited by the Berlin dentist Ewald Fabian. Fabian was involved with the German socialist doctors' organisation whose journal, *Der Sozialistische Arzt*, he also edited, and was keen that British socialist doctors set up a similar body. The SMA later repaid its debt to Fabian by sending funds in the summer of 1933 to help his journal out of its financial difficulties and by securing his release from a French internment camp at the beginning of the Second World War. Third, Brook was particularly incensed by a speech hostile to state medicine made by the Independent MP for London University, Sir Ernest Graham-Little MD. This prompted him to write to the Labour newspaper *The Daily*

Herald proposing the setting up of an organisation of left-wing medical practitioners.[1]

Webster adds a further possible factor by suggesting that the creation of the SMA might have been in response to the BMA's *A General Medical Service for the Nation*, first published in April 1930. There is no direct evidence of this in statements by Association founders. But certainly it would have been part of the general context described earlier, since at least one reason behind the BMA document was, as Peter Bartrip puts it, the desire to halt 'local authority "encroachments" on private practice ... and to pre-empt government plans for a service antipathetic to BMA priorities'.[2] It is important to bear in mind here that in 1930 a minority Labour government was in power and, as we have seen, individuals and groups within the labour movement were already agitating for some form of state medical service.

A meeting was held in September 1930, attended by around 20 left-wing medical personnel. It was chaired by Esther Rickards, a Labour LCC member who had been, according to Brook, victimised 'for her political views when she sought surgical appointments at London hospitals'. A sub-committee was formed to draft a constitution, and in this was aided by James Middleton, Acting Secretary of the Labour Party. The three principal aims of the new organisation (the name of which had been a matter of some debate) were to work for a socialised medical service, both preventive and curative, free and open to all; to secure the highest possible standard of health for the British people; and to propagandise for socialism within the medical and allied services. The proposed constitution was put to a further meeting in early November, and appointments to various offices agreed. The founding officials of the Association were Hastings (President); Alfred Welply, of the MPU (Treasurer); and Brook (Secretary). Brook, who was especially active in the early phase of Association history, also allowed his home to be used as its first office. Other members of the newly-created Executive Committee (EC) included Santo Jeger, soon to be an LCC member and later MP for South West St Pancras; and Alfred Salter and Robert Forgan – like Hastings at this time, MPs. Immediately after the first meeting, Brook told Fabian that: 'Much notice is being taken of our new organisation in the English press and we are being attacked by the Capitalist newspapers'. None daunted, Brook was convinced that 'ultimately we shall be very strong in numbers'.[3]

Because of its small membership, the Association initially decided to postpone applying for Labour Party affiliation. This did not mean, however, that it was inactive. The EC met regularly, and sub-committees on research and on education were set up. The secretary to the latter was the American doctor, Caroline Maule; and to the former G.P.

Blizard, an old associate of Hastings and also, once again, secretary to the PHAC. The research sub-committee was charged with devising 'practical measures for a free socialised medical service', and heard evidence from, among others, Henry Brackenbury of the BMA. As Brook points out, this was quite a coup for such a small and recently-formed organisation. A London and Home Counties branch was formed, a sub-committee of which prepared the document *Labour's Hospital Policy for London*, the basis of Labour's health policy in the 1931 LCC elections. London's importance to the SMA is discussed in Chapter Five. Contact was also made with foreign socialist medical organisations. As Webster suggests, the founding of the Association 'reversed the decline' in Labour Party discussion of health issues which had taken place in the mid- to late 1920s, creating a 'new forum for mobilising the expertise of socialist doctors'.[4] How effective this was remains, however, rather more problematical.

The first annual general meeting (AGM) took place in May 1931. Resolutions were passed on the need to amend Neville Chamberlain's 1929 Local Government Act to allow for free treatment in municipal hospitals; on health insurance; and, at Maule's instigation, on the need for municipal hospitals to provide medical education to both men and women on an equal basis. The last was henceforth a consistent feature of the SMA's programme. The meeting was addressed by Major Greenwood, Association member and Professor of Epidemiology at London University, who spoke on 'The Municipal Hospitals, the University, and Research in London'. Greenwood, whose 'profoundly social orientation' to medicine led him to join the SMA, was to be an important influence on Richard Doll, later prominent both in his own field and in medical politics. However, two other features of the AGM stand out as especially noteworthy. First, on the EC's recommendation the meeting agreed to seek Labour Party affiliation. Later in 1931 Brook and Hastings appeared before the party's Organisation Sub-Committee, and the Association was duly affiliated.[5] This political commitment distinguished it from earlier bodies such as the SMSA, and opened up the possibility that the SMA might have a real chance of seeing its programme put into action. The organisation's first delegate – Hastings – attended party conference in 1932, and the significance of this will be discussed in the next chapter.

Second, Hastings gave a key-note speech, 'The Medical Service of the Future'. This is worth analysing in some detail for the clues it affords as to what the SMA sought.[6] Seven basic principles were identified:

1. a preventive service;
2. the end of economic barriers to medical care;

3. the importance of hospitals;
4. the centrality of teamwork;
5. the revised role of the general practitioner;
6. free choice of doctor; and
7. professional freedom.

The starting place here is Hastings's notion of the 'team'. However well-informed any individual doctor, he or she could not know everything about rapidly expanding medical science, so in the future 'the team and not the individual doctor must be the unit'. The 'medical centre' (a synonym for 'health centre') would be the location of such teams, and would 'bring together in closest possible cooperation all the several spheres of clinical activity'. These centres were to be linked to hospitals, reorganised into a 'complete and coordinated ... system'. All this would facilitate the already-existing trend towards preventive medicine, which in turn would yield 'an increase in knowledge such as we have yet hardly dreamed of'. This sense of optimism about the possibilities of medical science was, rather unthinkingly, a characteristic of Association attitudes throughout the period of this study. In terms of administration, for Hastings the key institution was to be local authorities and their health committees. Implicit in this, therefore, was democratic control of the health services. Any other consideration aside, this was obviously seen as a direct contrast to the unaccountable voluntary hospitals ruled by the medical élite.

So far, Hastings was expressing ideas which had been around in reforming medical circles for some time, and elements of which can be seen in his own proposals of the 1920s and earlier. In his speech he also began to address what was to be one of the most problematic issues for the SMA in the coming years, the role of the 'independent' doctor, and particularly the general practitioner. Inherent in the idea of teamwork was, consciously or otherwise, the notion of a full-time salaried service. This was something of which GPs in particular were well-known to be deeply suspicious, their argument being that such a service would, among other things, undermine clinical independence and reduce them to the medical equivalent of civil servants. Hastings approached this from a number of different angles. First, he maintained that even in a system based on health centres the GP would be the 'most important link in the medical chain'. Second, there had to be 'professional freedom'. In other words although health services were to be democratically controlled (with all that this implied for the role of medical practitioners), nonetheless the autonomy of clinical judgement should be safeguarded. There was a clear tension here, which was to prove consistently problematical for the Association. In 1933, for example,

Hastings told an SMA meeting that there were four guiding principles in respect of doctors' control in a state medical service. It was certainly the case that medical appointments should be made by the appropriate public body. But doctors should also have direct access to administrators and elected representatives, both to remedy their own grievances and to give advice. The first, and crucial, principle was that 'medical staff must have the sole determining voice as to the type of medical treatment to be given to each individual patient'. Hastings had, at this point, a very low opinion of the average citizen's medical knowledge. As he put it on one occasion, the general public were 'extraordinarily bad judges of a doctor's worth'.[7]

This was, of course, unsurprising, given that Hastings also argued that medicine was now so complex that individual doctors themselves had great difficulty in encompassing it. But as will subsequently be shown, particularly after the capture of the LCC by Labour in 1934 democratic control by local authorities was consistently pushed as the model for health service reorganisation. Even so, Hastings in 1938 still emphasised that it was 'very difficult for the public to appreciate what is essential for the adequate treatment of disease'.[8] In effect, what the Association was encountering was the classic political dilemma of the role of professional bodies in democratic societies characterised by a high division of labour and specialised knowledge. This was an issue never fully resolved by the SMA perhaps because it is, ultimately, irresolvable. It recurs at various points, and in various contexts, throughout this work.

The third way in which Hastings addressed the GP issue in his speech was through the economics of health care. From the patients' point of view, he was clear that there should be no 'economic barrier' to the provision of medical services. Similarly, patients should have the right to choose which doctor they attended. Embryonically present here was another issue more explicitly dealt with in the debates of the 1940s, the citizen's 'right' to health. But the existing economic relationship between doctor and patient did not, Hastings further argued, benefit doctors either. Indeed the relationship could be one of dependence on the practitioners' part, 'undesirable' in a number of ways. These included the risk that the doctor might not give 'wholesome but unpleasant advice', and that he might become more concerned with 'mere externals' rather than an 'intimate knowledge of the science of his profession'. In other words doctors were, under the present system wherein some patients held the economic advantage through direct payments or through private or even state insurance, being put into positions which might ethically compromise them and which did not allow for the full development of medical skills and understanding. Clinical independence would, consequently, be enhanced rather than diminished by the kind of system Hastings proposed. The significance of these ideas, as further expounded in two important documents – *The People's Health* and *A Socialised Medical Service* – are returned to below.

Such arguments for a socialist medical system were, as will be evident, largely organisational. There was no questioning of the basis of scientific knowledge nor of the ability of doctors to employ such knowledge. Nonetheless, two points are worth emphasising about the ideas of its leading activists at the time of the Association's creation. First, medical practice at its best could provide a model for socialism, and this underpins arguments on matters such as teamwork and health centres. As Hastings told (no doubt bemused) medical colleagues in 1932, in principle at least, 'doctors more than any [other profession] practised socialism'.[9] Second, and as we saw in the last chapter, the proposals of some of its founding members were underwritten by a philosophy which found cooperation and harmony in the natural world. This provided an organic model on which both a socialised medical service and a socialist society could be built. Medicine was not, moreover, seen in isolation. On the contrary, it was clearly felt that the capitalist system, and the social conditions and inequalities it generated, was the ultimate source of the vast majority of ill-health.

Nor was health simply an individual concern. Illness had an impact not only on the lives of the sufferers, but also on society as a whole, to the detriment of both. Hastings wrote to the *Lancet* in 1932 on the subject of unemployment and health. There could be no question, he claimed, that many of the unemployed experienced considerable difficulties in gaining an adequate diet, and that existing welfare measures were in themselves insufficient – hence the urgent need to combat the physical degeneration certain to result from a deficiency of the proper type of food. It was, he continued, 'of the greatest importance that the standard of our national stock shall be maintained'. Nor did Association members doubt that the distribution of economic resources had a profound impact on individual and national well-being. As Stella Churchill remarked in 1935, it was 'one of the great anomalies in our civilization that matters of health receive far less State support than do those of Defence ... or business communications'.[10]

Health was therefore identified as a total package, an integral part of the wider society and thereby bound up with prevailing socio-economic conditions and political structures. This in part explains the SMA's continuous demand for a shift from curative to preventive medicine. Of course by this time there was nothing new, at least on the political left, in the idea that the capitalist system made you sick. Influential social democratic thinkers such as R.H. Tawney saw health inequalities as central to their moral condemnation of capitalism and possessive individualism.[11] What socialist medical personnel were able to contribute, however, was first-hand, professional experience of contemporary health care provision and analyses from both left-wing and medical perspectives. They saw the anarchy, instability, and inequalities of contemporary capitalism reflected in medical organisation. Services were provided on the basis of patients' income and the profit motive of independent contractors, distortions of medicine's true aims and purposes. At its best, medicine was altruistic; internationalist; geared towards patients' needs, not practitioners' profits; and carried out by teams of professionals – doctors, nurses, social workers and so on – working cooperatively. Moreover, health services should be controlled by *all* citizens rather than by medical élites: the right to health, therefore, implicitly involved more than the passive receipt of welfare.

These arguments put forward by the Association also fit in with wider trends in social democracy's history. In terms of policy formation the inter-war era was, Esping-Andersen suggests, the 'historical watershed in which the struggle for social citizenship became the linchpin of social democratic politics'; and when, as Howell puts it in the specifically British context, the Labour Party adopted a 'social democratic perspective'.[12] This was, however, highly problematic in that social democracy always faces the dilemma of whether to prioritise welfare provision or economic reconstruction. The SMA was on occasions forced to acknowledge this strategic choice; and that the broader labour movement did not always accept the priority it accorded to health care reform, nor the organisational structures which it proposed. But this should also be put in the context of the organisation's assertion that health was highly determined by social conditions and hence the need, for example, for a socialist government to devote significant resources to remedy poor housing conditions.

In 1931, however, when the central characteristics of the SMA programme were being put in place, these problems dwelt largely in the future. The Association had affiliated to the Labour Party – Brook's 'primary essential' – and had thus avoided what its founders saw as the main drawback of bodies such as the SMSA. The SMA had, from the outset, members already well-known in left-wing medical politics. Hastings in particular was important, through his membership of parliament and of party bodies such as the PHAC; through, according to Murray, his contacts with leading Labour politicians such as Christopher Addison and Arthur Greenwood; and in his already-emerging role as a prominent medical figure in London politics.[13] The Labour Party was, for the SMA, the vehicle for the achievement of socialism and, although it might not have yet recognized it, of a socialised medical service. What this might involve was laid down by Hastings at the first AGM. Before examining how the Association's ideas on medical reorganisation developed during the rest of the 1930s, however, it is necessary to look in more detail at certain aspects of its organisation. In particular, attention will be paid to the size and nature of its membership; and to the founding and role of its associated publications.

Membership and propaganda

In 1930 the SMA consisted of only a handful of committed individuals. According to Labour Party annual conference reports, membership throughout the 1930s was consistently 240, remaining so until the rapid acceleration recorded from the early 1940s onwards, dealt with in a subsequent chapter. This suspiciously precise figure almost certainly relates to Labour's requirement for minimum levels of affiliated membership so that an organisation be allowed a party conference delegate. Nonetheless the Association did expand in the course of the decade. The EC report for 1937–38, for example, noted the recruitment of 33 new members, thereby bringing the total to 190. The following year's report claimed five branches (London, Glasgow, Bridgend, Birmingham, and Rotherham) and a total membership of 242. One further point needs to be made about these figures. As the 1937–38 report also recorded, of the total membership of 190, approximately 150 lived and worked in or around London.[14] Having a membership concentrated in the capital had its advantages, particularly when it came to activities on the LCC. More generally, London is the location of national politics, and where pressure groups such as the SMA primarily conduct their business. Nonetheless, the low level of provincial membership was a clear Association weakness, and a hindrance in setting down deep roots in the labour movement as a whole.

If, concentration in London notwithstanding, the SMA was increasing in size by the late 1930s, there still remains the question of who made up the membership. There are two aspects to this, one political, the other occupational. In 1936, as a result of an EC-sponsored resolution to the AGM, the Association's constitution was altered to allow full membership to any socialist who subscribed to the organisation's aims; and who was a member of the medical or 'allied Professions', for example dentistry or nursing. Previously, only doctors accepting the rules of the Labour Party had been allowed full membership. The first of these changes effectively opened the door to members of the Communist Party. The timing here is significant for, as we shall see in Chapter Six, the Association was heavily involved in support for the Spanish

Republic. It therefore became, both practically and politically, a 'popular front' body, adopting a notably left-wing stance on a number of issues. However the acceptance of communists was, as will become apparent, a significant problem for the Association in the longer term.[15]

The admittance of other professions into full membership is also worth discussion. As Brook noted, despite this change doctors 'retained a controlling interest in the Association's governing body'. The Executive Committee of 1942–43, for example, contained 34 members, of whom the majority were medical practitioners or medical scientists. All the leading offices were held by doctors, a situation which prevailed through to the 1970s.[16] This hegemony had a further important dimension. In many ways, the SMA was keen to break down the middle class biases and prejudices of the profession, for instance in its campaign for a more broadly-based entry to medical education in terms of both gender and class. But it was also anxious to maintain professional standards and autonomy, and this attitude was clearly present in the potential tension between democratic control and professional rights.

Ultimately, though, and however much they agonised about it, the medical practitioners who led the SMA knew they were middle-class professionals. Hastings had issued a rallying cry to the middle classes in the early 1920s and in 1935 Brook invited Lawrence Benjamin to speak at the Association's AGM. Benjamin was the author of a Labour Party pamphlet on the role of the middle class in the coming of socialism. This noted that socialism was the 'scientific means' of solving problems of distribution, and that professional workers – including doctors, dentists, and nurses – performed the 'civilising work' of society. The position of such workers under socialism would, therefore, be guaranteed by the state. Moreover it was necessary, under capitalism and socialism, for professionals to organise themselves in associations. Hence Benjamin's urging of those suitably qualified to join bodies affiliated to Labour such as the SMA.[17] It is easy to see the attractiveness of this to the Association, and its intellectual debt to the Webbs. The appeal to science, professionalism, the public spirit ethos, and state guarantees were all matters with which SMA members could empathise. Benjamin was unable to accept Brook's invitation because of other commitments. He noted, however, that recruiting the middle class was of 'first importance to the Movement and specially since the Socialist Medical Association has organised itself for this purpose'. The aim of his pamphlet, he suggested, was to 'break down professional attitudes to Socialism'. This sort of approach is important in understanding the SMA. Its members were certainly socialists. But their aspirations were also motivated by professional ideals, as was the Association's behaviour as a pressure group.[18] This helps explain the continuing concern with clinical independence and the medical practitioners' retention of control within the SMA despite the widening of its membership base.

An important way of keeping in touch with these members was through propaganda and publications. At Welply's suggestion, the first edition of *Socialist Doctor* appeared in February 1932, taking on a new format in the summer of 1933. Its founding prompted a letter to Murray, installed as editor, from George Lansbury in which the Labour leader argued that state medical services were needed 'more than ever'. Health care, he continued, was an area of social organisation which had to be removed 'from the sphere of money-making', very much the sentiments of the SMA itself. *Socialist Doctor*, the 'official organ of the Socialist Medical Association', ran until 1936. It carried a range of material although much was contributed by Hastings and, in various guises, Murray. But as Brook later pointed out, owing to 'financial stringency ... and, eventually, through lack of support, it eventually petered out'.[19]

The indefatigable Murray, however, was not inclined to let matters rest. At the 1937 AGM he proposed the publication of a new journal, to remain the SMA's 'official organ' but widened to include 'all kinds of progressive thought'. Thus was created *Medicine Today and Tomorrow* (*MTT*), which continued until 1965 when it was replaced by *Socialism and Health*. In March 1938 the EC agreed that *MTT* be formally separated from the Association so as to facilitate its broader approach, and to this end a limited liability company was set up. Murray remained editor with the assistance of a sympathetic journalist, L.C.J. McNae. The journal, which first appeared in October 1937, was initially monthly, but once again financial constraints led it to becoming quarterly in 1939.[20]

Administrative complications aside, what is perhaps most noticeable in this story is the new publication's declared mission. As the *MTT* masthead put it, it provided

> a forum for expression of all forms of progressive thought within the medical profession, for discussion of the development of medical practice, and for focusing the attention on the place of the doctor in world affairs.

This certainly seems to have worked in that, according to Murray, contributions 'poured in' from those involved in medical politics from a broad range of positions. The first edition also noted that it had received greetings from important individuals on the left such as Labour leader Clement Attlee, and the advocate of 'social medicine' John Ryle.[21] Clearly, then, the journal sought to be a 'popular front' of medical opinion.

Medicine Today and Tomorrow was of prime importance to the Association, for two related reasons. First, it had an important role in, as Murray put it, keeping 'the SMA programme in front of an expanding audience'. It was therefore a major outlet for Association ideas, both as expressed by individuals such as Hastings and by the organisation as a whole. As internal correspondence in early 1938 makes clear, although technically Murray's responsibility as editor was to the publishing company's shareholders and not to the SMA, in fact the majority of these belonged to the Association. Furthermore, members still received a copy of *MTT* as a part of their membership, and the Association held shares in the publishing company in its own right. The separation of the Association and the journal was thus more formal than actual.[22]

Second, there was the presence of Murray himself. Murray claimed editorial autonomy on *MTT*, and on the creation of the independent publishing company resigned as editor to the SMA and consequently as an EC member. He was, however, soon back on the Executive, and remained a leading figure in the organisation and an important participant in policy formulation. Moreover Murray did not simply edit *MTT*. He was also one of its most frequent contributors, sometimes under pseudonyms such as 'Irwin Brown'. The central point here is that through *MTT* the SMA had the opportunity to thrash out, often in considerable detail, proposals for medical reorganisation. Murray was later to claim, 'with certainty', that 'most of the ideas later incorporated in the NHS, and many still being discussed after twenty years of that service, first appeared in *MTT*'. This view was broadly shared, much earlier, by Brook.[23] While an extravagant assertion, this did contain an element of truth. The journal also carried features on foreign health care systems; on issues such as nurses' pay and conditions; on the importance of environmental factors in ill-health; on the use of film in health education; and on the architectural criteria for efficient medical buildings. All this emphasises the Association's commitment to placing health in its broader social and political contexts.

Communication between the SMA leadership and members was further enhanced by the creation of the monthly *Bulletin*, first published in September 1938 with Dr Elizabeth Bunbury, the Association's Propaganda Secretary, as editor. Bunbury clearly saw her function as educational. As she told the left-wing scientist J.B.S. Haldane shortly after the *Bulletin*'s launch, 'I am trying gradually to introduce a more political and less exclusively medical attitude into the Association, on the basis that we are human beings before we are doctors'.[24] This is an interesting comment on Bunbury's view of her colleagues' political awareness. It implies that while the SMA leadership was highly politicised, this may have been less true of its ordinary members, most of whom were already heavily committed through the demanding nature of their work. The possible differences between leadership and membership are returned to in Chapter Ten. From a rather different angle, Honigsbaum argues that Bunbury's overtly political approach certainly tightened up the Association organisationally. But he also claims that it undermined the SMA's influence on the broader health debate, a further instance of the way in which its left-wing tendencies were, in the long run, a source of weakness.[25] For present purposes, what is important is that the *Bulletin*, like *MTT*, clearly saw itself as having a didactic role, and as dealing with medicine in its broadest possible sense. This is the context in which we now examine the issue which most preoccupied the Association in the 1930s: the need for, and proposed methods of, medical reorganisation.

The principles of socialised health care

The two key formulations of Association policy in the 1930s were *The People's Health* and *A Socialised Medical Service*. Particular attention will be paid to these, and to how their arguments were built upon in further statements by the SMA and its leading members. First, however, it is necessary to say something about their origins and status. In fact the 1932 pamphlet *The People's Health* was not an SMA publication. It was brought out by the Labour Party, with the disclaimer that it was not 'in any way a statement of official ... policy, and has not been examined or approved by the Labour Party as such'. Hastings was the principal author, assisted by J. Bacon, G.P. Blizard, Dr C. Parker, and Dr A. Salter, a 'group of members of the Labour Party particularly interested in public health'. The disclaimer was reinforced by a statement at 1932 party conference which noted that a number of educational texts – including that of Hastings – had come out, but could not be considered policy statements as they had not been discussed by the Policy Committee. This followed on a decision by the Research and Publicity Committee in May when it was agreed to publish the pamphlet but with a 'clear statement' that it was not necessarily official policy.[26] The party leadership's approach here was an early indication of the caution with which it was, ultimately, to deal with the SMA, and particularly its more radical proposals.

A *Socialised Medical Service*, which appeared in 1933, was by contrast an explicitly SMA publication. It too was not an unequivocally supported document. A policy statement had originally been prepared by the Association's research sub-committee and presented to the 1932 AGM, where it was the subject of a day-long debate. During this it ran into opposition from, especially, a dissenting member of the sub-committee, Dr Frank Bushnell. According to Murray and Brook, Bushnell objected to the document's 'reformist' tendencies, particularly regarding the control of a socialised service. This is an interesting – if rather obscure – remark in that Bushnell, at the 1930 ILP conference, had proposed a resolution arguing that in a socialised system the 'authority of medical science would be confined solely to its own sphere, where it would be unquestioned'. Wittingly or otherwise, he was raising an issue we have already noted, the tension between democratic control and professional autonomy. At the SMA meeting other members, less worried by reformism, expressed the need to proceed by stages towards a state medical service, particularly through extending health insurance. Despite these doubts and disagreements the document was subject to only minor modifications, and duly published.[27]

The wariness of the Labour Party leadership and the misgivings of some Association members are not without meaning. It is important to remember two broader issues. First, Labour had only recently suffered a catastrophic general election defeat. This was followed by a period of intense soul-searching and internal debate as to the way forward to a socialist society, with important sections of the party stressing the need to gain command of the economy as a first step. Ameliorative social reform was not necessarily precluded by such a strategy, but it was placed in an ambiguous position – the classic social democratic dilemma. Second, for its socialist critics at least the most obvious characteristic of the inter-war health care system was that it was hardly a 'system' at all. Rather, the provision of medical services was characterised by anarchy, inefficiency, and duplication. Although the SMA drew heavily on the ideas and experiences of earlier in the century, it still saw itself as, in effect, having to build from the foundations upwards. In such circumstances, it was the clarity and coherence of their vision which should be admired, rather than their disagreements and inconsistencies condemned. But what, more precisely, was this vision?

As Murray correctly points out, *The People's Health* and *A Socialised Medical Service* were not identical. Rather enigmatically, he suggests that 'there are just enough differences between the two to show that the author met some differences of opinion in one of the organizations to which the drafts were presented'.[28] Presumably the 'author' here was Hastings, and the 'differences of opinion' those expressed at the 1932 AGM. These notwithstanding, and they are relatively minor, in what follows the two documents are taken together to illustrate SMA thinking on medical reorganisation in the 1930s. Where appropriate, this will be expanded upon or modified in the light of subsequent policy and other statements. The themes under which this discussion is organised are hospitals; teamwork and health centres; and funding and remuneration.

SMA members had long had reservations about voluntary hospitals because they were autonomous and so not subject to planning or control, and because private philanthropy was thought an inefficient and inappropriate method of health care funding. The voluntary hospitals' situation was highlighted by the 1929 Local Government Act which permitted, but did not compel, local authorities to take over Poor Law institutions, and thereby began to bring some measure of order by way of an expanded municipal hospital system. As both *The People's Health* and *A Socialised Medical Service* argued, 'the ideal medical service will need to have associated with it a complete and co-ordinated hospital system', which was also 'a single hospital system'. The 1929 Act's significance was acknowledged, and it was proposed that a slight amendment would enable the full transference of Poor Law institutions to the local authorities which could then build a municipal system free from Poor Law stigma. This was to be a first step towards the abolition of all charges, a process which would be furthered by the repeal of clause 16 of the Act – 'a particularly odious clause' – which required authorities to pursue patients for payment. Municipal hospitals would thus become effectively free, and 'if their efficiency is insisted on by an active Ministry of Health, they will be used by an increasing number of the population'. The potential of the 1929 Act was therefore huge – hence Hastings's earlier noted admiration for Chamberlain's tenure at the Health Ministry, and his claim in 1934 that the Act was a recognition by the Minister that private enterprise in health had failed.[29]

Here, then, were emerging what were to be a number of Association preoccupations, notably the 'active' Health Ministry with, nonetheless, local authorities carrying out the responsibility of hospital provision; and free services, part of a 'complete and co-ordinated hospital system'. Where did these proposals leave the voluntary hospitals? In some respects, *The People's Health* and *A Socialised Medical Service* were relatively moderate here, not least when compared with what Brian Abel-Smith describes as the 'outspoken attack' on them by Hastings in 1931. This had included the suggestion that voluntary institutions would soon have outlived their usefulness, and that their absorption into a 'National or Municipal system seems ... certain within a comparatively few years time'.[30]

Both documents found it 'most undesirable' that a voluntary hospital could be set up anywhere without 'consideration of the existing facilities or the needs of the district'. Such institutions should therefore be licensed and registered, and no new ones founded without special need being demonstrated to the Health Ministry. Moreover the popularity of a free, expanded municipal service would almost certainly increase the charitable sector's current financial problems. In such circumstances, those voluntary hospital governors with the 'good of the community at heart' would realise the need for greater cooperation with the municipal system, and allow local authority hospital committees to take over their institutions. These would then become part of the municipal system, with existing governors being allowed to form up to one-third of the boards of managements during their lifetimes.[31] This was a gradualist approach, predicated on the increasing financial problems of the voluntary sector, with no implication of enforced takeover by local or central state. It is clear, though, that there was an inevitability to this gradualism, and no suggestion, for example, that the voluntary hospitals should be bailed out by government, national or local. Given the political circumstances of the 1930s, this gradualism is understandable enough. The National Government which took power in 1931 was disinclined, ideologically or for any other reason, to either challenge the position of the voluntary sector or to amend the 1929 Local Government Act in the ways suggested by the SMA.

Nonetheless the latter's critique continued unabated. Hastings, Brook, Rickards, and H.B. Morgan gave evidence to the Sankey Commission on voluntary hospitals in 1936, confirming that the SMA's 'ultimate policy' was for their absorption into a 'complete, unified and co-ordinated service'. Pending this, central coordinating offices should be established as a matter of urgency in London and in large provincial centres 'to facilitate speedy admission of emergency and urgent cases to all Hospitals irrespective of whether they are Voluntary or Municipal'. Specifically in the capital, this work should be handed over to the LCC, by 1936 an SMA stronghold. Brook saw their evidence as a 'notable success', with suggestions such as that for pooling beds in emergencies coming about with the wartime Emergency Bed Service for London.[32] The SMA's approach to the Sankey Commission was clearly to state its fundamental principles while pressing for immediate reforms which could, if implemented, bring the autonomous voluntary hospitals into something more resembling a planned system. The fundamental principles did, however, remain. As discussed in Chapter Five, Hastings and his LCC colleagues argued strongly against any council subsidy to the capital's voluntary hospitals. Pressing this point home, an *MTT* editorial in late 1937 suggested that for 'public money to be handed over to private enterprise' – that is the voluntary hospitals – would be 'the negation of democracy'.[33] The tactic was thus financial attrition; the strategy the replacement of an inefficient, ill-coordinated, and undemocratic 'system' with a socialised and municipally controlled health service.

The hospital scheme being proposed was not an end in itself. It was to be part of a comprehensive, unified service covering all aspects of health care, curative and preventive. Furthermore, given the complexity of modern medical knowledge, 'no one doctor, however clever he may be, can know all there is to be known about prevention, diagnosis, and treatment of *all* diseases'. Consequently, in the socialised medical service to come the basic unit must be the team rather than the individual doctor. Under the current state of affairs, as Murray further argued, it could not be suggested that 'the organization of the medical profession has reached its optimum efficiency'. British doctors did remarkably well by individual patients, but 'as a whole the work is unorganized, and the arrangements permit at one and the same time of much overlapping and of many gaps in the service'.[34] What was therefore needed was teamwork and integration, and the crucial institution which would ensure this was to be the health centre.

The idea of the health centre was embryonically present in the Edwardian era in the proposals of the SMSA and other left-wing reformers, and had also been part of the post-war Dawson Report. As we have seen, Murray was later to blame the decline of the SMSA partly on the mistaken belief of some of its members that the battle for health centres had, consequently, been won. This was despite the fact that, as far as Murray was concerned, the Dawson Report had not fully addressed the issue of what constituted a health centre. Moreover by the 1930s there continued to be widespread discussion of how, if at all, such institutions should be organised and controlled. The famous Peckham Health Centre, visited by Association members, provided one possible working model.[35] So it became important for the SMA to define what was meant by the term, and to agitate for the introduction of what it saw as 'true' health centres.

Unsurprisingly, therefore, these were questions which both *The People's Health* and *A Socialised Medical Service* addressed. In urban areas, the population was to be divided into units of around 60 000 people, each served by a health centre located, as far as possible, at the 'obvious natural centre of each unit'. Every centre would have a team of general practitioners, each responsible for between 2000–2500 patients. Patients would be able to choose their own doctor, as long as the doctor still had room on his or her list, and would be seen 'mainly by appointment' at the centre. Although the stated purpose of the GPs was to practise curative medicine, it was also clearly intended that they should have a preventive role. It was to be their duty to 'do their utmost to maintain and improve' their patients' health. General practitioners would therefore carry out periodic medical checks and various mechanisms were to be put in place to allow, for example, for the reporting of unhealthy domestic conditions. Finally, at least one of the GPs attached to each health centre was to be a woman.[36]

If, however, this was the sum of the SMA's proposals they would amount to little more than an advocacy of group practice. But in a socialised medical service, health centres were to have a much broader and more important function. Qualified pharmacists would be available to dispense drugs, while there would be departments and clinics specifically geared to such health issues as child welfare and 'the study and treatment of early mental disease'. Pathological laboratories were to be provided for it was important that 'pathology should not be divorced from clinical medicine', a proposal probably put forward by Murray, himself a pathologist. Centres would have an important role in record keeping, thereby enabling the maximum knowledge of each individual patient; and, again emphasising their preventive and didactic functions, would provide 'health education by lecture and demonstration'. Similar, if slightly more modest, proposals were also made for health centres in rural areas.[37]

The health centre, then, was to provide a comprehensive, integrated service – both curative and preventive – to the citizens of its designated area, and so act as the focal point of health care. Importantly, there was also to be a close relationship with hospitals, general or local. These would take patients sent to them by GPs, who would be encouraged to remain in contact with their hospitalised charges. Once again, this was part of the SMA strategy for bringing general practitioners fully into the health care system, thereby ending their professional and intellectual isolation. Hospital specialists – for example in tuberculosis and venereal disease – would also be attached to centres and have patients referred to them by GPs. Patients could thus receive both primary and more specialist care at or through the centre. As far as the relationship between hospitals and health centres was concerned, integration was clearly to be a two-way process.[38]

Health centres were central to the SMA's vision of a socialised medical service, although many of the details of their operation remained to be worked through. The Association did not have a totally static or fixed model, and matters such as the size of clientele and the precise nature of the services offered were to be the subject of considerable discussion and debate. The significance of health centres, however, was never in doubt, and it is clear that in their method of operation they were to embody the inherent socialism of medical practice. The idea of health centres continued to be pressed by the Association for the rest of the 1930s. In 1938, for example, in a piece devoted largely to a critique of the BMA's plans for a reformed medical service, Hastings stressed the need for local authorities to be encouraged to 'centralize in Health Centres in each locality their various clinical activities'.[39] One of the most important functions of health centres for the Association was, as has been suggested, the merging of all medical personnel into a comprehensive system. This was seen as particularly necessary in respect of general practitioners, as matters currently stood a highly autonomous and individualistic group. The integration of such medical workers in turn raised the issue of their conditions of service, including financial reward. This further raised questions as to how a socialised medical service was to be funded. As these matters were closely interlinked, they are dealt with together in the text.

One of the SMA's principal aims was that the whole population should have access to free medical care, irrespective of age, gender, or employment status. The health insurance scheme as it currently stood provided no coverage for groups such as the dependants of insured workers, and even they gained only limited facilities. The Association clearly felt that this system could not be expanded in such a way as to achieve the desired universality and comprehensiveness. In *The People's Health* and *A Socialised Medical Service* Hastings and his colleagues went into some detail in respect of the complexity of the issue, and the consequent need for a carefully planned transition to a socialised service. A shift away from insurance should be effected as 'soon as national finances make this possible', and medical services should be offered free to all who sought to take advantage of them. Hastings had gained considerable experience of the existing system through his part in drawing up Labour Party and TUC evidence to the Royal Commission on National Health Insurance in the mid-1920s. In 1939 he argued further that:

> Dr Cox (former Secretary of the BMA) had come down on the side of insurance, but he had not said whether he wanted it to be compulsory or voluntary. If compulsory, what was the difference between that and payment through the rates? If voluntary, the people who needed medical service the most would not take the trouble to insure.[40]

In short, universality could not be guaranteed or effectively implemented by the existing, or even an extended, insurance system.

Hastings's possible alternative of local taxation is also worth noting, for two reasons. First, the whole question of how to finance a state medical service was highly problematic given that, for example, the revenue derived from direct taxation was relatively small when compared with what it was to become during and after the Second World War. Raising funds locally, at least in part, may therefore have seemed an attractive option. Second, and rather more positively, Hastings and his colleagues assumed that any future socialised system would be administered primarily at local level. This issue had been made explicit in *A Socialised Medical Service* and *The People's Health*, both of which affirmed that the 'Health Service of the future will be administered by local authorities', although this was to take place under the general supervision of an enhanced Ministry of Health, with the latter having the power to compel 'reactionary local authorities to carry out their statutory duties'.[41] If, however, local authorities were to be given a substantial measure of control in a socialised service, this posed the dilemma of how doctors could be reconciled to such a system. Not only were GPs in particular hostile to the idea of a salaried service, they were also deeply antipathetic to any hint of supervision by local government bodies. How, with this tangle of issues in mind, did the SMA approach the matter of medical remuneration?

In the 1930s general practitioners were, effectively, independent entrepreneurs. They held property in the form of their medical practices, which could be bought and sold, and derived their income from a variety of sources. These included a combination of some or all of their fees from private practice; capitation fees from the health insurance system (the 'panel'); and fees for work undertaken for public bodies such as the school medical service. One effect of this was to institutionalise an inherent conflict between improving medical care and maintaining doctors' living standards. There was a further twist in that GPs, in the years before the Second World War, developed a strong sense of grievance over both their own income levels and the wide disparities in medical remuneration. They would therefore have been unlikely to welcome changes perceived, rightly or wrongly, as eroding their standard of living and economic autonomy. This was particularly so in the case of one crucial part of their earnings, that from panel patients.[42] This situation, whereby the nation's health was apparently being sacrificed to individual interests, was for the SMA a prime example of what was wrong with British health provision. It therefore argued that all medical personnel in a socialised health system, including doctors of all types, should ideally be salaried employees of the state. At least some of its members were uneasy about what was perceived as, in the words of one correspondent to Brook, the organisation's 'tendency to show a none too friendly attitude to the general practitioner'.[43] But the Association did realise the importance of not alienating GPs, many of whom were already feeling beleaguered, any more than was necessary. It was therefore anxious to stress the positive aspects of a particular form of relationship between doctors and the state.

This question was hardly a new one. It had been the subject of discussion by, among others, the Webbs and the SMSA in the Edwardian period, while the PHAC had called for doctors to work in teams, and for the funding of a state medical service through general taxation rather than insurance. Crucially, Hastings had, as we have seen, addressed the implications of the economic relationship between doctor and patient in his speech to the Association's 1931 AGM. Here he stressed the 'dependence' of many medical practitioners on their patients and, by contrast, the professional benefits which payment by salary could bring to doctors themselves. This idea that doctors would actually be liberated by a salaried service – for example through the economic security of a pension scheme, the true independence which an end to the cash nexus would bring, and the opportunity to pursue further medical education – became a central strand in the SMA's argument and an appeal to both the altruism and the self-interest of its fellow professionals. In turn such a rejection of individualism was part of a broader historical change. As Hastings again put it in 1931, in health private enterprise had failed 'lamentably'. The 'spirit of the age demanded collective action', and he therefore had no doubt that the already existing trend away from the family doctor to state medicine would continue.[44]

Consequently, these issues were very much the concerns of *The People's Health* and *A Socialised Medical Service*. Both emphasised that there should be no 'economic barrier between the doctor and his patient'. Both repeated, verbatim, Hastings's remarks about economic dependence, and stressed that a free and comprehensive state service must necessarily be staffed by full-time, salaried medical practitioners. Team work too was emphasised, again in terms very similar to those of 1931, for 'lacking in our health services to-day is above all else organisation and cooperation'. In short, the doctor was to be 'at the service of his patients'. Patients had, or ought to have, rights by virtue of being citizens in a democratic society. These rights were to include not only free access to medical care but also the right to have a say in how medical services were to be run, although once again the question of possible tension between this democratic right and doctors' professional rights remained unresolved. The overall message, however, was clear. A socialised service should be free to all patients, and doctors should be salaried employees of the state to the benefit of both themselves and society as a whole.[45]

The international character of medicine

So far we have traced both the organisation and ideas of the SMA as they developed from its foundation in 1930, focusing in particular on two early policy statements. Before placing these in the broader context of labour and medical politics in the 1930s attention needs to be paid to one further important influence on the Association's thought. The SMA was firmly committed to internationalism: medical knowledge was shared across national boundaries, and socialism was, by definition, internationalist. Part of the impetus for the Association's creation had come from a German colleague. In 1931 it sent delegates – Hastings and Dr V.H. Rutherford – to the first congress of the International Socialist Medical Association in Carlsbad, and Hastings and Brook became the British representatives on its Executive Committee. Hastings later recalled that he brought home a photograph of the participants in the Carlsbad conference which allowed him to identify refugee doctors in the years before the outbreak of war. When invasion of England seemed imminent, he took the sensible precaution of burying this photograph and accompanying documents in his garden, from whence he was able to retrieve them unharmed a few years later.[46] Chapter Six shows some of the practical implications of SMA internationalism, but here the influence of ideas from other medical systems is considered.

The Association had an ongoing interest in the health service provision of other nations – hence the regular *MTT* column, 'Medical News of the World'. In the 1930s Hastings in particular also visited various foreign countries. In 1931, for example, he and Salter travelled to the Soviet Union. Hastings subsequently praised that country's 'prophylactoria', or health centres, commending especially their apparent efficiency, medical division of labour, and preventive as well as curative functions. Despite the scepticism of some Association members about the Bolshevik regime, Soviet health care was often held up by the left as an example of what could be achieved in a socialised system – hence Harold Laski's invitation to Hastings, in the immediate aftermath of his journey, to join a Fabian Research Bureau committee on the USSR.[47]

Murray had no doubt that in qualitative terms British doctors were at least the equal of their Russian counterparts. But, he went on, the Soviet Union could 'teach us something of organisation and give us new ideas to ponder over'. In particular, it had shown that when doctors were 'freed from financial anxiety' and integrated into a comprehensive and free service, then they were able to give to patients the full benefits of modern medicine. Like Hastings and Salter, Elizabeth Bunbury visited the USSR. While finding it a 'paradoxical country', she was nonetheless impressed by a society where medicine was not seen as isolated, but as part of the 'social complex'. In England, doctors were continually hampered by the 'economic system', among the consequences of which were lack of income on the part of patients and lack of coordination and research on the part of doctors. In the Soviet Union, by contrast, there was 'a general plan for public health in which all forms of activity are correlated'. All medical workers could thus justifiably feel they were contributing to the general good.[48] Here Murray and Bunbury were clearly stressing the positive impact on both doctors and patients of a salaried service, as did Hastings.

Another important aspect of the Soviet system for Association members was its method of recruitment. The SMA, quite rightly, saw the British medical profession as being drawn largely from the middle classes, in part at least because of the expense of medical education. In the USSR, Hastings told an Association meeting in 1932, the full costs of education were met by the state, and students were 'for the most part recruited from the factories and collective farms'. Drawing trainee doctors from all parts of society meant, he continued, that students came to their studies 'with some knowledge and experience of the world as it really is'. This contrasted with the British situation, where the outlook of doctors was largely shaped by 'the nursery and public school'. It was clear from all this which system Hastings – a public school product himself – preferred.[49]

Idealised (and misguided) as such analyses of Soviet health care undoubtedly were, they clearly played a part in reinforcing SMA policy on socialised medicine. This process was almost certainly furthered by the publication in 1937 of Henry Sigerist's book on medicine in the USSR, the subject of a favourable review in MTT. Sigerist's work provided, for example, a detailed and generally positive description of health centres, and was dedicated to the 'young medical workers in whose hands the future of medicine lies'. It is perhaps from Sigerist that Murray took the title for one of his own books, The Future of Medicine, published in 1942. On the other hand, and as Honigsbaum again points out, the enthusiasm of certain leading members for the USSR would have done nothing to enhance the Association's reputation with the Labour leadership.[50]

But the USSR was not the only foreign country from which the Association could derive inspiration. Certain characteristics of social democratic Sweden's health provision were also much admired. Hastings visited Sweden in the early 1930s and reported that in terms of organisation and equipment its hospitals were 'the best in the world'. He was inspired enough by what he had seen to claim that at least in the sphere of health Sweden was 'solving to some extent the difficult problem of the transition from Capitalism to Socialism'. It seems likely that Hastings was particularly won over by the fact the Swedish hospitals were run by local authorities, another possible source of SMA inspiration on this issue. And as with the Soviet Union, he was also taken by the availability of a scholarship scheme for medical school.[51] In short, the SMA was internationalist in outlook, and prepared to draw lessons from the health systems of other countries and apply these to the British situation. As Hastings put it in 1933,

> What we want ... is a State Medical Service providing at the cost of the rates and taxes, the best that medical services can give for rich and poor alike. There is nothing unusual or extraordinary in such a service. They have it in Russia and they have it in Sweden. I have seen it working in both countries ... .[52]

This was a brief, but accurate, statement of the Association position. We will now examine the wider context in which the organisation operated, and the extent to which its proposals were gaining influence.

Notes

1. Murray, *Why a National Health Service?*, p. 17ff; Brook, *Making Medical History*, p. 1ff; DSM 1/1, EC Report, AGM 1934; and DSM 1/1, Report of the EC, May 1939–April 1940. The Hastings article was 'The Future of Medical Practice in England', *Lancet*, 1928, I, pp. 67–9.
2. Webster, 'Labour and the Origins of the National Health Service', p. 187; Peter Bartrip, *Themselves Writ Large: the British Medical Association 1832–1966*, BMJ Publishing Group, 1996, p. 215.
3. Brook, *Making Medical History*, pp. 3–4; Murray, *Why a National Health Service?*, pp. 21–2; DSM (2) 5, 'International SMA', Brook to Fabian 24 September 1930.
4. DSM 1/1, Report of the EC, 1930–31; Brown, *Back-Room Boys of State Medicine*; Brook, *Making Medical History*, pp. 5–6; Webster, 'Labour and the Origins of the National Health Service', p. 187.
5. DSM 1/1, Minutes of the First AGM, 10 May 1931; Report of the EC, 1931–32; Milton Terris, 'Epidemiology and the Public Health Movement', *Journal of Chronic Diseases*, 1986, 39, 12, p. 958.
6. *Lancet*, 1931, I, pp. 1115ff.
7. *Lancet*, 1933, I, p. 1324, and II, p. 1459.
8. Somerville Hastings, 'The First Steps towards a Socialized Medical Service', *MTT*, July 1938, p. 4.
9. *Lancet*, 1932, I, p. 838.
10. *Lancet*, 1932, II, p. 1185; Stella Churchill, 'Socialisation of the Medical Services', *Fabian Quarterly*, no.5, March 1935, p. 16.
11. Geoffrey Foote, *The Labour Party's Political Thought*, 2nd edn, Croom Helm, 1986, pp. 77–8.
12. Esping-Andersen, 'Citizenship and Socialism', p. 83; David Howell, *British Social Democracy*, Croom Helm, 1976, p. 47.
13. Brook, *Making Medical History*, p. 3; Brown, *Back-Room Boys of State Medicine*; Stewart, '"For a Healthy London"', pp. 419–20.
14. DSM 1/1, Report of the EC, 1937–38; and Report of the EC, 1938–39.
15. DSM (2) 6, document for 1936 AGM, 'Proposed Changes in the Constitution'; DSM 1/1, Minutes of the Sixth AGM, 24 May 1936. See also Honigsbaum, *Division in British Medicine*, pp. 259–60; and Brook, *Making Medical History*, p. 3.
16. Brook, *Making Medical History*, p. 3; DSM 4/2, Members of the Executive Committee 1942/3; Watkins, *Medicine and Labour*, p. 61, where it is

also noted that the shift to a predominantly non-medical membership resulted in the change of name to 'Socialist Health Association'.

17. Lawrence Benjamin, *The Position of the Middle-Class Worker in the Transition to Socialism*, Labour Party, 1935, pp. 11, 16, 17, 22.

18. DSM (3)/3, item 2; on the whole issue of professionalisation see Harold Perkin, *The Rise of Professional Society*, Routledge, 1989, *passim*.

19. DSM 1/1, Report of the EC, 1931/2; Report of the EC, 1932/3; AGM 1934, EC Report; DSM (2) 7, item g), Lansbury to David Stark Murray, 7 July 1933; Brook, *Making Medical History*, p. 7.

20. DSM 1/1, Minutes of the Seventh AGM, 9 May 1937; Report of the EC, 1937/8; and Murray, *Why a National Health Service?*, pp. 36–7.

21. *MTT*, no. 1, October 1937, p. 13.

22. Murray, *Why a National Health Service?*, p. 37; DSM (3) 14/25; DSM 1/1, Minutes of the Eighth AGM, 22 May 1938.

23. On Murray's life and ideas, see Stewart, 'The "Back-Room Boys of State Medicine"', *passim*; *idem*, 'David Stark Murray', in the forthcoming *New Dictionary of National Biography*, London and Oxford, British Academy/Oxford University Press, 2004; Murray, *Why a National Health Service?*, p. 38; Brook, *Making Medical History*, p. 7.

24. Murray, *Why a National Health Service?*, pp. 40, 46; DSM (3) 14/30.

25. Honigsbaum, *Division in British Medicine*, pp. 261–2.

26. Somerville Hastings, *The People's Health*, Labour Party, 1932, p. 2; Labour Party, *Report of the Thirty-Second Annual Conference*, Labour Party, 1932, p. 64; Minutes of a Meeting of the Labour Party Research and Publicity Committee, 18 May 1932, p. 2.

27. SMA, *A Socialised Medical Service*, SMA, 1933; DSM 1/1, Report of the EC 1931/2; Report of the EC 1932/3; and Brook, *Making Medical History*, p. 6; Murray, *Why a National Health Service?*, p. 26; DSM 4/1, 'Socialisation of Medicine: Independent Labour Party Resolution', by F.G. Bushnell.

28. Murray, *Why a National Health Service?*, p. 26.

29. Hastings, *The People's Health*, pp. 10, 18–19; SMA, *A Socialised Medical Service*, pp. 11, 18–19; Somerville Hastings, 'Socialism and Public Health', *Socialist Doctor*, vol. II, no. 3, May 1934, p. 12.

30. Abel-Smith, *The Hospitals, 1800–1948*, pp. 365–6.

31. Hastings, *The People's Health*, pp. 18–19; SMA, *A Socialised Medical Service*, pp. 18–19.

32. 'Submission to the Voluntary Hospitals Commission of the Socialist Medical Association of Great Britain', DSM (2) 5; also, *Lancet*, 1936, II, p. 353; Brook, *Making Medical History*, p. 10.

33. *MTT*, no. 3, December 1937, p. 13.

34. Hastings, *The People's Health*, p. 5; SMA, *A Socialised Medical Service*, p. 5; David Stark Murray, *Science Fights Death*, Watts and Co., 1936, p. 9.

35 Phoebe Hall, 'The Development of Health Centres', in Hall, Phoebe, Land, Hilary, Parker, Roy and Webb, Adrian (eds), *Change, Choice and Conflict in Social Policy*, Heinemann, 1975, pp. 279–80; Jane Lewis and Barbara Brookes, 'The Peckham Health Centre, "PEP", and the Concept of General Practice during the 1930s and 1940s', *Medical History*, 27, 1983; DSM 1/1, Report of the EC, 1935–36.

36. Hastings, *The People's Health*, p. 9; SMA, *A Socialised Medical Service*,

p. 9. The two disagree about the number of patients per doctor, the former arguing for 1:2000, the latter for 1:2500. This is one of the modifications alluded to by Murray, *Why a National Health Service?*, p. 26.

37. Hastings, *The People's Health*, pp. 9–10, 13; SMA, *A Socialised Medical Service*, pp. 9–10, 14. With respect to rural areas, the two works once again disagree slightly on the ratio of doctors to patients.

38. Hastings, *The People's Health*, p. 11; SMA, *A Socialised Medical Service*, p. 11.

39. Somerville Hastings, 'The First Steps Towards a Socialized Medical Service', *MTT*, no. 10, July 1938, p. 5.

40. Hastings, *The People's Health*, pp. 16–17; SMA, *A Socialised Medical Service*, pp. 17–18; *BMJ*, 1939, I, pp. 451–2; Earwicker, thesis, p. 177.

41. SMA, *A Socialised Medical Service*, p. 7; Hastings, *The People's Health*, p. 7.

42. Anne Digby and Nick Bosanquet, 'Doctors and Patients in an Era of National Health Insurance and Private Practice, 1913–1938', *Economic History Review*, 1988, 2nd series, 41, 1; Charles Webster, 'Doctors, Public Service and Profit: General Practitioners and the National Health Service', *Transactions of the Royal Historical Society*, 1990, 5th series, 40.

43. DSM (2) 6, E. Fairfield Thomas to Brook, 19 October 1936. Thomas in fact resigned over this issue.

44. Somerville Hastings, 'Can We Afford to Leave the Nation's Health to Private Enterprise', *Labour Magazine*, April 1931, p. 545; and *BMJ*, 1931, I, p. 470.

45. Hastings, *The People's Health*, pp. 4–5, 6; SMA, *A Socialised Medical Service*, pp. 4–5, 6.

46. Murray, *Why a National Health Service?*, p. 24; SMA *Bulletin*, no. 5, January 1939, pp. 1–2; DSH, File 3, 'International Socialist Medical Association', memo by Hastings on 'A New International Socialist Medical Association', 1948.

47. There are accounts of the Russian trip in Brockway, *The Bermondsey Story*, pp. 155–61; and in Somerville Hastings, *Medicine in Soviet Russia*, n.p. , 1932(?), reprinted from *Medical World*, January 1932; DSH, Bundle 1, General: Laski to Hastings, 6 January 1932.

48. David Stark Murray, 'Should Medicine be Just a Trade?', *Reynolds Illustrated News*, 26 December 1937, cutting in DSM (2) 4; Elizabeth Bunbury, 'An English Doctor in Russia', *MTT*, no. 7, April 1938, pp. 15–16.

49. *Lancet*, 1932, I, p. 1213.

50. Henry E. Sigerist, *Socialised Medicine in the Soviet Union*, Victor Gollancz, 1937, pp. 289–96, and dedication; review, by Philip Wiles, in *MTT*, no. 4, January 1938, pp. 5–6; Honigsbaum, *Division in British Medicine*, pp. 261–2.

51. Somerville Hastings, 'The People's Health in Sweden', *Socialist Doctor*, vol. II, no. 2, November 1933, pp. 2–3.

52. Somerville Hastings, 'When Sickness Comes', *The Chingford Advertiser*, October 1933, cutting in DSH, File 2, 'Articles'.

CHAPTER FOUR

The SMA, the Labour Party, and Medical Politics in the 1930s

The SMA's founders had come to view the State Medical Service Association's lack of political focus and identification as one of its principal weaknesses. Affiliation to the Labour Party was therefore perceived as a major breakthrough in left-wing medical politics, not least because it gave the Association a platform – the annual party conference – from which to address the wider labour movement. Hastings was conference delegate for most of the 1930s, and he and his organisation achieved their first major success in 1932. Hastings proposed a motion – seconded by Rickards, one of the London Labour Party delegates – seeking the introduction of a state medical service. As Hastings put it, the country's health needs

> can only be effectively provided by the establishment of a complete State Medical Service, giving everything necessary for the prevention and treatment of disease, free and open to all.

An investigation into the issue was also demanded of the party executive, and the resolution as a whole duly agreed.[1] The Association could therefore feel justifiably pleased at having made such an impact at the first conference at which it was represented in its own right.

But this was not an unequivocal triumph, and in this we can see once more the circumscribed place which the SMA held in the contemporary labour movement. In the wake of the electoral disaster of 1931 the Labour leadership was cautious about immediately committing itself to any specific policy until all options had been fully considered. As George Latham, conference chairman and NEC member, told delegates in 1932, he did not wish to be seen as offering any objection to the Association's motion. But, he continued, he would be failing in his duty if he did not point out that its implications were 'very far reaching'. The executive would examine the matter, and consult not only with the SMA but with 'everybody concerned'.[2] Such official caution was also, as we saw in the last chapter, evident in contemporaneous publication of *The People's Health*.

Consequently the Association was moved to write to party headquarters in mid-1933 asking what had become of the proposed inquiry into a state medical service, and in response was told that nothing could be done about this prior to annual conference. At this meeting Hastings further questioned why the previous year's resolution had not been acted upon. Herbert Morrison, a colleague of Hastings on the LCC and a leading figure in both London and national Labour politics, replied that it had been a busy year and that the NEC would address the issue as soon as possible. Hastings was careful to acknowledge that other socio-economic matters, for example bank nationalisation, might have to be considered first. But he argued that while a state medical service could not be achieved immediately, nonetheless 'we must have a mental picture of the service we want to develop'. To this end, and perhaps explaining Hastings's conciliatory tone, the party set up a Medical Services Committee which, as Murray suggests, was largely composed of representatives from the SMA. This body, which met four times in the course of the following year, was chaired by Association member and TUC medical advisor H.B. Morgan. Other SMA participants, of whom there were around eight out of the committee total of fifteen, included Hastings, Brook, and Rickards.[3]

The Medical Services Committee presented its report, A State Health Service, to 1934 party conference. The document acknowledged the complexity of the subject under discussion, as a result of which the committee had felt it best to raise the general issues at conference before going any further with its work. Nonetheless specific policy proposals were made, and a number of these clearly coincided with those of the SMA. It was suggested, for example, that a state service could be built in one of two ways: through an extension of health insurance, or through local authority health services. The latter was deemed 'the proper course'. This meant, effectively, that the existing panel system should come to an end, something to be welcomed given its 'very grave deficiencies'. The 'ultimate aim' was a unified service providing, through local authorities, universal, comprehensive, and free care. This could, however, only be achieved in stages, for 'financial and other reasons'.[4] Such arguments echoed very closely those put forward in documents such as The People's Health and A Socialised Medical Service. Similarly, A State Health Service identified three prerequisites for the development of a socialised service: the consolidation of all existing local authority medical services outside the Poor Law; the ending of local authority dealings with voluntary agencies, including voluntary hospitals, which ideally should be taken over; and the provision of a service under such a scheme at least as good as that provided to those covered by the insurance system. Suggestions were made as to the timing and prioritising of the transitional arrangements, although it was recognised that even before this much work had to be done, especially by local government. Emphasis was also laid on the need to develop health centres, designed not to replace the domiciliary service but rather to become 'the centre round which such attendance and the other facilities of the Public Health Service should evolve'.[5]

Finally, the report turned its attention to the medical profession itself. The panel system had created 'vested interests', in that panels were in effect a form of property which could be bought or sold. It should therefore be transformed as soon as possible into a non-transferable institution, effectively being absorbed into the public scheme to which doctors would be contracted on a part-time basis. In the longer term, the document continued, the 'aim would be to amalgamate part-time appointments into full-time public appointments'.[6] This was a rather convoluted way of proposing something approaching a full-time salaried service, but the general message was clear enough. The concept of 'vested interests', which we have already encountered in the writings of Edwardian reformers and which was consistently advanced by the SMA, is also worth noting. It encompassed the commercial insurance companies and, in particular, the organised medical profession as represented by the BMA. These, it was argued, had an interest in promoting sickness rather than health, and were thereby a block on medical progress. The rhetoric of 'vested interests' was to become especially pronounced in the 1940s.

The SMA's success in strongly influencing the form and content of this report should not be undervalued. However, while *A State Health Service* pressed some central Association preoccupations, unsurprisingly given the composition of the committee which produced it, it was also a deliberately cautious document. This was pointed out forcefully in the journal *Socialist Doctor*. An article, unsigned but almost certainly by Murray, welcomed the emphasis on the local authority model of administration. This was especially important for, as we shall see in the next chapter, by this time Labour had gained control of the LCC and Association members been given considerable powers over the capital's health services. But as a whole, the piece continued, *A State Health Service* would 'do nothing to further the case for a State Health Service'. It showed 'no comprehension of the whole problem' – for example in its lack of clarity 'as to how much of the wasteful voluntary system should be allowed to continue'. The exercise had been valuable, however, in prompting a critical reappraisal of the SMA programme.[7] This last comment is especially interesting, suggesting as it does the fluidity and complexity of the debates and discussions inside the organisation, as well as within the broader labour movement.

The report was discussed by conference itself. Hastings, again Association delegate, agreed that it was only a 'first step' and that he and the SMA would continue to fight for a free and comprehensive service, curative and preventive. He admitted that devising a socialised medical service was a difficult task, but pointed out that Labour was now 'getting hold of the local authorities' – undoubtedly a reference to the LCC – and that some sort of plan was necessary for advances to be made. These remarks should be seen in the broader context of Labour's tactic of seeking to undermine the National Government through the capturing of local institutions. Hastings was also at pains to stress the need for health centres; and to suggest that while patients should have a free choice of doctor, this was something which did not need over-emphasis. The report, and the associated passage in the policy statement *For Socialism and Peace*, were duly adopted. The Labour leadership, however, remained cautious. The Annual Report noted that the Medical Committee's proposals were 'preliminary'. Moving their acceptance on the NEC's behalf, Barbara Ayrton Gould also drew attention to the provisional nature of the committee's findings, and suggested that a more detailed document would be forthcoming the following year.[8]

The Public Health Advisory Committee

Nothing, however, came of this, at least in the form promised. Once again, therefore, the SMA can be regarded as having experienced mixed fortunes in its attempts to push the Labour Party towards its vision of a socialised service. It had clearly made the running in health terms from 1932 to 1934, both in its own right and through its influence on an official party committee. The 1935 EC Report remarked that the events of this period were 'an achievement of which the Association may be particularly proud', and its members were later to look back on the 1934 conference as the first major step in the creation of the National Health Service.[9] When added to SMA activities on the LCC, all this seems highly positive. On the other hand, the Labour leadership was clearly keeping its options open and not, as yet, committing itself to any specific form of health service reorganisation, and this must be seen as a qualification on the Association's successes. However, before suggesting what further constraints were operating on the SMA, both inside the labour movement and in the wider medico-political sphere, attention should be drawn to one of its most important domestic political achievements of the 1930s.

We have noted that the Labour Party's Public Health Advisory Committee, following a spasmodic existence after the First World War, finally expired in the early 1930s. This was despite offers of help from Brook, on behalf of the SMA, in late 1930. Although Hastings and his Association colleague Dr R.A. Lyster were coopted to the Local

Government and Social Services Sub-Committee specifically to help prepare a report on the 'Development of Public Health Services', the mid-1930s were a period of anti-climax for the SMA in respect of overt influence on the Labour Party, at least at national level. After the satisfaction in 1935 with the course of events inside the party, by the following year the EC was noting the failure of its conference resolutions to be taken on two consecutive occasions (on health matters at least, this was to continue to be the case at subsequent pre-war conferences); and suggesting the need, as a matter of urgency, for a reorganisation of conference machinery so that more resolutions could be dealt with.[10] Such complaints about conference organisation re-emerged in the late 1940s, suggesting that over the long term the Association did not feel that it had been especially well served by participation in these events. More generally, Labour itself was under the control of moderates anxious that the electoral gains of 1935 should not be jeopardised in the next general election, due in 1940, by any over-ambitious plans or rhetoric.[11]

However 1937 did see a significant development of the SMA's role within the Labour Party. At a meeting of the newly-created Home Policy Committee in November it was agreed to reappoint a number of subsidiary bodies. These included the Local Government Committee, one of whose own advisory sub-groups was to be the Public Health Committee whose purpose was the preparation of a 'comprehensive statement of public health policy'. It took a full year for the reconstituted PHAC to meet for the first time, but when it did it had a strong SMA presence. Of its sixteen members, at least half belonged also to the Association. These included Brook, Murray, Rickards, Lyster, Amy Sayle, and, in the crucial position of chairman, Hastings. Although the inaugural meeting made it clear that committee members were to act as individuals, not as representatives of any organisation, nonetheless the size of the SMA contingent must be viewed as a clear recognition of its place within the labour movement in devising plans for a reconstructed health service.[12] It was certainly the case that by the late 1930s the Association was becoming increasingly determined that greater stress should be placed by Labour on this issue. As an *MTT* editorial of January 1938 put it, the SMA had some years ago put forward what was in many ways a 'good plan' for medical reorganisation, but since then things had moved on, especially in local government. It was therefore necessary to devise plans

> for a full and complete State Medical Service, not a sketchy outline of hopes and aspirations to serve as policy, but a scheme complete in all its administrative details, ready for adoption by the first Administration with sufficient vision to put it into operation.

This was clearly a call to action for both the SMA and the Labour Party. The former had proposals for a socialised scheme which it was adapting in the light of experience, especially that of the LCC. The latter, however, was much less focused in its ideas, hence the need for enhanced Association input to party deliberations. Furthermore, as an article in the same edition put it, any new scheme should not be built on health insurance, 'that idol with the feet of clay'.[13] Much hope must, therefore, have been invested in the SMA's strength on the reconstituted PHAC, and in its various guises this body was to play an important role in the ensuing years in debating and formulating Labour's health policy.

However, one of the first issues the PHAC faced highlighted the complexities of creating a socialised system of health care, and the contested area in which the SMA was operating. In 1936 a Joint Committee on Medical Questions was set up by the TUC and the BMA, and its principal outcome in the pre-war era was suggestions for a national maternity scheme. The maternal mortality rate remained stubbornly high in the 1930s, and was thus in itself extremely important in driving health discussions. This was particularly so in the labour movement, and Labour Party policy statements frequently highlighted its significance. Furthermore, there was an ongoing debate over the respective merits of hospital and home deliveries; and the role to be played by specialists, midwives, and general practitioners. The Joint Committee scheme rested on the three related ideas of the primacy of GP care; a domiciliary service; and funding through an extension of insurance. As Earwicker points out, the acceptance of these principles was a 'complete capitulation by the TUC to the BMA point of view'. Considerable disquiet was voiced in the labour movement about these proposals, for example over the suggested control of such a service by the medical profession, with SMA members prominent in the objections.[14] The whole episode throws light on the kind of problems faced by the Association, even allowing for its influence on official Labour committees, and this is further illustrated by a brief account of the critique offered by its members.

The SMA attacked the BMA-TUC scheme through a number of routes: by its meetings and propaganda; on the PHAC; and, as Earwicker has shown, as individuals (notably Hastings and Sayle) in Labour Party delegations. In so doing, it drew on its own existing plans for enhanced maternity provision. These had been worked out in 1933–34, primarily by Rickards and Edith Summerskill, and despite differences – notably over home versus hospital deliveries – consensus had been reached on two vital issues. First, any maternity scheme should be part of, and integrated with, a more general state medical service, supervised nationally by the Ministry of Health and locally by local authorities. Second, and irrespective of whether delivery took place at home or in the hospital, the primary responsibility should rest with midwives. This was designed to move maternity care out of the hands of GPs and into those of specialists. In turn, this was a critique of GP skills, greed, and commitment to an essential public service. As Summerskill put it, the 'time has come when we must recognise only one interest – one that has been largely ignored – the interest of the expectant mother'. Brook was later to claim the Association's role in highlighting the problems of maternal mortality as the beginning of 'the campaign for safer mother-hood in Britain'. The SMA had also, by the mid-1930s, direct experience of the administration of maternity services through its activities on the LCC, especially in the wake of the 1936 Midwives Act.[15]

Drawing on these analyses and experience, the July 1938 edition of *MTT* described the BMA-TUC scheme as a 'negation of progress', and denounced the TUC for supporting the BMA's 'backward step'. In an internal Association document prepared primarily by Hastings it was pointed out that, contrary to the claims of the BMA and the TUC, many GPs disliked providing maternity services, were incompetent at such provision, and did so only in order to maximise their incomes. Explic-itly on this last point, it was argued that

> so long as doctoring remains a trade in a capitalist society, very
> many other factors beside the best interest of the patient are bound
> to enter in, little as the doctor himself may be conscious of the fact.

Furthermore, the conditions under which GPs worked had in them-selves contributed to the high levels of maternal mortality.[16] Here, then, were further instances of the economic barrier to health which disad-vantaged the patient and compromised the doctor, and of Association scepticism about current GP expertise.

The proposed scheme was also debated on Labour Party bodies. The Home Policy Committee noted its deviation from official party policy, and that it was to be discussed by the PHAC. These discussions, which took place at two meetings in November 1938, illustrate both the role being played by Association members in official party deliberations on health and the potential for dissension on such issues inside the broader labour movement. At the first meeting, the view was initially expressed (it is not clear from the records by whom, but very probably the committee chairman, Hastings) that the BMA-TUC proposals were con-trary to party policy as laid down in 1934, in particular because they would take away important functions from local authority clinics and hand them back to private practitioners. This would create – in a familiar phrase – 'enormous vested interests' which would be difficult to displace, but which would have to be destroyed with the coming of a state medical service. Nonetheless the scheme had its defenders, specifically in the persons of TUC medical advisor H.B. Morgan (also, of course, an SMA member) and J.L. Smyth, Secretary of the TUC's Social Insurance Committee, the two principal labour movement initiators of the Joint Committee. Among their arguments was that GPs should be given facilities to attend their patients while in hospital. This effectively meant that one doctor – the GP – should be solely responsible for the whole course of a woman's pregnancy. If implemented, this would institutionalise and consolidate the general practitioner's position, and thereby his income.[17] This position was attacked by, among others, Esther Rickards. She (reluctantly) agreed that Morgan and Smyth's argument might apply to rural districts, but claimed that it was 'undesirable and unworkable' elsewhere. In most big maternity units in modern hospitals, she continued, 'there was complete coordination and continuity of knowledge of a patient but not one doctor responsible for the case'. This was, she implied, the most efficient means of care in virtually all circumstances. The second meeting a week later equally failed to reach a consensus. Criticisms were raised over the lack of consultation with the Labour Party on the proposed scheme, and Lyster made the not especially helpful, but almost certainly heartfelt, point that 'the BMA represented the great vested interests of disease'.[18]

This was the last, inconclusive, discussion of the issue on the PHAC, although not entirely the end of the affair. The Home Policy Committee recorded in December 1938 that the Health Committee had debated the proposed maternity scheme on two occasions, and that 'negotiations with the TUC were under way'. A number of meetings, at which SMA members such as Sayle and Hastings were present as Labour Party representatives, duly took place. In the face of mounting criticism, and aided by the interruption of war, the BMA-TUC scheme went quietly to its grave. The PHAC itself lapsed into relative inactivity, apart from producing a rather vague document on *Labour and the Hospitals*.[19] The maternity episode provides, however, a useful way into assessing the SMA's position as the 1930s drew to a close.

The SMA and the wider labour movement

The first point is to re-emphasise the Association's success in gaining, in a short space of time, access to and influence on the Labour Party as a whole. It was affiliated to the party, the Fabian Society, and its London branch to the London Labour Party. The SMA had played an important part in driving Labour's discussions of health policy, initially through party conference, and had gained an important foothold on the PHAC.

It had also set up a 'memorandum of agreement' with another left-wing medical organisation, the Inter-Hospitals Socialist Society, whereby each body had two members who sat on the executive committee of the other.[20] To all this should be added the Association's position on the LCC, very much Labour's 'flagship' in the 1930s. Furthermore it was able to put forward a relatively coherent vision of what it wanted from a state medical service, and the method of its achievement. This was no mean feat, given the anarchy, overlap, entrepreneurialism, and lack of coordination of the existing health care 'system'. But, as will already be evident, it was certainly not the case that the SMA was the only player in this complicated game.

The Medical Practitioners Union, for example, was also part of the labour movement through its affiliation to the TUC in 1934. Two years later it too entered the maternity care debate. The MPU's policy statement was described by Brook to a correspondent as 'a most reactionary and in my opinion inconceivably stupid Memorandum'. The recipient of this letter was a St Helens councillor, Alderman Taylor. Taylor had sought Brook's advice on a forthcoming MPU delegation taking up the cause of local GPs who had been excluded from maternity provision, presumably in the municipal hospital. Brook commended the council on its stand; argued that the 'only proper method' for deliveries was attendance by specialists; and so suggested that the council not bother seeing the MPU deputation. Brook's hostility to the MPU proposals was based on factors such as its proposed expansion of opportunities for GPs to take on maternity cases, a point it had in common with the BMA-TUC plan. On the other hand, the MPU – unlike the Joint Committee – favoured a nationally rather than locally organised maternity scheme. This reflected the deep hostility which GPs, and an organisation of GPs such as the MPU, felt towards any move towards local authority, lay control. More generally, MPU ideas on a reformed health care system centred largely on an extension of insurance.[21]

What is important here is less the formal aspect of the MPU's affiliation to the TUC – the former was often ignored or treated brusquely by the latter, for example through exclusion from the Joint Committee – than the actual existence of a trade union oriented organisation concerned to promote its own ideas for a reconstructed health care system. Initially, relations between the SMA and the MPU were reasonably good, and throughout the period of this study there were overlaps in membership between the two organisations. As we have seen, Alfred Welply was a founder and first treasurer of the Association. Brook was elected to the MPU Executive Committee in 1929, a post he retained for at least five years, and was the first MPU delegate to TUC conference in 1935. He also wrote to SMA members urging them to join the MPU in early 1935, that is immediately after the latter had affiliated to the TUC. Even at this stage, however, not all Association members were as enamoured of the MPU and Brook records that he was effectively censured by the SMA leadership for his activities in 1935.[22]

Relations between the two organisations continued to deteriorate, for a number of reasons. First, as we shall see in Chapter Six, the Association was extremely hostile to the MPU's stand on medical refugees. Second, its EC passed a resolution in early 1936 recommending that SMA members not join the MPU, a decision Brook then communicated to the Labour Party secretary James Middleton. This resulted from MPU support for an 'anti-Labour' candidate in the Swansea municipal elections. Shortly afterwards Welply – who had resigned as Association treasurer in late 1935 – protested to Hastings about the Association's activities, claiming that the MPU's policy had always been 'non-party political', not a stance likely to endear it to the SMA.[23] Most importantly of all, however, were the different ways in which the two organisations saw the future of medicine. Brook's outburst over the MPU's maternity plans signals a number of the problems. Its proposals regarding general practitioner autonomy and a health system based on insurance, for example, were diametrically opposed to key SMA demands. Such differences also further highlighted another feature of the Association, namely the low opinion which many of its leaders held of GPs. As private contractors, these doctors had little time or incentive to acquire more specialised medical knowledge. To critics such as the SMA, GPs were also obsessed with economic issues such as the size of their 'panel' and with the right to sell their practices on retirement, the latter being viewed by individuals such as Hastings as especially morally repugnant.[24] Here, then, was another instance of 'vested interests' operating to the detriment of national health. These reservations may also have been an unconscious reflection of what was seen as a contrast between the political, and metropolitan, sophistication of Association members and the political, and provincial, backwardness of many GPs.

Of particular significance for this study, however, is the MPU's hostility to local authority control. The strategy of the SMA, by contrast, was to argue for reconstructed health care provision administered through local government, with the LCC's achievements being held up as an example of the efficacy of municipal socialism. As will become apparent, this was to prove a highly divisive issue in the labour movement. Indeed some SMA members, often those with some sort of relationship with the MPU such as Brook, were to break ranks with the Association's advocacy of the local authority model, partly on the pragmatic basis of its unacceptability to the mass of GPs. The MPU was not, furthermore, the only labour movement body sceptical of locally run health services. While this issue is dealt with more fully in later chapters, it is worth noting here a Fabian Society document produced in 1939. This argued that while the intention of the 1929 Local Government Act had been to leave local authorities 'as free as possible', this had in fact resulted in wide disparities in the level of services provided. These were caused not by the needs of the inhabitants, but rather by the rateable value of local property. The Ministry of Health had not taken on a positive role, for example through promoting the 'regional grouping of local authorities where they are individually too small to carry out particular schemes effectively'. It was thus concluded that such 'central planning will become an absolute essential when the hospital services are organised ... '.[25] In short, explicit and implicit criticism was being made of the local variations, and thereby lack of uniformity of provision, which came with administrative devolution. Even in the 1930s, therefore, there were differences inside the labour movement over the structure of socialised health service. This in turn suggests, at the very least, constraining factors on SMA power and influence.

A number of other organisational and historical factors exacerbated this situation. First, we have observed that the SMA was at this stage very much a small London-based organisation, which meant that its impact in the provinces, both on its potential political allies and more generally, was strictly limited. Second, the Association had a difficult relationship with one of the most important sections of the labour movement, the trade unions. In 1937, for example, a delegate to TUC conference suggested its inclusion on the BMA-TUC Joint Committee, to counterbalance BMA influence. He could, however, find no seconder for his motion. In such circumstances it is not surprising that, as Brooke puts it, the 'SMA was not yet completely convinced that Transport House supported a radical health policy', and that it was concerned that the TUC was being seduced by the BMA's proposals. As Hastings wrote to Brook in the summer of 1937, he found a recent speech by union leader Ernest Bevin favouring improvements in the panel system 'very serious. It looks as if the BMA were getting their tentacles into the TUC very strongly'.[26] From the other side, it seems likely that the Association's criticisms of the TUC-BMA maternity plan would have done little to recommend it to the leaders of organised labour. The strained relations between the SMA and the TUC were to continue in the 1940s, when the latter proved more accommodating to the sensitivities of the medical profession than to the Association's radical ideas. Overall, this tension must be seen as a serious hindrance to the SMA's ambitions, and will be the subject of further comment in subsequent chapters.

In fact, in the 1930s the Association was already aware of the problem of its standing with the industrial wing of the labour movement. In

1938 it sought affiliation to the London Trades Council, only to be rejected on the grounds that only trades unions were eligible. The following year, Brook wrote to TUC Council member George Gibson expressing the hope that one day members of the medical profession might have a 'proper Trade Union' affiliated to the Labour Party and to the TUC. Of the two main doctors' organisations, the BMA was powerful but hostile to the idea of trades unionism. The MPU, on the other hand, was a registered union but 'so reactionary and incidentally so weak in its influence that little can be hoped from it'. The position of most of the MPU on the question of a state medical service, moreover, was 'definitely more reactionary than the BMA'. Of course militant doctors alone would not be enough to constitute a powerful union body, so what was really needed was a federation of health workers. The SMA, while 'purely a political and propagandist organisation', had at least made some steps in the right direction, almost certainly a reference to the decision to expand its membership base.[27]

The third factor relates to the more general historical position and condition of the labour movement in the mid- to late 1930s. It is clear that the Association was making considerable advances in Labour policy and policy making on health matters. Nonetheless it remained the case that the party as a whole was, understandably given the circumstances of the 1930s, more concerned with economic planning and foreign affairs than with the complexities of health care provision. Labour had a general commitment, from 1934, to a state medical service, but continued to prioritise other issues. Thus while *A State Health Service* was duly passed by the 1934 conference, one of the decade's key policy statements, *Labour's Immediate Programme*, limited its remarks in this area to: 'Health Services will be extended and special measures will be taken to reduce maternal mortality'. The predominant emphasis in the Labour Party's strategy can be inferred from the Report for 1935, which noted that educational conferences had been held on Industry, Finance, and Foreign Affairs, with no mention made of health matters.[28]

On the level of ideas, the model of health care reform which the Association offered fitted in with a particular, and undoubtedly influential, ideological strand in contemporary Labour thought. This stressed popular democratic control, especially at local level and hence an activist, participating citizenry. Devolution of power and the accountability of social services were regarded by thinkers such as Tawney and G.D.H. Cole as necessary safeguards against an over-centralised and bureaucratic state, as well as being in themselves integral components of a socially responsible society. Intellectuals such as Tawney further stressed the need for professions to behave in a public spirited way, rather than simply to pursue pure self-interest.[29] Or, to put it in a slightly different way, the Association adopted in the 1930s what Peter Clarke describes as a 'moral' rather than a 'mechanical' reform strategy, based on the 'free will, spontaneous endeavours and democratic efforts of the citizens'. The 'irreducibility of the distinction between moral and mechanical means of change' is for Clarke a variant of the observation by Cole – which again bears strongly on the kind of programme being put forward by the SMA – that socialist thought was fundamentally divided in two ways: not only between reformers and revolutionaries, but also between 'centralisers and federalists'.[30] Cole's distinction thus reminds us that the labour movement contained not only proponents of devolved, democratic power such as Hastings and his colleagues. It also contained planners and 'centralisers', proponents of efficiency and uniformity who saw central government, with expert advice, as the best way of achieving such ends.[31] This was true in the 1930s and, as will become apparent, a case can be made that in the longer term it was the latter type of socialist who won out over the former in the creation of welfare institutions such as the NHS.

Other aspects of the Association's political views posed more immediate problems. We have already remarked upon the admittance of communists to membership in the mid-1930s, and the organisation's generally radical stance. Further instances of this came in 1937 when a resolution was passed objecting to the expulsion of the left-wing Socialist League from the Labour Party; and two years later when both the EC and the AGM protested at the expulsion of Stafford Cripps, the motion at the latter being proposed by Richard Doll.[32] In short, the Association was well to the political left, as its policies, actions, and the composition of its membership testify. At a time when the party and trades union leaderships were highly suspicious of any hint of communist penetration, this was hardly a point in its favour. The SMA's left-wing attitudes were to continue to put a distance between itself and the Labour Party and the TUC. For all these reasons, the Association had by no means a clear run inside the labour movement, despite its undoubted role in Labour's health policy formation.

The SMA and medical politics in the 1930s

Of course, the Association was operating and competing not only within the labour movement, but also in the broader medico-political arena. Here, once again, it had some positive achievements. The 1930s saw an intense debate about nutritional standards and the impact upon them of high levels of unemployment. Association activists played a prominent part in these discussions. A Scientific Committee was set up in 1933/34 to examine the effects of malnutrition, and more generally to consider all diseases seen as having socio-economic bases. These included tuberculosis, conventionally viewed on the political left as an illness exemplifying poverty and thereby the failings of the capitalist system. This committee subsequently produced a memorandum on 'The Assessment of Adequate Nutrition'.[33]

Particular concern was expressed over the impact of poor feeding on children, and not simply for altruistic or humanitarian reasons. As Leslie Haden-Guest, a doctor and MP associated with the SMA,[34] told the Commons in June 1938, malnutrition, which was related to unemployment and low levels of welfare benefits, was especially damaging to the young. There resulted

> a permanent injury, a permanent handicap, a reduction in their productive capacity, in their intelligence, and in their nervous stability, and a reduction in the most vital asset of the nation, which is, the children of the nation.

Haden-Guest concluded, very much in the spirit of the times, that if it was possible to have a five-year plan for rearmament, then the same could be done to 'improve the nutrition of the children of this country'.[35]

The idea of 'nervous stability' had already been picked up by Hastings, as previously observed a lifelong advocate of child welfare measures. In 1934 he argued that the present manifestations of 'mass-hysteria' in Germany were at least in part attributable to the 'mental and psychological effects of under-feeding during the war'. The message here was clear. A degraded, demoralised, and undernourished population, particularly a child population, resulted in a deformed and degenerate political system – hence the need for, as he put it, a 'national physiological minimum' and for the full exploitation of all existing social welfare measures to ensure adequate nutrition. The level of interest and expertise the SMA was able to bring to this issue resulted in its participation in labour movement investigations into health standards. It was asked, for example, to prepare a Labour Party leaflet on 'Nutrition', and Hastings, Salter, and Maule were invited to join a sub-committee on school meals for children of the unemployed set up by the party's women's section.[36]

Association members also became involved with non-labour movement pressure groups such as the Campaign Against Malnutrition, and Hastings, in part because of his experience as a school medical officer, was asked to chair the medical sub-committee of the Children's Minimum Organising Committee. The SMA's demand for adequate nutritional standards also led it to ridicule the National Government's 'fitness campaign' of the late 1930s, which it argued was a farce in the absence of proper feeding, especially of children; and to stress that modern medical knowledge now allowed that the 'science of dietics has become part of the science of preventive medicine'. The Association's emphasis on preventive medicine was thus further justified by the growth in scientific understanding itself.[37] SMA members therefore intervened to some effect in the nutrition debates of the 1930s, just as its views on the need for reconstruction of the health services were being brought to the attention of the wider medico-political world through, for example, its use of the Sankey Commission as a platform from which to broadcast its ideas.

Nonetheless, the SMA had rivals in the field of health care reform. One of the most famous, and subsequently influential, surveys of health provision in the inter-war period was that of the research group Political and Economic Planning (PEP). PEP was part of a more general movement concerned with 'planning' in the 1930s and which sought to create what Marwick describes as a 'middle opinion' located between the perceived extremes of unbridled capitalism and socialism. The PEP report on health was published in 1937 and was, it was later claimed, the subject of an 'extraordinarily favourable reception' from leading articles and commentary in national and provincial newspapers; professional journals such as the *Lancet* and the *BMJ*; and the BMA. Consequently, it was further claimed, the paperback edition had run into 25 000 copies by 1939 and the report itself was 'a sort of Bible at the Ministry of Health'. It was its health report which gave PEP, Daniel Fox suggests, 'for the first time, national status'.[38]

Although ambiguous in a number of areas, PEP's health strategy stressed the need for improvements in general practice and the greater planning and coordination of services, ideas with which the SMA could certainly empathise. The Association also picked up very explicitly on a particularly important aspect of the PEP analysis: the cost of the current health services. As *MTT* pointed out, a 'serious argument' against a socialised service would be removed

> if it could be shown that it would not cost more than at present, and the case for such a service would be strengthened if the possibility of a saving could be demonstrated.

This was, the article continued, exactly what PEP had uncovered. Estimated current expenditure of around £400 million was not being properly spent. On the contrary, the picture was one of 'overlapping, redundancy, and at the same time complete inadequacy'. The report also showed, *MTT* suggested, the wastefulness of the voluntary hospital system, and the impact on health of environmental conditions.

Consequently much of the illness that doctors were called upon to treat was 'caused by conditions which can and must be changed'. A socialised medical system would thus be more economically efficient than capitalistic anarchy, while a socialist society would tackle the socio-economic conditions which led to ill-health in the first place.[39]

The PEP report was an extremely useful tool for the SMA, in at least two ways. First, the quantitative approach to health service provision was one which the Association would draw upon and develop as it began, during the Second World War, to bring forward more detailed estimates of the cost of a socialised scheme. Second, the PEP findings appeared, from a politically 'neutral' point of view, to bear out many of the points which the SMA had been arguing for a number of years. However the report also showed up weaknesses in the Association's position. For one thing, PEP was able to call upon considerably more financial and other resources than the Association, whose members were trying to devise plans for a socialised health service while, in the vast majority of cases, holding down demanding full-time medical posts. The amount of publicity the PEP report engendered must have been the source of some envy to SMA members.

Moreover PEP was determinedly 'non-political'. Its aim was not that of the Association, a socialised service as part of the transition to a socialist society. PEP had no real quarrel with the capitalist system; rather, it wanted the more efficient allocation of resources and services. This 'non-political' stance was part of its broader appeal and gave authority to its pronouncements in a way less open to an overtly political body such as the SMA. Furthermore, in collecting its evidence PEP approached, according to Fox, 'members of every faction in medical politics except ... the Socialist Medical Association'. Nor, it transpired, did it seek the views of any other section of the labour movement. While it may have been that PEP was seeking to maintain its 'non-political' stance, it could also be that it thought the Association either too controversial or too marginal to the mainstream debate to be considered. Whatever the reason, this was a snub to the SMA. It is notable that Brook does not mention PEP in his history of the Association, and Murray does so only in passing, despite its report's undoubted significance.[40]

If – its failure to be consulted notwithstanding – the Association could at least draw some positive messages from the PEP report, this was much less so in respect of another significant health policy statement of the late 1930s. This was the BMA's revised *A General Medical Service for the Nation*, published in 1938. We have already noted that the publication of the first edition, in 1930, may have been one of the factors which prompted the SMA's creation, and that by the late

1930s the Association was deeply concerned about the relationship between the BMA and the TUC. There is no doubt that the SMA saw *A General Medical Service for the Nation* as a dangerous and reactionary text, exhibiting a number of the same erroneous arguments as were employed in the contemporaneous BMA-TUC ideas on maternity care.

An early response came in an *MTT* article which denounced the BMA statement as 'out of touch with both public and professional opinion'. The BMA sought to perpetuate the existing form of private practice, despite the fact that the public were becoming increasingly unhappy with treatment by an 'isolated "family doctor"'. The emphasis on the expansion of the insurance system was at odds with 'modern thought', which sought a service freely available to all. The document as a whole showed the BMA's determination to 'get its ideas accepted before anyone had time to consider them, and to make as few changes as possible'. It had therefore not taken the opportunity to put forward a 'revolutionary scheme designed primarily to serve the sick'.[41] This was all good knockabout stuff illustrating, among other things, the SMA's view of the BMA (and by implication the bulk of general practitioners) as at this stage profoundly conservative.

But this should not disguise the seriousness with which the BMA plan was treated as is witnessed by, first, an internal SMA document; second, the interventions of Association members at a New Fabian Research Bureau conference in late 1938; and, third, the publication of H.H. MacWilliam's 'Walton Plan'. The internal document was written by Hastings, and analysed the BMA plans in some detail. He first pointed out that the proposals under review were simply an updated version of those of 1930. While the kind of service recommended might have been acceptable a century ago, it was now 'completely out of touch with modern medical thought' which, Hastings suggested, stressed the need for specialisation and for teamwork. The BMA was further out of touch because of its failure to take into account the 1929 Local Government Act's impact on hospitals.

Hastings, like the *MTT* article, opposed any expansion of the insurance and panel system. Rather, what was required was a system controlled and directed by public representatives. Indeed, Hastings emphasised the idea of popular control more forcibly than had usually been the case previously. The profession should not be allowed to regulate itself, nor should advisory committees composed of doctors be set up, for these would act as a brake on the local authorities which should have the responsibility for health matters. This was not because doctors were inherently self-seeking or dishonest. Nonetheless, the medical profession was almost entirely middle class in origin, and had a 'predominantly conservative' outlook. In a socialised service, by contrast, the doctor must have a

> responsibility to the nation and must understand it. He must be something more than a tradesman whose sole duty is to please his customers, and whose practice and remuneration depend almost entirely on the way in which he succeeds in this.[42]

This was a further example of the 'economic dependency' argument noted in the previous chapter.

Similar themes were picked up shortly afterwards at the Fabian conference on the health services, another instance of the Association using all possible labour movement platforms to propagate its views. Murray, as usual pulling no punches, thought the BMA proposals 'a typical product of a conservative body ... not concerned with the interests of the mass of the population'. Brook, rather more positively, claimed that he could agree with many aspects of the scheme, but acknowledged its failure to address the question of which bodies controlled the hospitals. It was in fact, he continued, a plan concerned only with general practice, with little to say about hospitals despite the example set by an authority like London through its full use of the 1929 Act. Brook also found fault with the BMA's 'commercial spirit' and with any attempt to extend the insurance scheme. The arguments for this, he suggested, were the same as 'those used in the nineteenth century against the provision of free education'.[43]

The third notable response by the Association came with the so-called 'Walton Plan for a National Medical Service'. The Walton Plan – an historic document, according to Murray, and certainly a significant example of the sharpening of focus of plans for a socialised service – was devised by H.H. MacWilliam and published in *MTT* in March 1939. MacWilliam, Medical Superintendent of Liverpool's Walton Hospital, had been influenced early in his career by Benjamin Moore of the SMSA. This had been supplemented by 20 years at Walton Hospital, during which time he had ample opportunity to observe the workings of the hospital system.[44]

One of MacWilliam's initial points was that the BMA's advocacy of extended health insurance derived from its 'natural conservatism'. However, he continued, nowadays 'everyone knows that efficient modern medicine is the work of a team and *the BMA plan has the fatal defect that it is founded on the solitary individual practitioner*' (emphasis in the original). This led him into criticisms of the current form of primary care and of what he saw as the trend towards bureaucratisation in the existing municipal services. To this MacWilliam counterposed a national medical service based on the general hospital; or, as he put it, the 'real' general hospital. All services, including domiciliary care, were to be focused on this institution and detailed attention was given to the requirements of all departments. The emphasis throughout was to be on teamwork, with all staff having a say in the running and administration of the hospital. Medical practitioners were to be salaried, with a suggested upper limit of £1500 per annum. MacWilliam agreed that this was 'a low figure compared with the income of many men in practice now', but a salaried system would have important compensating advantages such as pensions, sick pay, and family allowances. He further expanded on one particular aspect of his scheme, maternity services, a few months later, again going into considerable detail over matters such as staff salaries and the ratio of health personnel to patients. Here MacWilliam was making a further contribution to the debate over the proper system of maternity care while re-emphasising the centrality of the hospital to his proposals.[45]

The Walton Plan explicitly restated a number of central SMA preoccupations, for example the hostility to the insurance system and the security for doctors of a salaried service. It did not entirely conform to the emphases of existing Association policy statements in that it did not, for instance, deal in any detail with how democratic control was to be exerted over the medical system, although MacWilliam did approach this obliquely by suggesting the need for local government reorganisation. Similarly, he was ambiguous about the extent to which the service was to be free to the consumer. Nonetheless his scheme was very obviously, and very deliberately, different from that of the BMA. And it was certainly the case that the Association saw the Walton Plan as yet another nail in the coffin of the existing system, and of the BMA proposals for health service reform. As Murray put it in 1939, the 'germ' of any socialised health service was to be found in MacWilliam's work which contained 'on close examination the ... only basis on which a socialized service can be built, the basis of the general hospitals'.[46] This was slightly misleading, in that the SMA had always tried to see a socialised health service as a totally integrated system, and not just a reformed hospital system, although it was clearly intended to counter what was viewed as the BMA's obsession with the general practitioner. Nonetheless Murray's comment is an indication of the Walton Plan's place in Association thinking on the eve of the Second World War.

The re-publication of A General Medical Service for the Nation was an important event in the SMA's early history. Although, rather surprisingly, Murray was later to say that it showed how the BMA 'had moved forward quite a long way', there is no doubt that at the time both that body and its plan were seen in almost wholly negative terms by the Association. Three related points in particular had been raised which were of concern to the SMA. These were, first, the failure of the BMA to address the central questions of control of the system and the place in it of hospitals. Second, the BMA's preoccupation with general practice, which was to continue in its present form in according to GPs sole and independent contractor status. In turn, this involved an ongoing emphasis on curative rather than preventive medicine. And, third, the BMA's commitment to the insurance system. Each of these was largely or totally incompatible with SMA demands or strategy.[47] As Chapter Six shows, the BMA was also at this time taking what the Association considered to be a highly reactionary stand on medical refugees and on the National Government's preparations for war. Nonetheless it was an inescapable fact that the BMA was a powerful organisation in its own right, which in addition had contacts with important sections of the labour movement. Of course some, although by no means all, SMA activists were eligible to join branches of the BMA through which they might seek to change its policy. But in the late 1930s hopes were not high. The British Medical Association was, therefore, a formidable opponent in both medical and political circles, and *A General Medical Service for the Nation* brought home very clearly its commitment to a certain kind of medical practice and organisation. The SMA's fight against what it saw as 'medical reaction' will be one central concern of the remainder of this book. What the present and previous chapters have endeavoured to show is that, on the one hand, the SMA was a forceful body which was developing clear and well thought out proposals for a particular form of socialised medical service. On the other hand, it was a small organisation in what was becoming, by the late 1930s, an increasingly crowded field, both in the labour movement and more generally. Rudolf Klein suggests, in a musical analogy, that the SMA had a 'radical treble' in contrast to the BMA's 'conservative bass drum'.[48] Having its voice heard at a volume it considered appropriate was a persistent Association preoccupation. We now go on to consider one area where it did enjoy considerable success in the inter-war period, the London County Council.

Notes

1. Labour Party, *Report of the Thirty-Second Annual Conference*, Labour Party, 1932, p. 269.
2. Ibid., p. 270.
3. Minutes of the Labour Party Finance and General Purposes Committee, 26 June 1933, p. 57; Labour Party, *Report of the Thirty-Third Annual Conference*, Labour Party, 1933, p. 141; DSM 1/1, AGM 1934, EC Report; Murray, *Why a National Health Service?*, p. 25; Labour Party,

Report of the Thirty-Fourth Annual Conference, Labour Party, 1934, p. 7.

4. Labour Party, *Report of the Thirty-Fourth Annual Conference*, Labour Party, 1934, Appendix VI, 'A State Health Service', pp. 256–7.

5. Ibid., pp. 257–8.

6. Ibid., p. 258.

7. *Socialist Doctor*, vol. II, no. 4, p. 1.

8. Labour Party, *Report of the Thirty-Fourth Annual Conference*, pp. 214–15, 9.

9. DSM 1/1, Report of the EC, 1934–35.

10. DSM (2) 5, 'Labour Party', correspondence between Brook and G.P. Blizard, October and November 1930; Minutes of the Labour Party Local Government and Social Services Committee, 14 July 1936; DSM 1/1, Report of the EC, 1935–36.

11. Martin Pugh, *The Making of Modern British Politics*, Oxford, Blackwell, 2nd edn, 1993, Ch. 13. I am grateful to John Macnicol for this point.

12. Labour Party Home Policy Committee, Minutes (unclassified material, Labour Party archives): Minutes of the Policy Committee, 15 November 1937; Public Health Advisory Committee Minutes, 1938–44 (unclassified material in three files, Labour Party archives): file 1, Minutes of the Public Health Advisory Committee, 23 November 1938.

13. *MTT*, no. 4, January 1938, pp. 12, 3.

14. Ray Earwicker, 'A Study of the BMA-TUC Joint Committee on Medical Questions, 1935–1939', *Journal of Social Policy*, 8, 1979, pp. 344, 347, and *passim*; for the development of the TUC's views on health policy, see Earwicker, thesis, Ch. 7. I am grateful to both Stephen Brooke and John Macnicol for reminding me of the nature and significance of maternal mortality.

15. DSM 1/1, AGM 1934, EC Report; Esther Rickards, 'A National Maternity Service', and Edith Summerskill, 'Hospitalisation as the Basis of a Maternity Service', *Socialist Doctor*, vol. II, no. 2, November 1933, pp. 4–7; 'Supplement: A National Maternity Service', *Socialist Doctor*, vol. II, no. 4, November 1934, pp. 9–12; Murray, *Why a National Health Service?*, pp. 27–8; and Brook, *Making Medical History*, p. 7; Stewart, '"For a Healthy London"', pp. 427–30. On the wider issue of maternal care, see Irvine Loudon, 'Deaths in childbed from the eighteenth century to 1935', *Medical History*, 1986, 30, 1–41.

16. *MTT*, July 1938, p. 7; DSM 4/1, 'Comments by Dr Somerville Hastings and Others on the TUC and BMA National Maternity Scheme', pp. 1–2.

17. Labour Party Home Policy Committee Minutes (unclassified material, Labour Party archives): Minutes of the Policy Sub-Committee, 5 November 1938; Public Health Advisory Committee Minutes, 1938–1944 (unclassified material in three files, Labour Party Archives): file 1, Minutes of the Public Health Advisory Committee, 23 November 1938; Earwicker, 'A Study of the BMA-TUC Joint Committee on Medical Questions, 1935–1939', pp. 338–40.

18. Public Health Advisory Committee, Minutes 1938–1944 (unclassified material in three files, Labour Party archives): file 1, Minutes of the Public Health Advisory Committee, 23 and 30 November 1938.

19. Labour Party Home Policy Committee Minutes (unclassified material, Labour Party archives): Minutes of the Policy Sub-Committee, 13 December

1938; Earwicker, 'A Study of the BMA-TUC Joint Committee on Medical Questions, 1935–1939', pp. 349–56; Brooke, *Labour's War*, p. 137.

20. DSM 1/1, Report of the EC, 1938–39; DSM (2) 5, 'Inter-Hospitals Socialist Society', memorandum 24 May 1936.

21. DSM (2) 5, 'Labour Party', Charles Brook to Alderman R. Taylor, 20 April 1936; Earwicker, 'A Study of the BMA-TUC Joint Committee on Medical Questions, 1935–1939', pp. 348–50, 338.

22. MSS.79/MPU/1/2/1, Minutes of Council, 18 July 1929; Brook, *Making Medical History*, p. 8; DSM (2) 5, 'MPU', Brook to SMA members, 2 January 1935.

23. DSM 1/1, Report of the Executive Committee, 1935–36; DSM (2) 6, Brook to Middleton, 9 January 1936; DSM (2) 5, 'MPU', Welply to Hastings, 21 January 1936; Honigsbaum, *Division in British Medicine*, p. 261.

24. See, for Hastings on the class composition of the medical profession and on the sale of practices, Stewart, 'Socialist Proposals', pp. 341, 345.

25. Fabian Society Papers, J41/2, memorandum on 'National Health Insurance' by the Health Services Sub-Committee of the Social Services Committee, pp. 9–10.

26. Earwicker, 'A Study of the BMA-TUC Joint Committee on Medical Questions 1935–1939', pp. 340–341; Brooke, *Labour's War*, pp. 136–7; DSM (2) 6, Hastings to Brook, 29 July 1937.

27. DSM (2) 5, 'Trade Unions', London Trades Council to Buckle, 6 September 1938; and Brook to George Gibson, undated but 1939.

28. Labour Party, *Report of the Thirty-Seventh Annual Conference*, Labour Party, 1937, Appendix X, 'Labour's Immediate Programme', p. 279; Labour Party, *Report of the Thirty-Fifth Annual Conference*, Labour Party, 1935, p. 25.

29. On the labour movement and active citizenship, see Steven Fielding, Peter Thompson and Nick Tiratsoo, *'England Arise': the Labour Party and Popular Politics in 1940s Britain*, Manchester, Manchester University Press, 1995, Chs. 4 and 5; and Abigail Beach, 'The Labour Party and the Idea of Citizenship, unpublished PhD thesis, University of London, 1996, *passim*; Nicholas Deakin and Anthony Wright, 'Tawney', in George, Vic and Page, Robert (eds), *Modern Thinkers on Welfare*, Hemel Hempstead, Prentice Hall/Harvester Wheatsheaf, 1995.

30. Peter Clarke, *Liberals and Social Democrats*, Cambridge, Cambridge University Press, 1978, pp. 5, 15, 65; *idem*, 'The Social Democratic Theory of the Class Struggle', in Winter, Jay (ed.) *The Working Class in Modern British History*, Cambridge, Cambridge University Press, 1983, p. 13 and pp. 262–3, note 23.

31. See, on economic policy, Elizabeth Durbin, *New Jerusalems: the Labour Party and the Economics of Democratic Socialism*, Routledge and Kegan Paul, 1985.

32. DSM 1/1, Minutes of the Seventh AGM, 9 May 1937; Report of the EC, 1938–39; and Minutes of the AGM, 14 May 1939.

33. DSM 1/1, AGM 1934, EC Report; and Report of the EC, 1935–36.

34. Frank Honigsbaum, *Health, Happiness and Security: the Creation of the National Health Service*, Routledge, 1989, p. 18.

35. Parliamentary Debates, 5th series, vol. 337, col. 1443ff.

36. Stewart, 'Socialist Proposals', pp. 349–53; and *idem*, '"The Children's Party, therefore the Women's Party"', pp. 176–80; Somerville Hastings, *A National Physiological Minimum: Fabian Tract 241*, Fabian Society, 1934, p. 8; DSM 1/1, Report of the EC, 1937–38, and Report of the EC, 1935–36; Minutes of the General Purposes Committee of the SJCIWO, 8 December 1932, p. 2, and Minutes of the SJCIWO, 12 January 1933.

37. DSH, File 9, 'School Medical Service', Marjorie Green to Hastings, 1 November 1934; *MTT*, no. 3, December 1937, pp. 14–15.

38. On planning, see Arthur Marwick, 'Middle Opinion in the Thirties: Planning, Progress and Political Agreement', *English Historical Review*, LXXIX, 1964; for the PEP report, see S.M. Herbert, *Britain's Health*, Harmondsworth, Penguin, 1937; Max Nicholson, 'PEP through the 1930s: Growth, Thinking, Performance', and Kenneth Lindsay, 'PEP through the 1930s: Organisation, Structure, People', both in Pinder, John (ed.), *Fifty Years of Political and Economic Planning*, Heinemann, 1981, pp. 45, 27; Fox, *Health Policies, Health Politics*, p. 68.

39. *MTT*, no. 4, January 1938, pp. 1–2.

40. Fox, *Health Policies, Health Politics*, p. 65; Murray, *Why a National Health Service?*, p. 35.

41. *MTT*, no. 2, November 1937, pp. 1–2.

42. DSM 4/1, 'Some Notes on the BMA Scheme For a General Medical Service For the Nation', by Dr Somerville Hastings, 18 October 1938.

43. DSM 4/1, New Fabian Research Bureau, 'Report of a Conference on the Health Services, held at the Royal Star Hotel, Maidstone, on October 22–3, 1938', pp. 12, 5–6.

44. Murray, *Why a National Health Service?*, pp. 7, 38–9.

45. 'The Walton Plan for a National Medical Service', *MTT*, vol. 2, no. 1 (New Series), March Quarter 1939, pp. 2–12; 'A Model Maternity Scheme', *MTT*, vol. 2, no. 3 (New Series), September Quarter 1939, pp. 3–7.

46. 'The Walton Plan for a National Medical Service', pp. 4, 12; *MTT*, vol. 2, no. 2 (New Series), June Quarter 1939, p. 20.

47. Murray, *Why a National Health Service?*, p. 39.

48. Klein, *The New Politics of the NHS*, p. 4.

CHAPTER FIVE

The SMA and the London County Council

It has already been noted that the SMA's membership in the 1930s was heavily concentrated in the London region. In the longer term, this was almost certainly a major structural weakness of the Association because of, for example, its relative failure to put down deep roots in the labour movement as a whole. But in the years immediately before the Second World War the organisation had a considerable influence on the LCC's health policies, in particular through its role on the Hospital and Medical Services Committee which it dominated in the wake of Labour's election victory in 1934. This was a period when the SMA came to seriously consider the council as a possible blueprint for a future health service; when, more generally, the local authority model of socialist organisation – including the administration of welfare services – formed an important strand in Labour ideology; and, related to the previous two points, when the Labour LCC was seen as a 'flagship' local authority by the broader labour movement. It is also the case, of course, that London is where much political activity takes place, and where pressure groups are usually located so as to more easily seek to influence ministers and officials. This chapter examines the SMA's role in London medical politics, and the lessons it drew from both its successes and its failures.[1]

'For a healthy London'

Even before the SMA's creation, and during the period when the LCC was controlled by the Municipal Reform Party (in effect, the London Conservative Party), a number of its founder members were already active in metropolitan political life. Alfred Salter was MP for Bermondsey and a member of the London Labour Party (LLP) Executive Committee as were, at various points, Hastings and Rickards. Hastings, Brook, Rickards, Churchill, and Jeger, all soon to become prominent in the Association, were from 1929 members of the LCC Central Public Health Committee and its various sub-committees, either by appointment or as elected LCC representatives.[2] This involvement with the council was particularly important in that it meant that SMA members participated from the outset in London's implementation of the 1929 Local Government Act which allowed, although it did not compel, local authorities to take over Poor Law infirmaries and transform them into municipal hospitals. The authority most active in taking advantage of this was the LCC. Poor Law institutions, as well as the hospitals of the Metropolitan Asylums Board, were appropriated. The carrying out of this legislation was to involve a significant change in attitude to the sick and a huge shift in the nature and volume of London's public health provision.[3]

The 1929 Act was, as we saw in Chapter Three, viewed by the SMA as a start in the dismantling of the Poor Law system of medical relief; hence, as we have also already seen, Hastings's praise of Neville Chamberlain for promoting this piece of legislation. In particular, the Act offered huge potential for a municipalised hospital system. Its possibilities were noted at the time of its passing by London's Labour councillors who saw in Chamberlain's measure the chance to build 'through the transferred hospitals one of the most comprehensive municipal services in the world'. According to the sympathetic historian of the Labour LCC, Brian Barker, the Labour group's positive suggestions in respect of municipalisation were largely ignored by the Municipal Reform majority, a factor in the latter's defeat in 1934.[4]

The Act's potential was consistently pressed by SMA members on all possible occasions. Two months after Labour's success in 1934, for example, Hastings told an SMA meeting that, rightly used, the Act was 'the key which would open the door to a complete and unified hospital system'. It had come into being because 'intelligent administrators were impressed by the wastefulness of two systems of treatment – one for poor-law patients and one for the public generally'. A clear echo of the Webbs' analysis can be heard here. If, Hastings continued, the legislation could be used further to end 'the equally wasteful system of dual hospital administration' then it would be 'of even greater value'. In consequence, where this strategy was being pursued the public was beginning to see the hospitals as their own, places where they could go 'by right of citizenship, and not as a charity'. Local authority control also meant that citizens 'had the right of protest through their elected representatives'.[5] These were significant comments, for two reasons. First, they are witness to Hastings's increasing emphasis on the desirability of a democratically accountable local authority model for a future health service, an idea clearly influenced by the LCC experience. Second, it will also become evident that Hastings and his LCC colleagues laid great stress on the idea expressed here that London's citizens should have access to health care as a matter of right, and free from Poor Law stigma. This fed into the more detailed articulations of the 'right to health' by Association members in the 1940s, discussed in Chapter Seven.

An SMA London and Home Counties branch was formed in mid-December 1930 with Dr Morgan Finucane as chairman and Dr Powell-Evans as secretary, and subsequently affiliated to the LLP in 1937. It was, unsurprisingly, to be the most active and influential branch of the Association, participating in a wide range of political and social activities within both the labour movement and wider medico-political circles. It built up, for example, close links with the organisation of left-wing lawyers, the Haldane Society; and as shall be seen in the next chapter, was active in supporting medical refugees and in criticising official preparations for war. The London branch put forward a successful motion at the Association's first AGM demanding the amendment of the 1929 Act so as to allow for free treatment at municipal hospitals, yet another instance of the faith placed in the possibilities opened up by Chamberlain's legislation. Around the same time Lewis Silkin, leader of the LCC Labour group, suggested that the Association prepare a health policy statement for the 1931 London elections.[6] A first draft, whose principal authors were Salter, Brook, and Hastings, was presented to the LLP Executive in January 1931. Ultimately this document was published as the election leaflet: *For a Healthy London: A Municipal Hospitals Policy that will Lessen Suffering and Disease*. This noted the current problems of both voluntary and municipal hospitals. The latter would suffer further if administered by a party, Municipal Reform, committed to keeping down the local taxes. By contrast, a Labour administration would finally break the link between hospitals and the Poor Law by fully exploiting the 1929 Act's potential. Patients would be admitted because they were London citizens – for whom only 'the best is good enough' – needing treatment. The aim was not only to make London's municipal hospitals the best in the world, 'but ultimately to make them free to all, rich and poor alike'. Labour also sought to develop municipal hospitals 'as the Medical Centres of the districts in which they are situated', so encouraging 'the home treatment of the sick poor being undertaken from these hospitals'. In short, this was an attempt to find an immediate and practical way of setting up a system of health centres. The leaflet concluded by arguing that for Labour the nation's health was of 'so great importance' that it was 'unsafe to leave it to private charity'. The moral was clear: 'Vote Labour for an Efficient Public Hospital Service.' In abbreviated form these proposals were incorporated in the 1931 Labour LCC manifesto.[7]

For a Healthy London, written by leading SMA activists, laid out the preoccupations of important members of the capital's medical left in the early 1930s. The period between the Association's foundation and Labour's victory in 1934 saw further considerable activity by its London members, with Hastings taking a leading role. In April 1933, for example, he told LLP conference that proposed cuts in public health expenditure by the Municipal Reform administration were 'an act in the class war' aimed at working class living standards. Hastings who, like both historical and contemporary Labour politicians, often stressed fiscal responsibility, agreed that economic efficiency was necessary. But it was wrong, he continued, that the 'first consideration' of health officials 'must be the saving of pennies' rather than the enhancement of communal health. There remained scope for improvement in the health of London's citizens, and however much standards did get better 'there will still be need for a service for the prevention and treatment of disease and the encouragement of healthy living'. Here is one instance of the Association's concern with preventive medicine, and its desire to have each citizen reach the optimum level of health, in part through their own endeavours. Specifically in respect of hospitals, Hastings explained the following month that a socialist administration would aim to create a 'great municipal system'. Clearly this had implications for the capital's voluntary hospitals, an issue returned to below.[8]

Further evidence of SMA activity in the early 1930s can be found on the LLP's Health Research Group, one of a number of such bodies set up by Herbert Morrison, now Labour's leader in London. Chaired by Silkin, this had eleven members, of whom five belonged to the Association. Given their professional expertise, it is reasonable to assume that this strong SMA presence was crucial in shaping the Group's findings. Its 1934 report, *The Public Health of London*, constituted a health manifesto for the impending elections. While noting the advances in public health, and their impact on the general death rate, the document also pointed to worrying trends in the capital, including rising maternal mortality and deaths from diseases such as cancer. Ill-health was the product of three factors – poverty; bad sanitation; and inadequate medical care and treatment. Municipal Reform's cost-cutting policies, particularly when directed at the social services, had caused a decline in the general standard of Londoners' health. Labour, by contrast, stood for every person's right to 'the best medical advice and treatment'; saw health as 'every bit as important as education' (an opinion often expressed by Hastings); and viewed popular physical well-being as 'the greatest asset a nation can possess'. It was therefore necessary to attack the causes of ill-health, for example by dealing with slum housing; to increase the number and improve the employment conditions of medical personnel; to provide better facilities and treatment for patients; and to continue to sever the link with the Poor Law. The lack of coordination between various parts of the medical services was also critically noted.[9]

The Public Health of London, as befits a document produced at election time, was relatively imprecise, thereby reflecting the LLP manifesto, described by Bernard Donoughue and G.W. Jones as a 'model of generalization'. However – and unsurprisingly – its priorities closely reflected those of the the SMA, and provided a platform from which Hastings and his Hospital Committee colleagues were to operate in the coming years. All this should also be put in the broader context of Morrison's strategy in 1934. One theme of his campaign, the most efficient Labour had carried out in London so far, was 'A Healthy London' and in this Association members played a vigorous part.[10]

Socialist medicine in London

The 1934 election result – a 'great victory', Clement Attlee was later to recall – was seen by the London Labour Party as an opportunity to expand and improve the hospital system. As *The Hospital* commented in the wake of Labour's success, the LCC had 'in its Health Service an instrument of the greatest potency'. This point was picked up by Morrison, who promised that 'the Hospitals and Medical Services of the county will be improved and expanded, so as to give our citizens a splendid civic service'.[11] It was therefore important that the election resulted in ten individuals closely associated with the SMA becoming LCC members. In the following years they served on a range of council bodies, the most important of which was the Hospital and Medical Services Committee where Association representation was nearly one-third of the total membership of 24.[12] At its meeting of 21 March 1934 Hastings, on the nomination of Jeger and Brook, was elected unopposed as Committee chairman, a post he held for the next ten years. Association activists were also members of various sub-committees of the main body – for example Blizard, Brook, Jeger, Rickards and Hastings served on the Hospital Management Sub-Committee – and on hospital boards to which the committee had the power of appointment. So, for example, Maule and Churchill were on the boards of, respectively, Archway and St Margaret's Hospitals.[13]

As the EC Report of 1934 put it, the SMA now had the opportunity to 'play a most important part in developing Labour's policy on public health and hospital services at the London County Hall'. This was significant not just administratively, but also in terms of the development of Association ideology. Murray pointed out in May 1934 that Labour's victory made the SMA look at the question of socialised medicine 'from an entirely new point of view'. Previously some form of national health care system had been envisaged. But the capturing of the LCC, which had the machinery to meet the demand for medical services run by a local authority, changed the picture. A socialised medical system might be reached by a route, the local, which 'we have not yet adequately explored'.[14] This was something of an exaggeration for, as we have seen, local control of welfare services was already a powerful strand in labour movement thought and in the proposals of previous socialist medical reformers. Nonetheless Murray's remark does highlight the LCC's importance for the SMA in terms of its opportunity to attempt to put into practice some of its central ideas and, in consequence, the further refining of its plans for a socialised service. On the other hand, it will become apparent in this and subsequent chapters that not all those on the medical left – including certain important Association members – were as impressed with the LCC experience as individuals such as Hastings and Murray.

The election of Hastings as Hospital Committee chairman was central to SMA influence. He had, it was later claimed, the respect not only of his Labour colleagues, but also of the LCC medical staff; his Conservative medical opponents; and the council's new leader, Morrison. The last point was important, for three reasons. First, Morrison was perfectly capable of keeping out of office those whom he did not trust, for example SMA member Santo Jeger (although this did not prevent the latter becoming vice-chairman of the Parliamentary Committee in 1935). Second, the paths of Morrison and the Association were from now on intertwined, most notably during the Labour Party debates over the organisation of the post-war NHS when both argued, unsuccessfully, for local government control. And, third, Morrison was prepared to allow his committee chairmen considerable latitude once entrusted with their positions.[15] This therefore offered Hastings and his colleagues scope to put their ideas into practice. The broader context should also be borne in mind here as 1934 was, as we saw previously, the year in which Hastings was instrumental in Labour Party conference's adoption of a proposal for a national health service.

The Hospital Committee was certainly active in expanding the volume of financial resources available for health. During the period 1934–40, hospital expenditure increased from £3.9m in 1933–34 to a peak of £5.3m in 1938–39, falling back slightly to £4.6m in 1939–40. This constituted between 13 per cent (1939–40) and 17 per cent (1938–39) of total council spending. Hospital expenditure increased more quickly than spending overall down to 1938, falling behind slightly thereafter, although it remained easily the third largest item after education and public assistance. Hastings encapsulated Labour's sense of achievement over the increased allocation of resources to hospitals in June 1939. Proposing the 1939–40 financial estimates, he suggested that it was 'with genuine satisfaction that I move these estimates. London has reason to be proud of its Municipal Hospital System'. This pride was shared by Morrison, who complained to the BBC if a London municipal hospital was mentioned on the radio without the prefix 'LCC', and who in 1936 described his council as the 'greatest hospital organisation in the world'.[16] Of course this investment was not an end in itself; it had particular aims and it is to what Labour in general, and the SMA's health professionals in particular, wanted out of improved medical services in the capital that we now turn.

As has now been noted on a number of occasions, left-wing analyses of health – including that of the SMA – tended to see ill-health as in the first instance a class problem, deriving from the inequalities of capitalism; the poor physical environment in which working people lived and worked; and the lack of resources for public services which should, by their very nature, be more widely available without punitive economic or social implications. Even the powerful LCC was not able, on its own, to fully address the first of these, the very essence of capitalism. But it could tackle much more directly at least part of the second factor through its housing policy, and this was to be seen as one of Labour's great achievements in London. For our purposes, however, it is the third factor – the allocation of resources to the social services, more precisely to health – which is of particular concern.

In 1935 Labour's health strategy for London was outlined in Herbert Morrison's pamphlet *London Under Socialist Rule*. This suggested that since 1934 decisions had been taken 'to enlarge, modernise, or otherwise improve, no less than 30 hospitals'. The numbers of medical, nursing and ancillary personnel had all been increased, and employment conditions enhanced. Behind this lay the Labour LCC's determination that the capital's 74 municipal hospitals would provide 'a service second to none, free from any Poor Law taint, which all classes of citizens will be proud to use'. Of course caution had to be exercised – partly to avoid any disruption of services through too-rapid expansion, partly for 'financial reasons'. And while payment for services had, since 1 July 1935, been taken out of the hands of the Poor Law's successor, the Public Assistance Committees, nonetheless charges still had to be made, although this was being done in a much less punitive way than previously. Overall, however, the tone was optimistic and the message positive.[17] Clearly it was felt that, even after only one year, Labour's policy on medical services had brought about significant change for the better, and had the potential to move further down this particular road.

The peacetime years of Labour rule saw Hastings and his colleagues continually seeking to advance medical reform. The continuing disassociation of health services from the Poor Law had already been addressed in February 1935. The Hospital Committee proposed the appropriation of four more institutions as the next step in its policy of 'taking all the hospitals under the Committee's management out of the scope of the Poor Law'. There were at least two factors behind Labour's desire to phase out Poor Law hospitals in London. First, to do so would take these institutions out of the control of the Ministry of Health and into that of the council. Second, while hospitals remained under Poor Law administration, technically every patient was a 'poor person', and had to gain admission by approaching the Relieving Officer. Ultimately, as Morrison was able to tell his fellow councillors, the 'only way a relieving officer could enter an LCC hospital was by becoming a patient', a clear indication of the aim of removing any stigma from hospitalisation.[18]

Municipalisation was central to the Committee's strategy, and Hastings spelled out some of its implications in April 1939. There were, he suggested, 'many advantages' to having a number of hospitals controlled by one authority 'as is the case with the LCC'. Specialist care, for example, could be expanded and coordinated, with those suffering from particular problems 'segregated under the care of doctors and nurses with exceptional experience, greatly to their advantage'.[19] This was clearly not only a positive claim on behalf of the LCC hospitals, but an implicit attack on the voluntary sector. The latter was not part of any planned or accountable scheme of hospital care, and thereby exemplified what Hastings and the Association saw as the overlap, inefficiency, and lack of coordination in the existing system.

Staff conditions too were, as promised, improved. In January 1937 Hastings reported that a new nurses' home, with accommodation for over 200 people, had been opened at Lambeth Hospital at a cost of £58 000. The same year saw the reduction of nurses' hours at 13 hospitals, and increases in medical and pathological staffs 'with due regard to the interests of the patients'. This was in line with the general improvement in LCC staff conditions under Labour. Supporters also argued that research flourished during Labour's rule. Barker claimed that 'many important discoveries in medical treatment have been made by workers in the LCC hospitals', so putting paid to the 'hoary calumny' that research would be stifled in a socialised medical service. On the contrary, London's 'great Municipal Health Service ... provided the scope, the opportunity and the resources for medical research on a scale which enabled rapid progress to be made in many fields'. Medical advances were due partly to the practice of grouping hospitals and to the creation of specialist units serving part or all of the metropolis, for example the cancer treatment centre at Lambeth Hospital which was able to employ the 'full scope of the latest x-ray and radium therapy methods of treatment'. Barker also highlighted the new pathology laboratories at Hampstead and Lambeth.[20]

Another area to which the Labour LCC, and Hastings and his Hospital Committee in particular, paid considerable attention was maternity care. We have already noted that in the 1930s maternal mortality remained high, and that this was an issue pursued in particular by Labour women through proposals for better organised and more easily accessible maternity care. Shortly after the Labour LCC victory the Hospital Committee reported that, as a result of considerable agitation on its part, the council had agreed in November 1934 to the ambulance service being extended so that under normal conditions all women could expect free provision as soon as they went into labour.[21] This is another significant example of the committee's attempt to introduce comprehensive services, free where possible, and without the stigma of pauperism. Further scope for development came with the 1936 Midwives Act which made local authorities responsible for the provision of a full-time, salaried midwifery service. The Hospital Committee, discussing the Bill in March 1936, regretted its omission of a number of issues. In particular, it did not allow for the limiting of medical aid to 'approved medical practitioners who would be specially qualified'. This concern very clearly coincided with the SMA position that maternity care should be provided by specialists, and thereby taken out of the hands of general practitioners. A deputation to the Health Ministry in January 1936 had, however, been unsuccessful in progressing such matters.[22] Nevertheless the Hospital Committee did not let the issue lapse. The following June it informed the Ministry that negotiations were under way with the London branch of the BMA for 'an approved list of practitioners to be available for the use of midwives' when they had to summon medical aid. It also asked the Ministry what action should be taken to ensure expert help in domiciliary maternity cases given that the LCC had, apparently, no powers to employ an obstetric consultant. The concern here was that the Act did not allow for the creation by the LCC of a 'flying squad' of specialist help for difficult confinements. These problems notwithstanding, in August 1937 Hastings reported the LCC's determination to use the Act 'to weld together the services provided by the Council, the Borough Councils, and the voluntary agencies'. The domiciliary scheme was not, he pointed out, the only option available to London mothers. Labour's commitment to better maternal care was already showing results, not least in the increased number of confinements in LCC hospitals, in itself a partial consequence of the 1929 Act.[23]

But it was the domiciliary service which attracted most attention. Hastings claimed in late 1937 that after 'months of hard work and repeated consultation with the many agencies concerned' the council now had in place a suitable scheme which was to come into force on 1

January 1938, with Ministry of Health approval. For women wishing to give birth at home, the LCC would have available nearly 50 full-time midwives. In addition, arrangements had been made with voluntary organisations so that, overall, London women would be able to call on the services of upwards of 200 midwives. Mothers would be charged £2 for a first confinement and 30 shillings thereafter, although mechanisms were available to have fees remitted or reduced. At this stage there was still no possibility of an LCC obstetric 'flying squad' for emergencies. This, under the Act, was a Borough Council responsibility, which in turn stressed the need for cooperation between all parties concerned in maternity provision. Indeed, some local authorities had already suggested that such specialist help would, in principle, be better handled by the London-wide authority.[24]

As Hastings acknowledged in 1937, there were still anomalies and overlap in the care London mothers might gain. Maternity and child welfare remained in Borough Council hands, while the domiciliary midwifery service was the responsibility of the LCC, which also provided 'a large number of hospital beds for maternity cases and young children'. Hastings returned to this issue in late 1945 – while the country awaited the NHS Bill – citing London's maternity provision as an example of the continuing lack of coordination of services. This was as absurd, he argued, as 'the presence of unconnected armies fighting one cause in a single area'. As we shall see, the Association was, during the 1940s, to repeatedly employ this sort of military analogy in the course of its 'battle for health'. However Hastings's tone and message in the 1930s were generally upbeat and optimistic, a position maintained by the LLP as a whole. Its 1938 annual report noted that the demand for council midwives had been such that three more had been employed in July 1938, with the engagement of a further five authorised as soon as need dictated. In the first seven months of operation, LCC midwives had attended nearly 2000 confinements, with a similar number of bookings arranged for the near future.[25]

The development of the LCC maternity services led Hastings to claim, in 1940, that its provision for expectant mothers since 1934 showed 'a better record (than) for any other class of people'. The new municipal midwives service was growing in popularity; the number of beds in maternity wards had almost doubled between 1933 and 1939; and more babies – over 21 000 in 1938 compared to just under 12 000 in 1933 – were being born in hospital. The result was a decline in maternal mortality at a rate of decrease faster than that of England and Wales as a whole. A post-war LCC publication made the same points, noting also the voluntary hospitals' deficiencies in maternity provision. This positive interpretation was shared by Barker, who suggested that under

Labour 'maternity services were, literally, transformed beyond recognition'. Before the war, he further claimed, under the auspices of the Council's Home Midwifery and Maternity Nursing Service 'over 10,000 mothers every year were receiving midwifery and nursing attention at their hands'.[26]

The SMA strategy in London should also be viewed in the broader context of its critique of the maternity plan proposed jointly in 1938 by the BMA and the TUC, and discussed in the previous chapter. As we have seen this scheme was, to Hastings and his colleagues, based on a number of erroneous, and medically reactionary, assumptions – principally that every general practitioner who undertook maternity work did so willingly and with adequate knowledge; and that every woman had a GP conversant with her medical history. On the latter, for example, Hastings claimed that 'as many as 95% of the mothers in one part of East London have no regular private doctor'. Consequently, in addition to the dangers inherent in unwilling or ignorant doctors attending childbirth, there could be no continuity of ante- and post-natal care. It was just such problems that the London schemes sought to avoid, by attempting to sidestep general practitioners through the provision of specialist care in the form of midwives and, more problematically, obstetricians; by stressing the availability of both domiciliary and hospital services; and by trying to ensure adequate ante- and post-natal facilities. Clearly making a political point as well as picking up on the contemporary controversies over maternity care, Hastings told a correspondent in 1938 that 'I can safely say that the BMA has not influenced the policy of the LCC in the slightest'.[27] On the other hand the concerns acknowledged by Hastings at various times undoubtedly suggested the need for a more comprehensive service in respect not only of maternity provision, but overall.

The SMA in London: a balance sheet

The creation of a fully municipalised, socialised system in London itself was clearly not unproblematic. In a review of hospital provision up until 1937, Hastings recognised the problems still obstructing the full achievement of his (and he stressed he was not talking on behalf of the LCC) plans. London suffered from 'the division of responsibility and multiplicity of authorities', and there was an 'almost infinite number' of voluntary agencies providing services of varying quality and coverage. Similarly, Borough Councils and the LCC could find themselves, because of arbitrary divisions in health functions, duplicating services and administration. This was, however, much less of a problem with

hospitals. Now only six were administered by the latest incarnation of
the Poor Law, and as soon as places were found for their inmates
needing accommodation 'for reasons other than sickness', these too
would be appropriated. The 'Poor Law spirit' had, nonetheless, not
entirely disappeared. Labour was thus determined that 'every possible
suggestion of charity, subservience, and general second-rateness' be abandoned, and that instead London's citizens should see the municipal
hospitals as their own. Everyone had 'every right to use them and
expect the best from them', a further example of the recurrent stress on
citizenship rights. The ultimate aim was to 'equal or excel' the larger
voluntary hospitals' high standards. Hastings warned that this would
take time, and that there was a long way to go before the LCC hospitals
could be seen 'as anything like perfect or complete'. Indeed it was
doubtful whether this was possible 'within the limits of existing legislation'.[28]

This was a significant remark suggesting that even Hastings, local
authority control's most fervent advocate, realised that substantial
changes were required before both the LCC could realise its full potential, and the LCC model be adopted elsewhere. While local control of
health services remained central to the Association model for a socialised service, the reform of local government was now also stressed in its
plans. Nonetheless the sheer scale of the LCC's medical services by the
late 1930s, and the SMA's role in promoting them, is worth emphasising. In 1937 its expenditure on centralised health services such as
hospitals had risen by a factor of nearly 20 since the immediate post-
war period. By this time London accounted, Roger Lee suggests, 'for
almost a quarter of national expenditure on centralised health care'.
This confirmed the capital's primacy 'as the major national centre of
hospital medicine'. Two years later Sir George Newman, former Chief
Medical Officer to the Ministry of Health, described the council as the
'greatest Local Health Authority in the Empire'. In numerical terms this
was certainly the case, the LCC being the largest single provider of
hospital beds in Britain, and probably the world. It was, moreover, the
municipal hospitals which bore the brunt of care for the long term and
chronic sick. And as Rickards pointed out in 1938, municipal general
hospitals provided over 22 000 beds for London's people. The voluntary hospitals, on the other hand, provided 15 000 'but only 9,000 of
these are available for the inhabitants of London, the remainder being
occupied by patients from outside the county'.[29]

By the late 1930s the work of Hastings and his colleagues was influencing events beyond London itself. Webster notes that Health Ministry
officials were both reacting to Labour policy initiatives 'and to developments taking place in London, associated with the rise of the LCC

hospital services and the decline of the voluntary sector'. This seems to have suggested to these civil servants that voluntarism might be on its last legs, and that the real choice for the future lay between municipalisation and nationalisation. The LCC position was certainly taken very seriously. One clear, forthright, and important exposition of this came in 1939. The SMA *Bulletin* noted in January an imminent conference of the Ministry of Health, the LCC, and the voluntary hospitals at which it was likely that the hospitals would ask for a grant from the council. This in itself was another indication of the voluntary system's failure, and hence 'the need for a unified municipal service'. The Labour LCC, the author continued, 'may be trusted to deal with the matter in such a way as to do nothing to make more difficult the coming of a socialised medical service'.[30]

At the meeting itself, of the ten LCC representatives two, Hastings and Rickards, were SMA members. Hastings argued that the council was the guardian of the ratepayers money, and continued:

> I am wondering whether one would have any justification in using the money of the ratepayers of London to support a system in which there is no unified system, no unified control and in which some of the work could be done more economically.[31]

The Ministry of Health official John Pater's description of the relationship between London's municipal and voluntary sectors in the 1930s as one of 'cold war', rather than the cooperation in principle encouraged by the 1929 Act, is therefore apt and in this Association members clearly had a part to play. The case of London also bears out Frank Prochaska's point that in the inter-war period the Local Government Act did 'more to unsettle relations between the voluntary and public hospital sectors than any other piece of legislation'.[32] In analysing the SMA, however, what is important was its influence on the LCC's health policy, and thereby its indirect input to the Ministry of Health's deliberations.

Such influence notwithstanding, questions still have to be asked about the actual extent of change under the peacetime LCC Labour administration. John Sheldrake suggests that the council's achievements were 'more in the realm of reorganization, rationalization and administration than in a massive programme of new hospital building'. As he points out, the number of beds available had actually declined by 1939, albeit as a result of increased efficiency of provision.[33] There were also political and structural barriers to a full realisation of the medical plans of organisations such as the SMA. The Labour LCC had to be sensitive to the feelings of Labour-controlled Borough Councils, which retained significant health functions. Such division of responsibilities between

London and Borough Councils was a cause of frustration to anyone seeking a coordinated system of medical care throughout the capital, as Hastings himself noted. Furthermore Morrison, while ambitious in his plans for London, was hardly fiscally reckless. He was also keen to prioritise housing. This had, of course, an important health function and the medical left, including the SMA, always emphasised that combating ill-health was not confined to the GP's surgery or the hospital ward. Nonetheless decisions still had to be made about resource allocation, and clearly medical services were not always accorded top priority. And as the 1930s drew to a close another competing call on municipal funds emerged in the need to prepare for the protection of the civilian population in the event of war – a topic on which, as the next chapter shows, the SMA had strong views.[34]

It may have been internal LCC strategic decisions of this sort, and perhaps also the more general bureaucratic constraints under which it operated, which prompted an outburst by Rickards in 1936. At a meeting chaired by Hastings she criticised the 'lack of formulative policy on the LCC Health Committee', and continued:

> They could run and build hospitals admirably, but when confronted with the necessity to provide a plan to combat measles or whooping cough they were up against a brick wall.[35]

Rickards's frustration was shared by Brook who, as we shall see, was to come out against local authority control in his submission to the wartime Medical Planning Commission. Indeed, as will also become evident, misgivings about the LCC's health care provision were not uncommon on the medical left, and during the 1940s in particular were to provide the basis of an alternative model for a socialised health service. Moreover the very scale and nature of what the Labour LCC sought to achieve in the health field was constrained by circumstances which it inherited or which were outside its control. As Sheldrake correctly argues, many hospitals were badly sited; certain special hospitals lay outside the administrative area of the LCC; and the voluntary hospitals, which in any case were not under council control, were largely concentrated in the capital's centre. A post-war retrospective on the London hospital system noted that many institutions taken over after 1929 were not in the best condition, and that the only solution was 'a long-term plan, spread over many years'. This was duly adopted, but the 'carrying out of these schemes of construction and reconditioning was of course disastrously interrupted by the war'.[36]

Another official post-war publication claimed that '[g]reat advances' had been made in the standard of treatment since 1930 but that, once again, 'progress was arrested by the war'. As Hastings himself later recalled, on the day that war broke out he was about to sign a contract for

> what I still think would have been the best Special Hospital that the world had ever known. But of course all this had to be scrapped. I shall never forget my grief.[37]

The LCC achievement in the 1930s was therefore based more on the refurbishment of existing buildings than on any massive programme of new hospital construction. Whether this would have continued to be the case had not war intervened is a matter for historical conjecture. But it is clear that in the 1930s not only did the unreformed system of local government pose problems for London health reformers, but structural and geographical factors likewise did not always operate in their favour.

What, then, should be our assessment of SMA influence on London's health services in the 1930s? Labour's 1934 LCC victory saw considerable power over the capital's peacetime health policy fall into the hands of the Association, an organisation committed to a socialised health service. It is no exaggeration to say that its members were instrumental in directing the capital's health policy after 1934, particularly through the Hospital and Medical Services Committee on which there was strong SMA representation, not least in the person of its chairman, Hastings. The Committee had dynamic plans for the future of, for example, London's hospital service. These involved not simply further building and renovation, important as these were, but also the appropriation of remaining Poor Law institutions; the improvement of employment conditions for all staff, medical and ancillary; and, ultimately, the integration of all hospitals into a unified, free service.

The ambitions and achievements of the hospitals system under the Labour administration in the 1930s were extremely important both to the Labour Party and to the SMA itself, and perhaps in particular to its key player, Hastings. One consequence of the London experience for the Association was, therefore, the further refinement of its model of health care provision. This stressed the need for democratic control by reformed local government bodies, centrally coordinated and supervised by the Ministry of Health. As we shall see in Chapters Seven and Eight Hastings was, for example, to press hard on the Medical Planning Commission for directly accountable health services, and this was to become official Labour policy by the end of the war. The direct significance of the LCC and its policies in the 1930s to the Labour Party, given its problems at a national level and the strand in its ideology strongly in favour of the devolution of political power, should likewise not be underestimated. And as we noted in the last chapter, by the late

1930s Labour's PHAC had been revived, with a significant Association presence. Although this was again in a state of limbo by the outbreak of war, it was later reconstituted, with the SMA once more in a powerful position. There was thus a direct link between the organisation's proposals for a socialised service put forward on Labour Party policy bodies and the experience of its members on the LCC.

Association thinking on the nature of a socialised health service was therefore further focused by its actual experiences of health service administration. Equally, however, there were a number of constraints to municipal expansion in the 1930s. Some of these, for example the distribution of health functions between the LCC and the Borough Councils, might have been resolved in time by appropriate national legislation. Others, and most obviously the coming of war, were clearly matters way beyond the control of even the powerful LCC. In consequence, some projects were fulfilled, but others frustrated in whole or in part. This must make us qualify the achievements of Hastings and his colleagues. Even the improvements in maternity provision introduced after 1934 were not as unified and comprehensive as might have been desired. This is not, of course, to belittle its contribution to the decline in maternal mortality, but simply to suggest that at an organisational level what was desired was not always achieved. In turn this suggests that important as London was to the SMA, it also had before it the task of persuading both the Labour Party as a whole and others on the medical left of the validity of its plans for a socialised medical service. Its attempts to do so are examined in detail in later chapters.

Overall, therefore, the Association's LCC involvement was important on the level of ideas, while at a more practical level was a story of qualified success which might, under different circumstances, have had significantly different outcomes. In an era when the various forms of health care provision were so complex, competitive, and overlapping as to hardly constitute a 'system' at all, even the most vigorous organisation might have found it difficult to do much more than the Hastings-led LCC Hospital Committee, given the circumstances in which it found itself. Credit should therefore be given to the Labour administration, and particularly to the SMA, for achieving as much as they did.

Notes

1. An earlier version of this chapter is to be found in John Stewart, '"For a Healthy London": the Socialist Medical Association and the London County Council in the 1930s', *Medical History*, 41, October 1997: Copyright the Trustee, The Wellcome Trust, reproduced with permission. On

the continuing significance of local politics to the Labour Party in the inter-war period, see Beach, thesis, p. 134 and Ch. 4 *passim*.

2. Brockway, *Bermondsey Story: the Life of Alfred Salter*, Chs 9 and 10; LCC/MIN/2207, 28 November 1929; on the composition of the LLP Executive in the 1930s, see Acc2417/A/2, Minutes of the Executive Committee of the London Labour Party, 1931–39.

3. John Sheldrake, 'The LCC Hospital Service', in Saint, Andrew (ed.), *Politics and the People of London: the London County Council 1889–1965*, Hambledon Press, 1989, pp. 187–94; Geoffrey Rivett, *The Development of the London Hospital System 1832–1982*, King Edward's Hospital Fund for London, 1986, p. 199ff.

4. Brian Barker, *Labour in London: a Study in Municipal Achievement*, George Routledge and Sons, 1946, p. 64.

5. *Lancet*, 1934, I, p. 1136.

6. For a sense of the London branch's activities, see DSM (3) 14. DSM 1/1, Report of the EC, 1930–31, and Minutes of the First Annual General Meeting, 1931; Murray, *Why a National Health Service?*, pp. 24–5.

7. Papers presented to the Executive Committee of the London Labour Party, Acc2417/A/15, folios 4397, 4400, 4479; *London News*, February 1931, pp. 1 and 8 – Salter was one of the authors of this manifesto.

8. *London News*, April 1933, p. 7, and May 1933, p. 8.

9. Bernard Donoughue and G.W. Jones, *Herbert Morrison: Portrait of a Politician*, Weidenfeld and Nicolson, 1973, p. 190; London Labour Party Health Research Group, *The Public Health of London*, London Labour Publications, 1934, pp. 3, 7, 9, 10–13. The SMA representatives were Salter, Hastings, Esther Rickards, Amy Sayle and A.J. Gillison.

10. Donoughue and Jones, *Herbert Morrison*, p. 190; London Labour Party Conference Papers, Acc2417/G/2, The Work of the London Labour Party, 1933–34, p. 9.

11. Clement Attlee, *As It Happened*, Heinemann, 1954, p. 81; *The Hospital*, December 1935, p. 320; Acc2417/O/34, offprint of Herbert Morrison, 'New Era for London', *Labour*, May 1934, p. 197.

12. DSM 1/1, AGM 1934, EC Report. Those concerned were full members Brook, Gillison, Hastings, Homa, Jeger, McClements, and Rickards; and associate member Sayle. Two other associate members became Aldermen: William Bennett and G.P. Blizard. The latter had served with Hastings on the Labour Party's Advisory Committee on Public Health; Brook, *Making Medical History*, p. 2; Minutes of the London County Council, 20 March 1934, and subsequently.

13. LCC/MIN/2211, 21 March and 26 April 1934; Minutes of the London County Council, 19 November 1935; DSM 1/1, AGM 1934, EC Report.

14. DSM 1/1, AGM 1934, EC Report; *Socialist Doctor*, vol. II, no. 3, May 1934, p. 1.

15. Donoughue and Jones, *Herbert Morrison*, pp. 192–4.

16. Donoughue and Jones, *Herbert Morrison*, p. 656 and p. 200; *London News*, June 1939, p. 3; quoted in *The Daily Telegraph*, 9 November 1936 – cutting in LCC General Hospitals Division Official Cuttings Book.

17. Herbert Morrison and D.H. Daines, *London under Socialist Rule*, Labour Party, 1935, pp. 7–9; see also London Labour Party, *Socialist Planning in London*, London Labour Party, 1935.

18. LCC/MIN/2212, 28 February 1935; Barker, pp. 138–9.

19. *London News*, April 1939, p. 8.
20. *London News*, January 1937, p. 5; London Labour Party Conference Papers, Acc2417/G/3, 'The Work of the London Labour Party, 1936–37', p. 35; Donoughue and Jones, *Herbert Morrison*, p. 196; Barker, *Labour in London*, pp. 140–143.
21. For the broader context, see Lara Marks, *Metropolitan Mortality*, Amsterdam, Rodopi, 1996, *passim*; LCC/MIN/2212, 14 March 1935.
22. LCC/MIN/2213, 26 March 1936; on Hastings's attitude to professional care and maternity services, see Stewart, 'Socialist Proposals', pp. 346–7.
23. LCC/MIN/2214, 10 June 1937; *London News*, August 1937, p. 5.
24. *The Labour Woman*, November 1937, pp. 168–9.
25. Somerville Hastings, 'The Municipal Hospitals of London: What They Are and What They May Be', *MTT*, no. 1, October 1937, p. 3; DSM 5/1, cutting from *Municipal Journal*, October 1945; London Labour Party Conference Papers, Acc2417/G/3, 'The Work of the London Labour Party, 1937–38', p. 28.
26. *London News*, June 1940, p. 3; London County Council, *The Hospital Service*, p. 6; Barker, *Labour in London*, pp. 148–9.
27. DSM 4/1, *Comments by Dr Somerville Hastings and Others on the TUC and BMA National Maternity Scheme*, 18 October 1938; DSM (2) 5, 'BMA', Hastings to Norman Bartlett, 18 June 1938.
28. Hastings, 'The Municipal Hospitals of London', pp. 3–6.
29. Roger Lee, 'Uneven zenith: towards a geography of the high period of municipal medicine in England and Wales', *Journal of Historical Geography*, 14, 3, 1988, 260–80, pp. 269, table 4, 268; quoted in Sheldrake, 'The LCC Hospital Service', p. 195; Rivett, *The Development of the London Hospital System 1823–1982*, p. 202; Esther Rickards in *The London News*, September 1938 – cutting in LCC General Hospitals Division Official Cuttings Book, London Metropolitan Archives.
30. Webster, 'Labour and the Origins of the National Health Service', pp. 190–191; Webster, *The Health Services since the War*, p. 22; SMA, *Bulletin*, no. 5, January 1939, p. 1.
31. MH 79/513, notes of a conference held at the Ministry of Health 27/1/39 between representatives of the LCC, Ministry of Health, and the Voluntary Hospitals of London, pp. 36–7.
32. Pater, *The Making of the National Health Service*, p. 16; Frank Prochaska, *Philanthropy and the Hospitals of London*, Oxford, Oxford University Press, 1992, p. 111.
33. Sheldrake, 'The LCC Hospital Service', p. 188.
34. Donoughue and Jones, *Herbert Morrison*, pp. 199, 206–7.
35. DSM (2) 5, 'Inter-Hospitals Socialist Society', typescript of a joint meeting of the SMA and the Inter-Hospitals Socialist Society, 31 January 1936.
36. Sheldrake, 'The LCC Hospital Service', pp. 195–6; London County Council, *The LCC Hospitals: a Retrospect*, London County Council, 1949, p. 59.
37. London County Council, *The Hospital Service*, London County Council, 1946, p. 3; DSH File 1, 'Articles' – 'Thirty Years on the LCC', n.d., but 1952.

CHAPTER SIX

Fascism, Medicine, and War

So far we have traced the early history of the SMA through activities such as its participation on the LCC. The Association did not, however, confine itself to domestic matters. It engaged with international affairs, both rhetorically and practically, for the following reasons. First, socialism was, by definition, internationalist. The Association itself had been created partly on the initiative of the German socialist dentist Ewald Fabian, and had affiliated to the International Socialist Medical Association shortly after its foundation. Second, if socialism was international, so too was medicine. Doctors traditionally had access to all medical knowledge, whatever its country of origin. *MTT* argued, during the diplomatic crisis of spring 1938, that medicine was 'international in the highest sense of the word'. Fascism involved the abnegation of 'the universal spirit that has developed in the medical profession during the past centuries'. Every doctor aware of medicine's debt to 'men of every race, of every religion, and of every shade of opinion' should condemn fascism and work for the spread of 'a true international spirit'. Furthermore, medicine's internationalism could, Murray argued at the height of the Second World War, make it the basis and inspiration of a global system prioritising citizenship over nationality.[1]

Third, medical organisation could benefit from other countries' experiences. We have already noted *MTT*'s regular feature on 'Medical News of the World', and how SMA ideas drew on the health care systems of nations such as Sweden. Fourth, in war it was the medical profession which had to repair human damage, and so knew best its human costs. Doctors therefore had a particular duty to agitate for cooperative solutions to international problems. In this, they would be aided by their 'greater influence over the community than any other profession'. Paradoxically, though, war could also have positive outcomes. In September 1941 *MTT* acknowledged the depth of the crisis facing Britain. For medicine, however, both technically and organisationally, the time was 'as potentially fruitful as any in history'.[2]

Finally, doctors were also scientists, and here too could play an important part in informing the public about issues with both domestic and international dimensions. Racist ideology, for instance, was 'not only inimical to progress', but based on 'false theories that every medical student knows are genetically wrong'. For the SMA, doctors were therefore both qualified and obliged to comment on matters other than the strictly medical. Not to do so could have catastrophic effects, as a German colleague pointed out in *Socialist Doctor* in 1934. Germany's medical profession had failed to provide any leadership during Hitler's rise to power, and lack of 'firm convictions' had facilitated the spread of fascism: 'Few withstood the lies and stupidity or fought against the loss of freedom of thought and the enslavement of a whole people.' It was thus doctors' duty to help shape public opinion. This notion of medicine's and of science's social responsibility was widespread among the medical and scientific left in the 1930s. Murray's statement on the unscientific basis of racism, for example, echoed that of a group of prominent Cambridge scientists in 1936.[3] This chapter now analyses the Association's practical expression of its internationalism through its support for medical refugees; its response to the Spanish Civil War and the British government's official preparations for war; and the debate within the organisation over its stance on the outbreak of World War II. As will become evident, the SMA saw these issues as not just important in themselves, but also as further illustrating the need for medical reconstruction.

Medical refugees

With the advent of the Nazi regime, and its subsequent territorial expansion, those hostile to, or demonised by, Hitlerism began to leave fascist-controlled Europe in considerable numbers. It is estimated that between 1933 and 1939 some 50 000 Germans and Austrians entered Britain, of whom 90 per cent were Jewish. It is further calculated that around 1200 German and Austrian Jewish doctors came to Britain from 1933 onwards and it was to medical refugees that, understandably, the SMA paid particular attention.[4] As is well-known, the main professional bodies, supported by sections of the popular press, were hostile to foreign doctors practising in Britain. This derived from concern over an allegedly 'overstocked' medical labour market, particularly among hard-pressed GPs; and racialism, overt or covert. The Association found such hostility particularly galling in the case of the MPU, which developed a notoriously anti-semitic standpoint, partly because of the impact of economic depression and the debt in which many GPs consequently found themselves. This was, in turn, blamed on Jewish moneylenders.[5] When combined with the conservatism of the main professional bodies, this indicates what the SMA was up against.

Individually and collectively, the Association rejected the analysis and prejudice of organisations such as the MPU. Major Greenwood, for instance, was an early and important member of the Academic

Assistance Council (later the Society for the Protection of Science and Learning – SPSL), a body specifically set up to aid members of the academic community forced to flee their own countries, many of whom came from medical faculties. Greenwood was highly active in this field, exploring ways in which, for example, individual refugee medical scientists might be found university posts. He was therefore part of one of the 'vital networks' which Paul Weindling identifies as significant in aiding refugee scholars in the 1930s.[6]

At an organisational level, we find the SMA questioning, from 1933, the approach of the General Medical Council (GMC) to refugee doctors. This required that even the most highly qualified foreigner undertake a further course of study in Britain. Such lobbying continued throughout the 1930s, after January 1939 being the particular responsibility of the newly-formed refugee sub-committee. This had Dr Mary Gilchrist and Professor J.R. Marrack as joint secretaries. Gilchrist, an embodiment of the Association's internationalist beliefs, later became secretary of the China Medical Aid Committee which, among other activities, sought to recruit medical personnel to help the victims of Japanese aggression in the Far East. The setting up of the refugee sub-committee was precipitated by increasing SMA activity on the refugee question in 1938–39, the era of the Kristallnacht, the Austrian Anschluss, and the end of the civil war in Spain, all of which increased the volume of refugees seeking asylum in Britain. This was also the time of Munich and the dismemberment of Czechoslovakia, both of which the Association viewed with considerable foreboding. Its concern over medical refugees was mirrored in the broader labour movement's fears for political refugees, both being enraged by what was perceived as official and professional apathy, and even hostility.[7]

Practical measures were taken by the SMA to help medical personnel fleeing fascist persecution. In 1933 a fund was set up to aid German doctors, particularly the vulnerable groups of Jews and socialists. This resulted from an AGM resolution condemning the persecution of doctors 'for political or racial reasons'. In November the same year, Hastings wrote to his fellow Association members that 'almost daily' he met German socialist and Jewish medical refugees, including at Labour Party conference when he had been approached by a 'German Socialist Doctor who was in charge of a stall of toys, made by refugees'. He concluded with a plea for financial aid, since 'we, as Socialists, cannot avoid some responsibility for the welfare of our colleagues who are now suffering for their Socialist principles'. To place this in context, in the same month Lord Dawson of Penn, President of the Royal College of Physicians, told the Home Secretary that the number of medical refugees who could be 'usefully absorbed or teach us anything could be counted on the fingers of one hand'. Consequently the Home Office agreed to consult the main professional bodies over the issue, a situation which continued throughout the 1930s, much to the disadvantage of medical workers seeking refuge in Britain.[8]

SMA aid to doctors victimised by the Nazis took a variety of forms. One particularly poignant example came in November 1938. In response to Kristallnacht, the secretary of the London branch wrote urgently to the London Labour Party. Were the LCC, he suggested, to give hospital employment to as many doctors and nurses as possible, then 'the great suffering of jewish and progressive doctors in fascist countries would be to that extent ameliorated'.[9] The activities of Association members on the LCC on behalf of medical refugees is discussed further below, but the urgency of the situation in 1938 is indicated by the SMA official's willingness to countenance lower-grade employment for refugee doctors, something it for the most part opposed. This tactic was repeated in a letter from Association secretary D.F. Buckle to the Labour Party Secretary James Middleton. Buckle pointed out that his EC had recently agreed that were refugee doctors to be employed as nurses their suffering would be lessened, particularly as there was currently a nursing shortage. He therefore appealed to Middleton to use his influence with Labour local authorities to further this proposal.[10]

The SMA's attitude is particularly significant in the broader context, since by 1938 the MPU was steadfastly against any further medical immigration, no matter what the situation. Indeed, by the summer of that year Association antipathy to the MPU's stance prompted it to complain to the Labour Party. Brook, writing on behalf of the EC, pointed out to Middleton that the number of refugee doctors practising in Britain was statistically insignificant; and that such doctors had, despite their existing qualifications, to undergo a further two years study before being allowed to practice. By offering assistance to refugees, Brook pointed out, 'we can promote goodwill and unity among Anti-Fascists of all countries, and this should prove a powerful force in checking the present world-wide onslaught against socialist principles'. The attitude of the MPU, a TUC-affiliated organisation, was therefore to be deplored. The following year, Middleton received more correspondence from the Association on this matter. Buckle claimed that the MPU was employing 'blatantly pro-fascist propaganda' over the refugee issue, even to the extent of circulating British Union of Fascist material. Middleton counselled caution over such claims, and pointed out that in any case there was little the Labour Party could actually do, although he agreed to send the SMA's findings to the TUC.[11]

The setting up of the refugee sub-committee was, therefore, a response to events both abroad and at home. One of its initial tasks was to provide funds for foreign medical workers who had aided the ill-fated Spanish Republic, now wished to enter Britain, and might offer their services in China. Arrangements were made for 15 nurses and doctors from Spain 'to enter this country for a short stay'. The Association was 'instrumental' in this, and in securing their release from internment camps in France. It was hoped that at least some of these refugees would go on to work with the Chinese Red Cross. This did happen, although not without problems. Association members were also encouraged, by the social committee created explicitly for this purpose, to meet medical refugees personally. In at least one case this hospitality extended to housing a refugee doctor, Dr John Kiszely, a Hungarian who had worked with the republican forces in Spain. In 1939, he was being put up by SMA member Kenneth Sinclair-Loutit, another Spanish Civil War participant. Kiszely was to be invited to a dinner for doctors recently returned from Spain provided, as yet another SMA veteran of Spain put it, 'there is no danger of the home office discovering ... his past history'.[12]

One particularly telling and significant example of the SMA's agitational activity came in the late summer of 1940. In August it approached a number of organisations, including the SPSL, with a view to holding a joint meeting on the refugee issue. The rationale for this was explained in a letter from Association treasurer, L.T. Hilliard:

> Government policy with regard to refugees, as set out in Cmd.6217 makes internment the rule rather than the exception ... We think ... that further letters to newspapers will do little good and therefore suggest that a public meeting of protest should be organised by various professional bodies and held as soon as possible.

This was indeed the case, the government in June 1940 having issued an order for the dismissal and internment of all alien practitioners. The SPSL turned down the SMA proposal on the basis that the 'Home Office has adopted many suggestions we (the SPSL and other refugee organisations) have made, as is shown by the latest concessions of which we heard last Thursday'.[13] Consequently the SMA went ahead and organised, without the SPSL, a joint meeting of nine organisations involved with medical refugees, some of whom 'were unaware of each other's existence'. Those participating included the Medical Department of the German-Jewish Committee; the Czechoslovak Medical Association in Great Britain; and the International Solidarity Fund, Austrian Section. An earlier survey by Marrack had suggested that around 130 internees were foreign medical personnel. Information exchanged now revealed that 'several hundred' such individuals remained interned, and that of those who were not, only the 'fortunate few' who had obtained British qualifications were able to practice. The skills of the others were going to waste, as in the case of one doctor employed as 'a workman in a cocoa factory'. Various proposals were made to better utilise the abilities of the 2000 refugee doctors claimed to be in the country, for instance by pressing for the recognition of Czech medical qualifications.[14] As *MTT* put it in late 1940, it was the 'height of folly' for the government to be bound by rules 'so open to criticism as those of medical registration'. It was therefore urged that all suitably qualified foreign doctors be allowed to practice. An element of compromise was introduced by suggesting that the contract issued could be for 'the duration of the war without any further implication than that we recognise their ability to assist in vital medical work'.[15]

The Association's willingness to go ahead without the apparently more cautious SPSL should be put in the context of the point made by Louise Burleston, that with the ending of the 'phoney war' the early summer of 1940 was a particularly fertile period for anti-foreigner sentiment. Moreover, the Home Secretary at this time was Sir John Anderson, an individual the Association viewed with considerable distrust. It was only in October 1940 that Anderson was replaced by Herbert Morrison. Morrison was to prove much more liberal in his attitudes to foreign refugees, thereby improving the political environment in which organisations like the Association operated. Nonetheless the MPU remained troublesome, for example in its warning to the socialist Minister of Labour, Ernest Bevin, that he should resist an SMA proposal to use interned medical refugees in industrial medicine. To do so, it suggested, would introduce a fifth column into British industry. The MPU's stance therefore remained anti-refugee, and we again find the Association publicly protesting about its behaviour and attitudes in 1941.[16]

The SMA itself viewed medical refugees positively. Victims of political or racial discrimination, they thereby qualified for special treatment by more humane and tolerant societies. Many were also eminent in their own fields, and should be welcomed into the British medical system, where their skills could be usefully employed. Consequently the Association was prepared to lobby on the refugees' behalf, as well as providing practical help and comfort. There was a further dimension to this. Professional antipathy to refugee medical personnel derived partly from the belief that they would add to an already overstocked job market. The SMA was not insensitive to this argument, as a close examination of the impact of Austrian refugees shows. Even prior to the Anschluss, Austria was of considerable concern to the SMA. From 1934 complaints were made about the right wing government's treatment of socialist doctors who had, as in Germany, a large political organisation led by the prominent anatomist Professor Tandler. To this end Hastings was part of a deputation to the Austrian embassy in London, and wrote to the medical press along similar lines.[17]

Fears over the situation in Austria were heightened by the German occupation. This led *MTT* to suggest, in April 1938, that Europe was facing the 'greatest crisis in history'. The journal expressed concern over the imprisonment, suicide, and emigration problems of Austrian doctors. Specifically it believed, wrongly, that Sigmund Freud had been imprisoned; and noted that 'Dr Baumgartner and Dr Herz, heads of the biggest municipal hospital in Vienna, and Professor Edmund Nobel, specialist in diseases of children' had taken their own lives. Among those who had actually managed to flee the country was Karl Breitner, a retired Jewish dentist from Vienna. Breitner had reached London's Croydon airport, only to be detained by the police and then repatriated. But *MTT* also suggested that, given current levels of unemployment, refugees did pose problems in potential host countries, and this was as true in medicine as elsewhere. No one advocated the 'immediate acceptance' of all those doctors compelled to leave Austria, although the utmost sympathy should be accorded those 'whose qualifications command our respect'. In this context the already noted hostility of the MPU is important, as is the observation by the socialist journal *New Statesman* that if all medical refugees were admitted British doctors would become 'roaring anti-semites'.[18]

Within weeks, however, when left-wing and Jewish doctors had become 'a particular butt for Nazi spleen', such reservations had been abandoned. Medical refugees, Murray argued, would not 'make a livelihood here only at the expense of others'. Rather, they would contribute to 'the common fund of knowledge which makes for a good medical service'. Later the same year, Murray condemned those in the medical profession pretending 'allegiance to liberal ideas' while demanding that Britain refuse entry to 'a single Jewish doctor'. Disclaiming racial prejudice, such individuals proffered the excuse of an already overcrowded profession. This was, however, a 'camouflage for a fear that the average income of doctors might be lowered'. In fact what was necessary was 'many more qualified men and women both here and in the Dominions'; not 'fewer doctors, but a new system'. In similar vein Edith Summerskill raised the issue of Austrian doctors in the Commons in July 1938. Was it not the case, she asked Home Secretary Sir Samuel Hoare, that 'many doctors in this country believe that the Austrian doctors are making a helpful contribution to the medical knowledge of this country?'. Hoare agreed, going on, rather ambiguously, to argue the necessity of judging each case on its merits.[19]

Two important points arise here. First, at this very time Hoare was being urged by the BMA – itself under pressure from the MPU – to

severely restrict the number of Austrian medical practitioners entering
the country. The BMA 'adamantly refused' to allow the admission of
more than a few such individuals, and a committee set up to monitor
the situation later reported its success on imposing a 'severe limitation'
on medical refugees. Around the same time the foreign secretary, Lord
Halifax, intervened personally on behalf of three Jewish doctors from
Danzig. These had been admitted by the Home Office, again in the face
of BMA opposition. The SMA was therefore responding, in a more
sympathetic and humane way than many of its professional peers, to
domestic and foreign events affecting medical refugees. Ironically, or
tragically, it was from around mid-1938 that the government began to
adopt, in general terms, a more liberal policy towards refugees. The
notable exception remained, as a result of the professional bodies'
intransigence, medical practitioners.[20]

Second, Murray's statement encapsulates a key Association demand,
that the health services be increased and rationalised. The commonly-
held view that the medical labour market was already overstocked was
the exact opposite of the real situation. Consequently, medical refugees
were not just victims but also had a positive role, both qualitatively and
quantitatively, in health care provision. This idea was expanded upon
when war actually came about, and when the inadequacies of the
current system became widely apparent simultaneously with the prospect of constructive change. In such circumstances medical refugees
could contribute to the defeat of the very forces – anti-scientific, anti-
humanist – which had expelled them from their own countries. In
March 1941 MTT argued that their enlistment would help defeat Hitler
and 'destroy completely those unscientific and debased conceptions of
race' on which his regime rested. A few months later, the Association's
AGM noted that an appeal had recently been made for a thousand
doctors from the USA, and a decision taken to employ fourth- and fifth-
year medical students as house officers. In such circumstances it therefore
strongly protested against official failure 'to make use of the medical
services of the anti-fascist refugee doctors in this country'. Less than
one-tenth were being allowed to use fully their medical skills and training, and the process of registering and employing eligible foreign doctors
should, it was argued, be speeded up.[21]

When circumstances dictated the SMA could be pragmatic, but generally took a morally and politically principled stand on medical refugees.
At the end of 1940 – as noted, a year when refugees' circumstances had
been particularly difficult – MTT summarised the Association's position. Among those 'cruelly and wrongly interned' by the Home Secretary
of the previous administration – that is Sir John Anderson of the Chamberlain government – were 'many doctors with world-wide reputations'

who had come to this country 'to be of some service in the fight to save democracy'. These, when added to doctors from defeated allies, constituted a large number of practitioners prepared to help Britain. What was preventing them from doing so was 'not lack of medical proficiency but lack of a British qualification'. In a passage which could hardly have been further from the anti-immigrant attitude of other professional bodies, the article continued:

> So long as the conception of individual states, each setting up its own standards, remains with us these men and women must be lost to democracy. But when democracy is recognised as the basis for the Europe of the future there will be no need for artificially preserved standards in medicine or anything else.[22]

The admission and official recognition of medical refugees was therefore a matter of justice and democracy, as well as medical and, implicitly, military efficiency. Here, then, was a truly internationalist, and socialist, approach to medicine.

Of course the SMA was not above criticism in what it did for medical refugees. In late spring 1938, just as the impact of the Anschluss was beginning to be felt, Greenwood wrote to the SPSL general secretary, Walter Adams, noting that he and D.N. Pritt had been asked to address the joint dinner of the SMA and the Haldane Society. Greenwood sought some hard data on the number and situation of refugees, and whether there were any significant left-wing donors to the Society. He was hoping, he explained, to emphasise the 'truth that if they talked a little less about intellectual liberty, and subscribed a little more to our funds, they would be doing more essential service'. The response from Adams suggested that while left-wing bodies often sought information from his office, funds from the left were 'negligible' – not even Pritt was a donor. Left-wingers were on the whole, in this context, 'liabilities instead of assets'. Greenwood himself, as Weindling points out, was on the one hand deeply committed to the cause of refugee scholars while on the other having reservations about medical refugees practising, and ambiguous attitudes towards Jews.[23]

Equally problematic is the SMA's role on the LCC. In November 1939 the council noted that the Hospital Committee had 'agreed to opportunities being afforded to refugee medical practitioners of attending practice at the Council's hospitals'. This was, however, on the understanding that they would have no responsibility for the treatment of patients, and that they would not receive accommodation or food. Furthermore, since at least 1937, the Association had been active in using its influence on the LCC to place refugee nurses, or doctors who were prepared to work as nurses. In August of that year, for example, Ewald Fabian wrote to Brook asking if employment could be found for a well-qualified German nurse wishing to leave Berlin. Brook replied that the LCC was prepared to take on 'girls' of other than British nationality – not least because of the current nursing shortage – and that the individual concerned should write to the Matron-in-Chief, mentioning his or Hastings's name. In February 1939 Fabian told Buckle that Miss Dr Jacoby, a German doctor currently in Prague, was looking for a nursing post in England, and had written to the LCC's Matron-in-Chief, mentioning Brook's name. Poignantly, Fabian ended his correspondence with the remark: 'There are letters from everywhere and we can only help a little.'[24]

The employment of refugee medical personnel became a particularly acute issue in 1940 and 1941. In June 1940 the LCC's Medical Officer of Health, W. Allen Daley, issued a 'Secret, Confidential and Immediate' order to the 'Heads of Certain Establishments under the Management of the Hospitals and Medical Services Committee'. This required that the 'services of all German, Austrian or stateless aliens are to be terminated forthwith'. In turn, this was a response to Health Ministry circular 2026, shortly thereafter partially reinforced by circular 2045. The Hospital Committee itself further addressed the refugee issue in late 1940 and 1941. In September 1940 the employment or re-employment of non-enemy aliens was, other circumstances allowing, agreed. At this point, the matter was left in the hands of the chairman, Hastings. In January 1941, the employment of enemy aliens, once again circumstances allowing, was agreed by the committee, with specific mention being made of Austrian and German refugees. Later the same year, steps were taken to recognise their qualifications, and in November around 100 nurses, mostly it would appear German or Austrian, had their probationary periods shortened and salary scales adjusted upwards accordingly. As a recognition of the part being played by refugee medical personnel, in autumn 1942 Austrian nurses in council employ were allowed to attend a public meeting of the Austrians for Britain Campaign in uniform.[25]

A number of points are worth making here. First, although the records are ambiguous, it would seem that such positive measures as the Hospital Committee was able to take in respect of refugees applied primarily to nursing staff. Second, although a certain amount appears to have been done for them, at various points restrictions were placed on their activities: they could not, for example, work at hospitals receiving injured forces personnel. Third, and as might be expected, it is clear from the records that the Hospital Committee was not working in an administrative or political vacuum. On the contrary, it was bound by the regulations and policies of the LCC; of various other interested LCC committees; of the Home Office; and of the Ministry of Health.

Furthermore, although Association activists were central to the Hospital Committee, they had also to take into account the attitudes of their fellow members. More generally, London was bearing the brunt of the blitz in the winter of 1940–41, and even the enthusiasts of the SMA were no doubt unwilling to push the rights of 'enemy' alien medical personnel too far, at least to the public at large. Political and bureaucratic realities, therefore, almost certainly constrained their council activities for refugees.

However, criticisms such as those of Adams, at least as far as the SMA was concerned, were unfair. The Association continuously lobbied and criticised the government over its, and the professional organisations', attitude to medical refugees. This was in marked contrast to bodies such as the BMA, which retained its opposition to refugee doctors until 1941; and the MPU, which maintained an anti-semitic line. SMA members worked both as part of their own organisation and in person to lobby officials and ministers. In August 1940, for example, Hastings wrote directly to Malcolm MacDonald at the Ministry of Health urging the compilation of a register of refugee doctors and their specialisms so that they might be readily used in emergencies such as invasion. Similarly, Greenwood corresponded with the Ministry regarding the anomalous position of Polish military doctors.[26]

Consequently MTT welcomed, in late 1940, the Health Ministry's withdrawal of a number of restrictions on the employment of foreign doctors. This was almost certainly due to the perceived labour shortages of the period, but the pressure of organisations such as the SMA must also be taken into account. In the summer of 1941 Hastings was part of a deputation to the Ministry on the refugee issue which resulted in 'important concessions'. The same year saw the number of refugee medical practitioners allowed to contribute to the medical services rise significantly, not least because of the already-noted moderation of the BMA line around the same time. The relaxation in official attitudes was applauded by the SMA, MTT recording its 'considerable gratification' that the Health Ministry had ordered the GMC to allow the registration of medical refugees, which would be to the benefit of British medicine. Although a few issues continued to need attention – for example, the inclusion in the scheme of Spanish doctors, with the eminent surgeon Joseph Trueta being specifically mentioned – it is clear that the Association felt that considerable progress had been made.[27]

So 1941 saw something of a watershed in attitudes to medical refugees. Thereafter the SMA was also, understandably, rather more preoccupied with its proposals for post-war reconstruction. The refugee sub-committee seems to have fallen more or less into abeyance although a Refugee Secretary, Dr D. D'Arcy Hart, was appointed in May 1941 and appears to have taken his brief seriously. The fate of medical refugees did not, therefore, entirely disappear from Association concerns and activities, and the topic will be returned to briefly in Chapter Nine. It is also clear from SMA records that medical refugees were among those joining the organisation during the 1940s, and this says something about both their own political tendencies and the principled stand which the Association took on their behalf. An EC meeting in summer 1941, for example, noted that among the applicants accepted for membership were five refugee doctors.[28]

Clearly, the more tolerant attitude displayed towards medical refugees was in large part due to the demands of the wartime medical labour market and the recognition by bodies such as the BMA that they would have to modify their previous intransigence. Nonetheless the activities of the SMA were important. The Association put pressure on government, in parliament and through lobbying ministers and civil servants; argued against its more conservative fellow-professional organisations; continually propagandised for better treatment of foreign medical personnel; initiated campaigns and meetings; and gave assistance of a practical and immediate kind to individual refugees. Moreover, its profile in labour movement and medical politics was rising in the late 1930s and early 1940s, as we shall see in the next two chapters.

Such a widening of influence almost certainly helped the Association's advocacy of the refugee case, particularly after Labour became part of the wartime coalition in 1940. The appointment of Morrison, well-known to leading SMA members because of their mutual involvement on the LCC, was seen by the organisation as a positive move in aiding medical refugees, and such personal contacts should not be underestimated in influencing official policy. This was exemplified, albeit rather ambiguously, by the case of Dr Hans Kaiser. Kaiser had been denied both registration as a doctor and employment by the LCC by the Home Office, apparently in the person of the Home Secretary himself. The Association wrote to Morrison protesting against this and, when this seemed to fail, Hastings indicated that he would approach him personally to intimate that the LCC was prepared to employ Kaiser. There was no clear resolution to this episode, but the important point is that Hastings and his colleagues clearly felt that they could approach Morrison with direct personal appeals.[29]

The SMA's attitude to medical refugees was underpinned by a genuine belief in the internationalism of medicine and socialism; a wholehearted opposition to fascism and racism on scientific, political, and humanitarian grounds; and a conviction that those from other countries would enhance the health service with their talents rather than drive British doctors out of work. Unlike other medical organisations it therefore took a positive attitude towards foreign medical personnel wishing to enter Britain, and actively sought to make the conditions of their admission easier and to ensure that medical refugees, once in Britain, were treated with dignity and with respect to their medical aptitudes and qualifications. Honigsbaum even suggests that without the skills of medical refugees Bevan might have had problems in starting the National Health Service. Although a debatable point, this nonetheless implies that the SMA, which had campaigned hard on their behalf, can be credited with an – at least indirect – influence on the shaping of the NHS. Honigsbaum also suggests that no other British medical organisation 'did nearly so much for those who were persecuted by the Nazis'.[30] Despite the problems encountered by the Association in its generally principled campaign on behalf of medical refugees, this is a judgement with which it is ultimately difficult to disagree.

Spanish medical aid, and preparations for war

The Spanish Civil War too had an impact on left-wing medical politics. The SMA, like others on the left, moved quickly to give practical aid to the Republic. Most notably this was through the creation, in late summer 1936, of Spanish Medical Aid, largely on the initiative of Charles Brook. The Association dominated Spanish Medical Aid. Its president was Christopher Addison; its chairman H.B. Morgan; its vice-chairman Hastings; and its honorary secretary Brook – all prominent SMA members. Originally conceived as a supplier of medical aid and equipment to the democratic forces in Spain, the positive response to Spanish Medical Aid allowed it, Brook later recalled, to initiate a 'far more ambitious project – the dispatching of a fully-equipped and adequately staffed Medical Unit to the battle front'. This was the First British Medical Unit, which served on the Aragon front.[31]

Practical activity abroad was complemented by agitational and propaganda work at home. Addison, 'contrary to the advice tendered by some people in high places', chaired a large meeting at the Albert Hall in support of Spanish Medical Aid. On a rather smaller scale, Dr Cedric Hill, previously in charge of a front line dressing station in Spain, organised an appeal for funds for pro-Republican German and Spanish doctors stranded in France. Edith Summerskill and Stella Churchill were among the sponsors of the 'National Women's Appeal for Food for Spain', while in 1938 the Glasgow branch devoted its energies to canvassing doctors and chemists for medical supplies for Spain. And, returning briefly to medical refugees, Spanish Medical Aid successfully brought to Britain professionals who would have been in danger had they remained in Spain. These included Joseph Trueta, who had worked during the Civil War in a Catalan hospital. The experience he gained and the skills he developed were later to be used extensively in the Allied armies, a further example of the 'beneficial' effects of war for medicine. He left Spain for Britain in 1939, published a number of articles on the impact of civilian bombing based on his experiences in Barcelona, and in 1949 became Nuffield Professor of Orthopaedic Surgery at Oxford.[32]

The Association was actively involved in providing practical help to the Spanish Republic, and perhaps because of the nature of such aid seems to have avoided the sectarian conflicts which bedevilled the rest of the labour movement.[33] It also drew two particular lessons from the war. The first concerned blood transfusion. In MTT in late 1937 Sinclair-Loutit, administrator of the First British Medical Unit, described the new technique of having available chilled blood, ready for transfusion. From such surgical advances, he went on to make more general points. Despite the war, research continued, with surgeons free from the 'tyranny of the Old Men'. The experience of a year at the front illustrated how 'medicine, given freedom, and support from the State, has surged ahead'. Even in war, it found 'time and peace to make the world richer by its research'. The significance of chilled blood was not missed by the Spanish Medical Aid Committee, which sent three refrigerators to the British Unit in autumn 1938.[34]

Another SMA member who had served at the front, Reginald Saxton, took up these points. In spring 1939 he gave detailed plans, based on his Spanish experiences, of the requirements of a blood transfusion service should Britain become involved in war. The current situation, however, gave little cause for optimism. The authorities had 'learnt little from our experiences of actual war'. A national blood transfusion service prepared for the onset of conflict while augmenting peace-time arrangements, was required. Only then would experience gained in Spain 'enable us to make of it something of inestimable value in the practice of modern surgery'. Saxton continued to emphasise these points, for example in August 1940 when deploring the authorities' slowness in adopting methods which had proved 'invaluable in Spain'. In later recollections of Saxton's plans, both Murray and Hilliard credited him with the formulation of the service which the government adopted and integrated into the NHS.[35]

Second, the Civil War illustrated key features of modern warfare, particularly attacks on civilians. Even before the impact of the Spanish conflict was felt this was something to which the Association had turned its attention, for example in a 1936 report on the dangers of gas attacks. The BMA too had expressed concern on this issue, their May 1936 meeting condemning 'unreservedly' the use of poison gas in warfare. However what Spain – and the contemporaneous conflict in China – revealed was the danger not of gas, but of high-explosive, deep-penetrating bombs. *MTT* noted the scale of civilian losses in Barcelona and Shanghai and suggested that the 'fate facing civilization ... is nowhere better demonstrated than in the conduct of the hostilities in Spain'. Saxton supplied a graphic example of this, the destruction by aerial bombing of the original British Medical Unit and hospitals on the Madrid front.[36] What was needed, therefore, was a policy of constructing deep shelters. This was cogently argued, at the height of the blitz, by Murray. From the first, *MTT* had demanded the provision of deep shelters as the only safeguard against aerial bombing, and alone insisted that these 'be so constructed that people could spend long hours in them in comfort'. Shelters should be built not only to protect against bomber attack, but also to prevent the spread of disease. Bacteria and parasites were 'foes of the human race' in which 'Hitler has a weapon more potent even than his bombs'. In larger shelters at least, doctors should be present to deal with both injuries and disease. Modern warfare needed modern preventive measures for highly vulnerable civilian populations, as Spain, China, and the British blitz amply demonstrated. But the Association was not content simply to describe the horrors of aerial bombing, and further discussion of its air-raid shelter policy leads into its critique of official war preparations.[37]

The Association had long been concerned not only with the impact of mass bombing, but with preparations for such an event. The first *MTT* suggested that current air-raid precautions were 'entirely illusory' and noted the 'sensation' caused by the report of the left-wing Cambridge Scientists' Anti-War Group. This had effectively demolished government claims about proposed safety measures. An article in April 1938, a time of high international tension, argued that the government was concentrating on gas while ignoring high explosives – again the example of Spain was cited – and had done little towards the needs of children. Regarding the latter Marrack had recently given a talk to a teachers' conference where he had criticised the Board of Education's evacuation circular. Such was SMA concern that the EC put forward, in September 1938, an emergency resolution to Labour Party conference urging the need for deep shelters and organised evacuation in the event of war. Otherwise the medical services would be unable to cope with the 'mass of casualties'. This became part of a composite resolution, seconded on the SMA's behalf by Hastings, which sought, *inter alia*, the development of suitable health and social services, especially in potential evacuation areas; and measures to protect the civilian population against heavy bombing, 'as in Barcelona and Valencia'. Hastings argued that two things were necessary for success in war: 'to do as much damage as possible to the enemy, and to prevent him doing the same to you'. Suitable defence measures might even act as a deterrent, although they should not cut into social service budgets. The resolution was carried unanimously.[38]

SMA concern was almost certainly heightened by its own investigations. In autumn 1938 Elizabeth Bunbury attempted to discover what ARP arrangements existed for London. Little came to light save, alarmingly, that London Medical Officers of Health had met separately with the Home Office and the Ministry of Health and been given two conflicting pieces of advice. Shortly afterwards, an Association internal circular noted the unevenness of preparations in the capital, one instance of which was the relatively high level of organisation of LCC hospitals compared to the lack of coordination of voluntary hospitals. Given the SMA's already hostile attitude to the latter, this presumably came as no surprise. Association misgivings about official preparations were echoed in the wider scientific community. By the late 1930s, William McGucken suggests, British scientists were frustrated and upset by developments in warfare and the lack of official response to them, sentiments certainly shared by the SMA.[39]

SMA campaigning on civilian defence reached a climax with the outbreak of war against Germany. Public meetings were organised, and leaflets such as *The Casualty Services* and *Health and Shelters* produced. Moreover the SMA had on its EC an acknowledged authority on civilian defence, Dr G.B. Shirlaw. Drawing heavily on his experiences in Spain, a 'prelude to and practice for the future war against this country', Shirlaw pointed to the confusion and inadequacy of existing services and the 'fifth column of inefficiency and maladministration'. In the event of invasion, he stressed, the enemy's 'main blows' might be more against 'the civilian population and its vital services' than the military. Shirlaw published extensive and comprehensive proposals for adequate civilian protection, the need for which he had been urging since at least 1938.[40]

The onset of the blitz confirmed the failings of official policy. In December 1940 *MTT* claimed that until recently shelter policy had involved population dispersal, a 'callous attitude of merely attempting to reduce the incidence of inevitable deaths rather than of securing that all deaths are prevented'. The public had realised this approach's inadequacies hence their utilisation of, for example, the London underground. In the same edition, Murray berated the Ministry of Health's 'half-hearted' attempts to come to terms with the problems posed by shelters, and the BMA's failure to give any professional lead. The government had also not taken seriously the provision of deep shelters. The attack on the BMA was unsurprising for, as shown below, the SMA was suspicious of its previous behaviour over war preparations. Moreover although other professional publications, such as the *BMJ*, had discussed the threat of air-raids, much of this dealt with what to do after raids had taken place, rather than preventive measures to avoid large-scale casualties in the first place.[41]

Association scepticism over official policy for air-raid protection was part of a wider uneasiness over government plans for war, not least because of BMA complicity in these since 1935. This was most obviously so regarding the BMA's 1937 questionnaire seeking its members views on how they would react to a 'national emergency'. The SMA's response pointed to the lack of definition of a 'national emergency', and the role of the Committee of Imperial Defence in initiating the survey. This 'census of the profession' was designed to bring doctors 'blindly behind' the government in any catastrophe arising from its domestic or foreign policy. The government was also seeking to persuade the public of the efficacy of its air raid precautions by demonstrating the support of a large proportion of the medical profession. A subsequent *MTT* editorial added that this was the first peacetime attempt to organise the medical profession on 'a military basis', and that it required 'little imagination to perceive to what this might lead'. For those lacking such imaginative gifts, a 1939 AGM resolution clarified the matter, suggesting that in 'the hands of the Chamberlain Government conscription will be used not against the Fascist aggressors but as the first steps to the introduction of fascism in Britain'. Hostility to this form of centralised control continued into the war itself. An EC resolution in spring 1940 urged that there should be no 'conscription' of doctors until a national plan had been worked out which took account of the needs of both the civilian population and medical practitioners, and which met the needs of both by an 'equitable distribution of medical personnel'.[42]

The SMA was deeply uneasy about both the government's attitude to the medical profession and the adequacy of its actual plans. Services for women and children were described in March 1940 as being the subject of 'almost criminal neglect'. The Labour Party was urged to ensure the provision of milk for under-fives and expectant mothers, 'urgently necessary in time of war to protect the health of future generations'. The war itself was having a profound effect on national well-being. While the press printed 'sunshine stories' that health was unimpaired, evidence showed that vitamin deficiencies were beginning to have an impact, and such problems would increase as the war went on. The post-First World War influenza epidemic had shown how a weakened population could suffer from disease. Hence the maintenance of health was 'even more fundamental ... than the reorganisation of the medical services'. This sense of a nation's health under attack was evident in a resolution sent to party conference seeking the 'preservation and improvement of the standard of living of the people, especially as regards nutrition'; and the 'complete restoration and further extension of the social, health and medical services'. Such issues were, in fact, widely discussed at the 1940 conference. Although there appear to have been no direct interventions by SMA members, the speech of NEC member Harold Laski in particular was deeply redolent of Association preoccupations.[43]

A further example of the inadequacies of the Chamberlain administration lay in the creation of the Emergency Medical Service (EMS) and the Casualty Medical Service. Both had, *MTT* suggested, many deficiencies. These arose from the government's attempt to retain and expand the role of voluntary hospitals. Indeed, all medical services were 'full of anomalies, surrounded by ancient prejudices and modern red-tape'. Such was Association concern that a deputation to the Health Minister in January 1940 presented a memorandum deprecating the 'chaos in the medical services', and in particular the failings of the EMS. This did not produce any very productive discussion, with the Minister refusing to accept 'most of the points made'. However, widespread publicity in both lay and medical press, and in a radio broadcast of 19 January, was one positive outcome.[44]

The coming of war had produced, as Ritchie Calder put it to the Association's 1941 AGM, 'convulsions of the medical system'. The SMA statement of autumn 1940, *Medicine Tomorrow*, claimed the switch from fighting overseas to defending Britain itself meant that 'a metamorphosis in medicine appears inevitable'. War had not only shown the existing system's problems, but also made it desirable to 'set out a standard by which any service introduced may be judged and by which the development of the service on acceptable lines may be influenced'. Acceptable lines, for the SMA, involved a state medical service and this was to be found, embryonically, in the institutions and organisations already thrown up. War had forced many changes, and made it apparent that the crucial developments would derive from the setting up of the EMS. The much criticised EMS, therefore, contained within it huge potential. Such were the changes wrought by war that 'medical practice as it has been known in the last thirty years may largely disappear'. The time was ripe for reform, something agreed on by more and more doctors and laypersons. This was very much in line with the contemporary comment that more had been achieved in medical reorganisation in the early part of the war than in the previous 20 years, and with the sense among the left in general that with the outbreak of the European conflict socialism was now the only alternative to fascism.[45] The

Association's belief in the potential of the wartime situation is developed further in the next chapter.

Medical reorganisation had, however, to be carefully implemented. If the EMS embryonically contained a new form of organisation, and new plans were now being debated, nonetheless any proposed scheme must involve 'strong safeguards against the introduction of fascism into the medical profession, and ... avoid the evil effects of bureaucracy'. Written in late 1939, this was a reaction to the nation being led into war by the Chamberlain government, for the SMA a deeply discredited administration, and reinforces the earlier point about the perceived dangers of medical 'conscription'.[46] As shall be seen in Chapter Eight, Association members were also to go to considerable pains in the 1940s to make clear what they meant by 'state medicine', and how their proposals differed from the sort of corporatist model of medical organisation offered elsewhere.

Internal dissent

There remained, however, the fundamental question of what attitude the SMA should adopt to the coming of war. One of its founders, Alfred Salter, was a convinced pacifist and among the small group who opposed the war in the Commons. By contrast, others had participated in the Spanish Civil War, while others still had been active in organisations such as the Medical Peace Campaign, which had argued for collective resistance to fascist aggression. There was, therefore, a range of views towards the conduct of international affairs. As Murray later recalled, for those on the left the period after September 1939 was extremely confused, particularly with regard to the position taken by the Soviet Union, since at this stage the war was confined to western Europe and the Nazi-Soviet Pact still held. Like other left-wing organisations – including to some extent even the Labour Party – the SMA was internally divided.[47]

On the other hand, almost all Labour Party members in the Association welcomed the break up of the Chamberlain administration in 1940 and its replacement by Churchill's Coalition. The SMA, as we have seen, had been deeply suspicious of the National Government because of its attitude to medical refugees and to medical 'conscription'; to appeasement; and to preparations for war. The Coalition, however, contained Labour ministers and the Association could therefore reasonably hope that, as an affiliated organisation, it could help shape Labour's input to any future government proposals for post-war medical reconstruction. But, as we saw in a previous chapter, the Association had also

– in marked contrast to the Labour Party itself – from the mid-1930s allowed Communists to join the organisation; and by 1940 one of these, Brian Kirman, was honorary secretary. The presence of a Communist faction explains the main internal division within the SMA over the war. This was evident in, for example, Murray's public criticism in 1940 of those who had been prepared to help Republican Spain, but were now refusing support to Finland on political grounds in the wake of the Soviet Union's attack on that country. Clearly, this was aimed at Communist Party members and supporters.[48]

Disagreement surfaced in a particularly dramatic way at the May 1940 AGM. A motion was put that the war was neither in the British people's interest nor being fought for democracy or the rights of small nations. The Association should oppose it, and demand instead the extension and reorganisation of medical services. Uproar ensued. Murray, seeking to pre-empt the original proposal, put forward an emergency motion claiming that the 'preservation of the health of the nation must be regarded as second only to the necessity of defeating Fascism'. This was not accepted at this point, on the grounds that the original motion had first to be dealt with. Similar attempts to put forward a pro-war position, stressing the need to preserve democracy and defeat fascism, were equally unsuccessful, and the anti-war motion was passed by 19 votes to 12. The meeting did agree unanimously, however, to ballot the whole membership before acting further on the anti-war resolution.[49]

Association members were duly consulted, and given the views of Murray; Hastings on behalf of the EC; and the surgeon Ruscoe Clarke, proposer of the anti-war resolution. For Clarke, the organisation needed a 'clear political orientation'. Socialism would not be advanced by supporting the Allies, and while a Nazi victory would be appalling, the alternative was a victory for Anglo-French capitalism, a 'new Versailles', the subjugation of central Europe, the continued enslavement of India, and, possibly, a war against the Soviet Union. The choice was clear: either support for a 'government and a class that will sell us out to Hitler at the slightest sign of difficulty', or a struggle against that government and class 'for a workers' government that is capable of making a just peace. There is no middle road'.

Murray took a very different view. The original resolution had been formulated when Chamberlain was still prime minister, and with the belief that an end to the fighting would see the German people overthrow Hitler. This was now highly unlikely, given the recent attack on Holland and Belgium. Opposing the war would lead to the imposition of fascism in Britain, and the consequent destruction of socialist organisations such as the SMA. Continued support for the resolution would also cut the Association off from the mainstream labour movement.

The organisation's duty was to 'defeat Fascism but to do so without losing sight of the necessity to preserve democracy and to safeguard the health of the nation'. Hastings adopted a similar position. The SMA's disaffiliation from the Labour Party, one outcome of letting the resolution stand, would diminish its influence, which Hastings anticipated would increase in the likely event of a Labour election victory. What neither Hastings nor Murray specifically mentioned, although it was clearly a crucial part of the political context, was the formation of the wartime Coalition. Events seemed, in other words, to be moving in the SMA's direction, provided it retained its link with the Labour Party. Having considered the various arguments, 54 members voted against the anti-war resolution, 24 for. Although a turnout of less than half the membership, by this stage of the war political activity in general had reached a low point, partly because of population movements, partly because of electoral truces and postponements.[50]

In any event, the issue was now resolved in the leadership's favour, although some members did resign over the issue of communist activities. One, Frank Garratt of Pembroke, wrote that he had 'no wish to be associated in any way with a Society that has not the "guts" to expel such contemptible and stupid individuals as Ruscoe Clarke'. However with the Communist Party's change in policy following the invasion of the Soviet Union in 1941, near-consensus emerged over the necessary prosecution of the war. The Association in August 1941 sent its 'warmest fraternal greetings' to Soviet medical and health workers in their fight for 'the maintenance of Socialism against the forces of Fascism'. Some members even volunteered to work in the Soviet health services. This was turned down, although it was agreed that refugee doctors might be taken to the USSR when this became logistically possible. Unanimity in the organisation was followed by a sixfold rise in membership between 1941 and 1945, an indicator of optimism about the war's outcome and consequences and a trend reflected in the labour movement as a whole.[51]

The events of 1940–41 simplified matters for the Association. The Chamberlain government's demise, and its replacement by the Churchill coalition, gave the SMA the possibility of real influence in government circles. The Soviet Union's entry into the war unified left-wing support for the conflict. This was important for the SMA given the increasing level of Communist Party membership; because Soviet health services provided a model of health care provision attractive to both Communist and non-Communist Association members; and because it removed a potentially embarrassing problem with the pro-war Labour Party leadership. The war was to be prosecuted by all 'progressive' forces, with one of its outcomes the institution of state medical services, part of a move towards a socialist society. However a note of caution does need to be sounded. All these were certainly positive factors for the Association in the short term. What needs to be constantly borne in mind, however, is that the SMA's internal problems and politically heterogenous membership did little to endear it to the Labour Party and trades union leaderships, which had no doubt about the need to prosecute the war and every doubt about the virtues of the Communist Party. This is the context in which the organisation's apparent advances, described in the next two chapters, must be viewed, and the repercussions of admitting communists to the Association will be further picked up in the concluding chapter.

By 1941 the Association could feel at least partially satisfied over its international concerns. Medical refugees were beginning to be dealt with in a more humane and satisfactory way, and in part this must be attributed to SMA agitation. The refugee issue had also allowed the opportunity to denounce Nazi racial ideology and the backward attitude of many British doctors and their organisations; and to address the question of medical reorganisation through analysis of the medical labour market. The Spanish Civil War had hardly reached a satisfactory conclusion, but valuable lessons could be learned. This conflict brought important advances in medical technique as well as alerting the world to the nature of modern warfare, especially for civilians. Hence the SMA's continuing emphasis on the issue, and the acknowledged expertise in the field of some of its members.

Such concerns were evident in the Association's scepticism about the National Government's plans for war. The proposals for medical organisation in the event of a national emergency were perceived as having hidden agenda, at worst leading to the introduction of bureaucratic or even fascist methods. The collusion of the BMA in such plans only served to heighten left-wing medical suspicion. As the European crisis deepened and turned to war, the question of the future of the medical services took on greater urgency. For the SMA, wartime institutions such as the EMS were important for three reasons: first, they showed clearly the inadequacies of existing health care provision; second, they did, however, point the way towards a state medical service, part of wider social reconstruction; and, third, they showed the crucial role to be played by the state, rather than voluntary or piecemeal activity, in effecting these changes. The outbreak of the war itself had posed a serious political problem for the Association, but at least in the short term this appeared to have been resolved. As the conflict progressed, medical reconstruction became an ever more important item on the political agenda, and we now go on to analyse the Association's role in these debates and discussions.

Notes

1. 'Medicine and the Crisis: A Lesson from International Medical Research', *MTT*, no. 7, April 1938, pp. 3–4; David Stark Murray, 'International Health', *The Left News*, no. 85, July 1943, cutting in DSM (2) 4.
2. *MTT*, no. 1, October 1937, p. 13; no. 6, March 1938, p. 12; *MTT*, September Quarter 1941, pp. 1, 4.
3. *MTT*, no. 8, May 1938, p. 1; *Socialist Doctor*, vol. 2, no. 4, November 1934, p. 6. On the scientific left, see William McGucken, *Scientists, Society, and the State*, Columbus, Ohio, Ohio State University Press, 1984, and Gary Werskey, *The Visible College*, Free Association Books, 1988.
4. Bernard Wasserstein, 'The British Government and the German Immigration 1933–1945', in Hirschfeld, Gerhard (ed.), *Exile in Great Britain*, Leamington Spa, Berg, 1984, p. 65; Paul Weindling, 'The Contribution of Central European Jews to Medical Science and Practice in Britain, the 1930s-1950s', in Mosse, W.E. (ed.), *Second Chance: Two Centuries of German-speaking Jews in the United Kingdom*, Tübingen, J.C.B. Mohr, 1991, p. 243. A paper on the SMA and medical refugees was given at the Wellcome Unit for the History of Medicine, University of Oxford, in March 1996, and I am grateful for the useful comments it elicited. In particular, I wish to acknowledge the help of Paul Weindling.
5. Honigsbaum, *Division in British Medicine*, p. 275ff.
6. Society for the Protection of Science and Learning Papers, 20/7 folio 314; Weindling, 'The Contribution of Central European Jews', pp. 246, 245, 250.
7. *Socialist Doctor*, vol. 2, no. 1, August 1933, p. 7; DSM 1/1 Minutes of the AGM, 21 May 1933; Murray, *Why a National Health Service?*, p. 41; A.J. Sherman, *Island Refuge: Britain and Refugees from the Third Reich*, Frank Cass, 2nd edn, 1994, pp. 27, 179–80.
8. *Socialist Doctor*, vol. 2, no. 1, August 1933, p. 7; DSM 1/1, Minutes of the AGM, 21 May 1933; DSM (2) 5, 'Refugees', letter from Hastings 1 November 1933; Sherman, *Island Refuge*, p. 48.
9. DSM (3)/14/32.
10. DSM (2) 5, 'Labour Party', Buckle to Middleton, 3 December 1938.
11. DSM (2) 5, 'MPU', *passim*.
12. DSM 1/1, Report of the EC, 1938–39; SMA, *Bulletin*, no. 52, February 1943, p. 1; DSM 1/1 Report of the EC, May 1939–April 1940; DSM(3)/14/33.
13. SPSL Papers, 125/5 folios 470, 469; Weindling, 'The Contribution of Central European Jews', p. 251.
14. SMA, *Bulletin*, no. 24, September 1940, p. 2, no. 32, May 1941, p. 2 and no. 28, January 1941, p. 3. The other organisations attending were: the International Jewish Refugee Organisation; the Germany Emergency Committee; the Medical Department, Bloomsbury House; the Youth Relief and Refugee Council; and the National Joint Committee for Spanish Relief. By nationality, the refugee doctors were broken down as follows: 1600 Austrians and Germans; 270 Czechs; 340 Poles; and 40 Italians.
15. *MTT*, vol. 2, no. 8 (new series), December Quarter 1940, p. 12.
16. Louise Burleston, 'The State, Internment and Public Criticism in the Second World War', in Cesarani, David and Kushner, Tony (eds), *The*

Internment of Aliens in Twentieth-Century Britain, Frank Cass, 1993, pp. 102–3; Donoughue and Jones, *Herbert Morrison*, pp. 302–3; Honigsbaum, *Division in British Medicine*, p. 269; MTT, vol. 3. no. 1, March Quarter 1941, pp. 16–17; DSM 1/6, EC Minutes, 14 August 1941.

17. DSM 1/1 Minutes of the EC, 22 March 1934, Minutes of the AGM, 13 May 1934, Report of the EC, 1934–35; *Lancet*, 1934, I, p. 709.

18. MTT, no. 7, April 1938, pp. 3, 5, 13; quoted in Honigsbaum, *Division in British Medicine*, p. 276.

19. MTT, no. 10, July 1938, p. 12; and no. 8, May 1938, p. 9; Irwin Brown (David Stark Murray), 'Yesterday, A Surgeon – Today, A Jew', MTT, no. 12, October 1938, pp. 5–6; cutting from *The Times*, 15 July 1938, in MH 58/332, 'Alien Doctors, Nurses, etc.'.

20. Kenneth Collins, *Go and Learn: the International Story of Jews and Medicine in Scotland*, Aberdeen, Aberdeen University Press, 1988, pp. 143–4; Sherman, *Island Refuge*, pp. 123–4, 134; Louise London, 'Jewish Refugees and British Government Policy, 1930–1940', in Cesarani, David (ed.), *The Making of Modern Anglo-Jewry*, Oxford, Blackwell, 1990, p. 177ff.

21. MTT, vol. 3, no. 1, March Quarter 1941, pp. 16–17; SMA, *Bulletin*, no. 34, July 1941, p. 1.

22. MTT, vol. 2, no. 8 (new series), December Quarter 1940, p. 12.

23. SPSL Papers, 20/7ff. 426–30; Weindling, 'The Contribution of Central European Jews', p. 246; Marion Berghahn, 'German Jews in England', in Hirschfeld, Gerhard (ed.), *Exile in Great Britain*, p. 293.

24. Minutes of the London County Council, 21 November 1939; DSM (2) 5, 'International', Fabian to Brook, 17 August 1937, Brook to Fabian, 30 September 1937, and Fabian to Buckle, 3 February 1939.

25. MH 58/333, 'Alien Doctors', letter from W. Allen Daley, 1 June 1940; and circulars 2026 and 2045. Circular 2193 partly eased the restrictions on the employment of refugee medical personnel; LCC/MIN/2217, 10 September 1940; LCC/MIN/2218, 21 January 1941, 17 June 1941, and 4 November, 1941; LCC/MIN/2219, 8 September 1942.

26. MH 58/333, 'Alien Doctors', Hastings to MacDonald, 5 August 1940; and Greenwood to Professor F.R. Fraser, Ministry of Health, September 1940.

27. MTT, vol. 2, no. 8 (new series), December Quarter 1940, p. 6; Weindling, 'The Contribution of Central European Jews', p. 251; SMA, *Bulletin*, no. 35, August 1941, p. 2; Collins, *Go and Learn*, p. 152; MTT, vol. 3, no. 1 (new series), March Quarter 1941, pp. 16–17.

28. DSM 1/6, EC Minutes, 8 May 1941, and EC Minutes, 10 July 1941.

29. DSM 1/6, EC Minutes, 8 May and 10 July 1941. The final mention of Dr Kaiser comes in the Minutes of 9 October 1941, when the Refugee Secretary agrees to check his present circumstances. It is not entirely clear what this means.

30. Honigsbaum, *Division in British Medicine*, pp. 313, 260.

31. Brook, *Making Medical History*, p. 11; Murray, *Why a National Health Service?*, pp. 32–3; Spanish Medical Aid Committee, *British Medical Aid in Spain*, Spanish Medical Aid Committee, 1937. On the British left and the Spanish Civil War, see Jim Fyrth, *The Signal Was Spain*, Lawrence and Wishart, 1986; and Tom Buchanan, *The Spanish Civil War and the British Labour Movement*, Cambridge, Cambridge University Press, 1991.

32. Kenneth and Jane Morgan, *Portrait of a Progressive*, Oxford, Oxford University Press, 1980, p. 229; DSM (3)/14/33; Labour Spain Committee Archive, LSPC1/6; SMA, *Bulletin*, no. 4, December 1938, p. 1; Murray, *Why a National Health Service?*, p. 32; Josep Trueta-Raspall, *Joseph Trueta: A List of his Appointments, Distinctions and Publications*, Oxford, n.p. , 1967.

33. Buchanan, *The Spanish Civil War, passim*.

34. Kenneth Sinclair-Loutit, 'Spanish Medicine Triumphs over War', *MTT*, no. 2, November 1937, pp. 7–8; *MTT*, no. 12, October 1938, p. 9.

35. R.S. Saxton, 'Wanted – a National Blood Transfusion Service', *MTT*, vol. 2, no. 1 (new series), March Quarter 1939, pp. 19–22; *BMJ*, 1940, I, p. 335; Murray, *Why a National Health Service?*, p. 32; SMA, *The SMA and the Foundation of the National Health Service*, SMA, n.d. but 1980, p. 3.

36. SMA, *Gas Attacks – Is There any Protection?*, SMA, 1936; McGucken, *Scientists, Society, and the State*, p. 103; *MTT*, no. 5, February 1938, p. 12; and no. 7, April 1938, p. 4; Reginald Saxton, 'Bombs Over Spain', *MTT*, no. 5, February 1938, p. 9.

37. The Editor, 'Britain Underground – New Conception of Shelter Policy Needed', *MTT*, vol. 2. no. 8 (new series), December Quarter 1940, pp. 2–6; the broader context can be found in Joseph S. Meisel, 'Air Raid Shelter Policy and its Critics in Britain before the Second World War', *Twentieth Century British History*, vol. 5, no. 3, 1994, which also notes the significance of Spain for this issue.

38. *MTT*, no. 1, October 1937, pp. 13, 24; Werskey, *The Visible College*, pp. 225–33; *MTT*, no. 7, April 1938, pp. 6–7; DSM 1/1 Report of the EC, 1938–39; Labour Party, *Report of the Thirty-Eighth Annual Conference*, Labour Party, 1939, pp. 307–9.

39. DSM (3)/14/30; DSM 4/1, 'Medical Aspects of ARP', p. 5; McGucken, *Scientists, Society, and the State*, p. 127.

40. SMA, *Bulletin*, no. 24, September 1940, pp. 3–4; no. 28, January 1941, p. 1; G.B. Shirlaw, *Casualty: Training, Organisation and Administration of Civil Defence Casualty Services*, Secker and Warburg, 1940, pp. xv–xvi; G.B. Shirlaw and Clifford Troke, *Medicine versus Invasion*, Secker and Warburg, 1941, pp. xix–xx; L. Crome, R.E.W. Fisher and G.B. Shirlaw, 'Casualty Organisation in Air-Raids', *Lancet*, 1939, I, pp. 655–8. Crome also fought in Spain.

41. *MTT*, vol. 2, no. 8 (new series), December Quarter 1940, p. 1 and *MTT*, vol. 2, no. 8, The Editor, 'Britain Underground – New Conception of Shelter Policy Needed', pp. 2–3; P.W.J. Bartrip, *Mirror of Medicine: a History of the BMJ*, London and Oxford, BMJ/Oxford University Press, 1990, pp. 245–6.

42. Bartrip, *Mirror of Medicine*, p. 246; DSM (3)/14/11; *MTT*, no. 3, December 1937, p. 12; DSM 1/1, Minutes of the AGM, 14 May 1939; SMA, *Bulletin*, no. 19, April 1940, p. 1.

43. SMA, *Bulletin*, no. 18, March 1940, p. 1; SMA, *Bulletin*, no. 32, May 1941, p. 1; and no. 18, March 1940, p. 1; Labour Party, *Report of the Thirty-Ninth Annual Conference*, Labour Party, 1940, p. 144ff. There is circumstantial evidence that Laski was close to certain SMA members – the copy of Brook's *Making Medical History* in the British Library of Political and Economic Science is dedicated to Laski by the author.

44. *MTT*, vol. 2, no. 3 (new series), September Quarter 1939, pp. 1–2; vol. 2,

no. 6 (new series), June Quarter 1940, p. 9; DSM 1/1, Report of the EC, May 1939–April 1940; *MTT*, vol. 2, no. 5 (new series), March Quarter 1940, p. 23; SMA, *Bulletin*, no. 17, February 1940. This edition in the Hull archives also contains a copy of the memorandum, which was to become the SMA publication, *The Medical Services in War-Time*.

45. SMA, *Bulletin*, no. 35, August 1941, p. 3; *MTT*, vol. 2, no. 7 (new series), September Quarter 1940, p. 2; and vol. 3, no. 4 (new series), December Quarter 1941, p. 1; Webster, *Health Services since the War*, vol. 1, p. 22; Brooke, *Labour's War*, p. 270ff.
46. *MTT*, vol. 2, no. 4 (new series), December Quarter 1939, p. 3.
47. Brockway, *Bermondsey Story*, p. 219ff; Murray, *Why a National Health Service?*, p. 42; on the situation in the Labour Party, see Henry Pelling, 'The Impact of the War on the Labour Party', in Smith, H.L. (ed.), *War and Social Change*, Manchester, Manchester University Press, 1986.
48. *MTT*, vol. 2, no. 5 (new series) March Quarter 1940, p. 1.
49. DSM 1/1 Minutes of the AGM, 26 May 1940, pp. 1–2.
50. SMA, *Bulletin*, no. 22, July 1940, pp. 1–4; and no. 23, August 1940, p. 1; Pelling, 'The Impact of the War', p. 133.
51. DSM (2) 6, letter from Frank Garratt, 6 July 1940; SMA, *Bulletin*, no. 35, August 1941, p. 1; DSM 1/6, EC Minutes, 14 August 1941, p. 1; SMA membership figures can be found in Labour Party annual reports; Pelling, 'The Impact of War', p. 134; Brooke, *Labour's War*, Ch. 4; Webster, *The Health Services since the War*, p. 24.

CHAPTER SEVEN

'Health of the Future'

The wartime era saw Association members involved in a wide range of activities, in addition to their own demanding work. These activities included the publication of a significant volume of literature, an already existing characteristic of the organisation and in itself a reflection of the literate, educated nature of its membership. Among these texts were contributions by Murray and by Aleck Bourne to the famous 'Penguin Specials'. This series, which during this period focused especially on proposals for post-war reconstruction, was later seen as an important contributory factor in Labour's 1945 election victory. The books by Murray and Bourne were published in 1942, when considerable debate over plans for medical reform was taking place. Murray's work laid particular emphasis on, in the words of two chapter titles, 'The Chaos Which is the Medical Service Today' and 'A Possible Form of Medical Service'. Bourne, on the other hand, concentrated rather more on the nature and causes of ill-health. Both, however, captured in their titles – *The Future of Medicine* and *Health of the Future* – the medical left's optimism about the potential being opened up for reform of the health services.[1]

Nor was this the only form of political engagement in which SMA members were involved. Immediately prior to the meeting between an Association delegation and the Minister of Health in early 1943, discussed further below, Bourne participated in a radio debate with Charles Hill, the 'Radio Doctor' and leading BMA figure, and an unidentified GP. The question under discussion was: 'Should All Doctors be State-Employed?'. Bourne stressed the benefits to medical practitioners of a salaried service, and medicine's vocational nature. He dismissed fears about bureaucratisation, and highlighted the achievements of the LCC, including the improvement of London's hospital service 'out of all recognition'. Around the same time Hastings, in the first of a series of lectures organised by the Association and aimed primarily at medical students, claimed that previously the SMA had been 'largely a propaganda organisation'. Now, however, it was attempting to 'give students the facts of social medicine and public health'. Having reviewed the history of British health legislation, he concluded that there could be no 'reasonable stopping place between the first interference by the State in health matters and a complete State medical service'.[2] As shall become apparent 1943 was a particularly important and active year for the SMA.

The SMA also came to an accommodation with the MPU, albeit an uneasy and shifting accommodation. Despite their previous disagreements, the two bodies met and exchanged documents at various points throughout the war, and especially in the period 1940 to 1941. Although differences emerged – the MPU remained, for instance, consistently hostile to any suggestion of local authority control – a joint statement was produced early in 1941 stressing the need for a 'whole time salaried medical service, free to the public, without direct contribution or income limit, and including all doctors willing to join'. Such a service was urgently needed at 'this time of national emergency'. Both organisations agreed that this should form the basis of a joint delegation to the Minister of Health, although it is not clear whether such a meeting ever actually took place. What is clear, however, is that the Ministry nonetheless knew of the SMA's views. Reviewing the arguments for a salaried service, the civil servant John Pater noted that it was supported, on the grounds of promoting efficiency and medical cooperation, by 'certain branches of the profession e.g. the Socialist Medical Association, and (it is understood) by a number of the younger members of it'.[3] The idea that younger doctors were more inclined to a socialised medical service was shared by the Association, and an important component of its critique of the BMA leadership's policy stance.

The Association was, in short, prepared to explore and exploit all possible avenues in its attempts to have its plans heard by as broad an audience as possible. This chapter examines this strategy and these proposals in the light of its position in the early phase of the war; its participation on the BMA's Medical Planning Commission; its response to William Beveridge's scheme for post-war reform of the welfare services, a landmark in British social policy and the source of great inspiration to the social democratic left; and two meetings with Ministers in 1943. The following chapter continues this analysis, focusing on the Association's activities in the labour movement, the government's 1944 White Paper on the future of the health services, and the SMA's position as the war in Europe came to an end.

The upheavals of war

We have seen that Association members were horrified by the course of international affairs in the 1930s while retaining a belief that war could, paradoxically, bring significant medical progress, both technically and organisationally. This was one theme of a further policy statement issued shortly after the start of the conflict, *Whither Medicine?*, which reviewed existing proposals for health service reform, including those of MacWilliam and of the BMA; described a number of attempts at some form of medical reorganisation, such as the so-called 'Highlands and Islands Scheme'; discussed certain foreign health care systems, with that of the USSR gaining a particularly favourable notice; restated the SMA's fundamental principles; and argued the significance of the outbreak of war. The consequences of the EMS, for example, were potentially so great 'that medical practice as it has been known in the last thirty years may disappear'.[4]

Similarly, during a Commons debate on 'The Health of the Nation' in October 1940 – just after the beginning of the Blitz and some five months into the life of the Coalition government – Edith Summerskill told her parliamentary colleagues that within the last few weeks a 'tremendous change has taken place in the medical service'. Doctors with panel practices in London's East End had seen their security disappear, while Harley St physicians had had to call on the help of the state-supported EMS. Even doctors not currently suffering financially remembered the 'long lean years of peace', when in order to make ends meet they had been obliged to 'prostitute science and magnify symptoms of a patient in order that the illness may last a little longer'. This was a clear allusion to the alleged economic hardship of GPs in the 1930s; to the SMA charge that existing economic arrangements resulted in compromises in treatment and diagnosis; and implicitly to the Association argument that a salaried service would benefit doctors as well as patients. What was needed, Summerskill claimed (unsurprisingly), was a state medical service. In the preceding seven weeks, she concluded rather optimistically, 'not only have doctors' houses been bombed, but with this material destruction the prejudices of generations have been destroyed'.[5]

Moving from the general to the particular, Murray noted in 1941 that his own field, clinical pathology, had made great strides as a consequence of World War I, and there were indications that at least in this case history might repeat itself. He stressed the need to end the current preoccupation with 'rare or intricate cases', and for pathology to move out of the laboratory and into the broader medical and social spheres. Each pathologist should be seen as part of a team serving the whole community, rather than as an individual concentrating on one particular set of problems. The clinical pathologist could thereby become 'one of the most valuable liaison officers between the different parts of the medical services'. Murray went on to outline the 'four cardinal principles' of a fully socialised service – 'completeness, universality, unification and regionalism'. The last of these, he was at pains to point out, was not the same as the 'regionalisation' of the EMS or of the Nuffield Trust since neither involved the 'true democratic control' of a

system constructed to both doctors' and patients' benefit. The potential
of regionalisation is discussed further below. As to the third principle, if
the medical profession was to be shaped into 'one service with inter-
changeable personnel' characterised by the 'rapid dissemination of new
methods and ideas' and with a 'basic standard below which no part
may be allowed to fall', unification was essential.[6]

The Medical Planning Commission

Total war therefore opened up avenues for change in practice, attitudes,
and ideas. An important opportunity for the SMA to exploit this potential came with the formation of the BMA's Medical Planning Commission.
The Medical Planning Commission (MPC) was, Webster explains, from
the moment of its conception in late summer 1940 an attempt by the
BMA to 'update its image and seize the initiative', and hence an acknowledgement that *A General Medical Service for the Nation* was
increasingly out of date. The BMA had, in other words, identified the
need to be seen to be participating in contemporary debates over post-
war social reconstruction. Peter Bartrip further points out that although
the MPC was a BMA creation, and dominated by that organisation, it
did involve representatives from other bodies, for example the Royal
Colleges and the Society of Medical Officers of Health. To this we
might add the SMA. It is important to note, however, that the Commission was not welcomed by all members of the BMA itself. On the
contrary, there was internal dissent and criticism, prefiguring the fate of
the MPC's Interim Report and the medical profession's retrenchment in
the face of the Beveridge Report.[7]

The MPC first met on 7 May 1941 with a brief to 'study wartime
developments and their effects on the country's medical services both
present and future'. It had in the first instance 66 members, including
Hastings, MacWilliam, Murray and, from shortly after its first meeting,
Brook. More ambiguously, Leslie Haden-Guest MP was also on the
MPC, representing the BMA's Parliamentary Committee. As Honigsbaum
points out, Haden-Guest managed to be associated with the SMA while
remaining acceptable to the BMA. Nonetheless as Honigsbaum also
remarks, the Association was the only medico-political group given a
place on the Commission in contrast to, most noticeably, the MPU.
Another MPC member – in this case of its General Practice committee –
close to the Association was John Ryle, Regius Professor of Physic at
Cambridge University. Ryle, an individual to whom Ministry of Health
officials paid particular attention, was a prominent advocate of a socialised service wherein, for example, physicians would be salaried

employees. Like the SMA, Ryle believed that this would bring positive benefits to medical practitioners, including the opportunity to further their medical education. More generally, Ryle was Britain's most famous exponent of 'social medicine', a number of whose tenets were close to Association preoccupations.[8]

The Commission then sub-divided into six committees of between 20 and 40 members each, one with a coordinating function, the rest concerned with matters of medical organisation. These, and their Association representatives, were: General Practice (Haden-Guest, Hastings, subsequently Brook); Special Practice (Murray); Public Health (MacWilliam and Murray); Hospitals (Hastings and MacWilliam); and Teaching Hospitals (Hastings). Prior to the first meeting some 17 documents, the 'More Important Reports and Opinions on the Development of Medical Services', were brought together, and of these five were from the SMA, including *Whither Medicine* and *Medicine Tomorrow*. The proportion of the material supplied by the Association is indicative of both its relentless propagandising during the previous decade and its attempts to come up with detailed plans for a socialised service.[9]

The Association viewed the setting up of the MPC with guarded optimism. Murray, in an *MTT* leading article in March 1941, welcomed its formation while having reservations about the representativeness of the BMA itself. Nonetheless, he continued, public opinion was moving in favour of a socialised service, not least because the EMS had demonstrated the existing system's inadequacies. Murray argued that there was a need for more doctors. The profession was *not* overcrowded – contrary to the 'overstocked medical market' argument used to oppose the entry of medical refugees. Murray concluded that the MPC's work would show that the profession could not stay out of politics, for 'every problem has its medical aspect'. The *Bulletin* agreed that the Commission's findings would be greatly influenced by current public opinion as well as by the extent of social and economic progress in the near future. But it also warned against the 'tremendous opposition' to socialisation in the profession, especially among consultants. Presciently, given their later behaviour, it was claimed that many of the more intelligent of these were fearful of the ongoing development, and increasing efficiency, of municipal hospitals, which in turn would further undermine the voluntary hospitals' position. This explained the proposals of some consultants for cooperation between the two sectors, for example through regionalisation, an effort to 'get in on the State service before it gets too far'.[10]

The SMA was thus sceptical about the motivation behind the MPC and its likely outcomes, but nonetheless prepared to use it as a means both to persuade medical colleagues and reach a wider audience. The

Association's analysis at this point – early in the war and at the time of the MPC – is usefully examined through the revised edition of *Medicine Tomorrow* and Elizabeth Bunbury's *Health and the Medical Services*, both published while the Commission was deliberating; and Hastings's Fabian pamphlet of late 1941, *The Hospital Services*. Capturing the mood of the times for the medical left, *Medicine Tomorrow* suggested that socialised health care was now 'no utopian scheme'. On the contrary, detailed proposals and financial estimates were presently available and there had already been adequate experimentation, in Britain and elsewhere, to ensure the success of an appropriate plan. The Association clearly felt that it had made much of the running in thinking through the practical details.[11] Here, as in other contemporary SMA statements, the transformative effect of the war is evident.

Bunbury noted the pre-war financial difficulties of many voluntary hospitals. Appeals to local authorities had been largely unsuccessful since, given that the charitable sector was unwilling to accept local government control, this would have gone against one of democracy's fundamental principles – 'no taxation without representation'. War and the EMS had, however, significantly changed the situation. The medical profession itself now realised that 'radical alteration' was needed to the health services, and socialists had the 'duty and the right ... to ensure that any changes made are progressive ones'. As for the SMA's plan, one key constituent of this could be summarised as follows:

> There would be a central hospital for each area: surrounding the hospital, at places convenient to the population, there would be a ring of clinics or health centres: and working at the health centres would be general practitioners (or family doctors) and nurses, who would see patients at the clinics or visit them in their homes.

All medical personnel, including doctors, would be full-time, salaried employees.[12] Bunbury's proposed scheme was therefore fully unified and fully integrated.

Hastings, looking specifically at current hospital services, noted the 'slavish consideration' shown to voluntary hospital interests under the EMS, and that organisation's lack of unified control. Remedying this fully might be difficult in the short term, but after the war the positive aspects of the EMS should nonetheless be built upon. In the post-war era, access to hospitals must be 'free to all, so that no financial consideration may prevent any person from seeking early treatment for disease or from continuing it until cure is complete'. As to administration, and above all else, hospitals 'must be under the control of the elected representatives of the people through the Ministry of Health and the Local Authorities'.[13] Hastings's experience of, and commitment to, the LCC model is once again evident here.

The official Association line therefore remained that democratic local authorities should have a central role in the running of a socialised service. In turn, this was related to an 'activist' view of citizenship – as noted in Chapter Four an important strand in labour movement thinking at this time – whereby members of the community not only benefited from, but also played a controlling role in, a socialist society. It is therefore worth digressing to look in more detail at the SMA's version of the 'right to health'. One member who devoted particular attention to this issue was Bourne. Addressing Cambridge students in 1941, he argued for 'good health as a right of the citizen, comparable to the right of being policed and defended'. While the State had recognised the right to universal education, it had not done so in respect of health, 'inasmuch as many known causes of ill health are still tolerated'. Citing a recent experiment in the Rhondda Valley where supplying vitamin supplements had halved the maternal mortality rate, Bourne claimed that much illness was due to social conditions, and that proper feeding and housing would do more for the nation's health than curative doctoring. The 'right to health' included, although Bourne did not make the distinction all that clearly, the right to health care and the right to an optimum state of physical well-being – health. It was, in turn, part of the wider right to social justice.[14] However it also involved, in a truly socialised service, participation, operating on at least two levels. First, as Bourne explained, 'we can go beyond the idea of the "right" of the individual and claim that the community should regard it as the *duty* of every citizen to keep himself well ...'. Preventive medicine was not, therefore, only an issue for the public authorities. Each citizen also had responsibilities towards his or her own body, for both their own and the wider social good. This hints at a rather more authoritarian approach to health than is usually associated with the SMA, and the implications of this do not appear to have been fully thought through during the 1940s. Second, as Association evidence to the MPC put it, if the state had a duty to preserve health, it was 'equally the responsibility of the citizens who constitute the State to play their part in the health services'.[15] The immediately obvious way this would operate was through democratically accountable local bodies.

Such were the Association's views around the time of the MPC. Murray's scepticism notwithstanding, as the Commission began its deliberations SMA representatives struck a positive note. At the preliminary meeting Hastings urged that members 'put aside all preconceived ideas'. The MPC should, in order to be sure of the basis on which it would make its recommendations, take account of the 'trend of the profession'; and seek more information on current working conditions in, for example, the EMS and general practice.[16] Here, once again, we can discern the sense that war had brought new opportunities for a complete revision of health care provision, as well as a hint of scepticism about the ability of the BMA to speak for the medical profession as a whole.

When the various sub-committees began their work, Association members forcefully advanced their views. Hastings told the General Practice Committee in August 1941 that there were two 'fundamental' principles in medical reorganisation: first, that income should be no barrier to care; and second, that GPs should be part of the 'bridging of the gap between preventive medicine and treatment'. Similarly, he argued on the Hospitals Committee the following month that the bodies set up to administer a socialised hospital service should be controlled by 'ratepayers and the charitable public' rather than by doctors, since to have the latter would raise the suspicion that 'medical men were there only to further their own interests'. Murray, in a memorandum to the Public Health Committee of which he was a member, suggested that at their best health centres would operate as 'the basis of a complete medical service', and that one implication of this was a unified hospital service. While the system as a whole should be centrally monitored, actual control should rest with 'popularly elected bodies governing a wide region'.[17]

The idea of the 'region' is worth noting here. A number of plans had been put forward advocating the 'regionalisation' of the health services, and especially the hospitals, and the EMS was organised on a regional basis.[18] In some respects, this seemed to offer a way through what was generally acknowledged – including by the Association – as the muddle of existing local government. However, as we have already seen with Murray and his rather strained distinction between 'regionalism' and 'regionalisation', SMA members realised that what the voluntary sector meant by the latter was very different from the kind of health service they themselves envisaged. Equally, the EMS model was rejected because of its lack of democratic control. Nonetheless, the idea did hold possibilities. As Murray put it in *The Future of Medicine*, published in 1942 and therefore a distillation of his ideas at the time of the MPC, 'we must free ourselves from centuries-old boundaries which bear no relation to the changes wrought by the growth of industry'. He further noted that the Ministry of Health had accepted regionalisation as the basis of post-war reconstruction, but further cautioned that the term had as yet no agreed definition. Murray himself stressed the need for a uniform pattern of administration throughout the country, with a coordinating role for the Ministry. But if one impulse behind reorganisation was to be efficiency and rationalisation, the other must be 'intensely democratic, responsive to the needs and wishes of every individual

citizen, and directly concerned with its own neighbourhood'. It is notable too how Murray evoked here a highly altruistic and organic ethos
which would inform the socialised service – he suggested, for example,
that at local level 'it will be for the doctors ... to inspire the system with
the spirit of service which will make it a living thing'.[19]

Murray's scheme must also be seen as a contribution to the much wider
labour movement debate identified by Abigail Beach. Sections of the left
were expressing concern over the centralising tendencies of war, with
regional administration seen as devolved central government rather than
a democratic or accountable expression of local or regional feeling. The
EMS was, as Murray suggested, an obvious example here. Decentralised,
democratic control was therefore not simply an SMA preoccupation, but
part of ongoing contemporary discussions in which a particular form of
regionalism was seen as the solution to both the problems of existing
local government and as the counterbalance to a potentially over-
powerful central state.[20] This in turn has to be put in the context of the
war itself, which was being waged against what were seen as the epitome
of centralised state power – Nazi Germany, fascist Italy, and authoritarian Japan. As we shall see in the next chapter, the SMA was extremely
careful to clarify what it meant by 'state medicine', and how this differed
from medical organisation in totalitarian societies.

The official Association evidence to the MPC came in a memorandum subsequently published (after the Interim Report) as a further
policy statement, *The Socialist Programme for Health*. This identified
ten general principles, the first of which was that: 'Health is a national
asset, and it follows that its promotion and preservation must be recognised as a responsibility of the State.' The other 'principles' built on
this, emphasising the need for a comprehensive and unified service
permeated by the 'scientific basis of much of our medical knowledge'. It
was also acknowledged that control was important, and that national,
local, and professional demands and aspirations must be satisfied. Consequently there should be

> a national plan centrally controlled, modified to suit local condi-
> tions by democratically elected authorities, and allowing doctors
> and other health workers a considerable say in the administration
> of the health unit.[21]

Again there is evidence here of a rather uneasy compromise between
popular and professional rights, a recurring problem for the SMA, but
the demand for some form of democratic control is clear enough.

The MPC produced its only official document, the Draft Interim
Report, in the summer of 1942. Webster describes it as a 'liberal', if
'disjointed', text, which none the less attracted 'widespread interest'.

Similarly, Honigsbaum finds the Report evidence, at this point, of medical 'radicalism' – albeit, in the last resort, a 'deceptive radicalism'. Perhaps the most obvious example of the apparent change in medical attitudes came with the Commission's acceptance of what had long been a key SMA preoccupation, health centres. This was incorporated in the Interim Report following a protracted discussion on the General Practice Committee in late summer 1941. In turn, this derived from statements made to the committee by Hastings, Brook, and a non-SMA member, Professor Mackintosh. Two prominent Association activists were, in other words, in a position to shape the terms of the committee's debate. Both Hastings and Brook emphasised the importance of health centres and, after 'much discussion', a resolution was agreed, the wording of which was almost identical to the relevant section of the Interim Report.[22]

This endorsement of health centres was undoubtedly a significant achievement for the SMA. It is therefore reasonable to claim that it did, particularly in this area, have a positive influence on the Commission. The SMA's ability to have some of its ideas inserted in the Interim Report was a victory for the intellectual power of its proposals, and an embodiment of the mood for change characteristic of the wartime period. The MPC also shows Hastings in a favourable light, testament to his growing status in medical politics. His role in promoting discussion on the General Practice Committee, although not a GP himself, is notable throughout the record of its proceedings. This positive view, from the SMA's standpoint, of the Report is further enhanced by the interest it engendered, so spreading more widely the general idea of medical reconstruction as well as more specific proposals endorsed by the Association. The Association must also have been relatively – although not entirely – pleased with the Interim Report's stance on hospital reorganisation; preventive medicine; and the need for an end to economic barriers to health care. However it is also evident that the SMA was far from having all its ideas accepted by the MPC's various committees. Again to use the example of the General Practice Committee, a majority – but certainly not including the SMA members – agreed that a new system should be based on an extension of health insurance.[23] Such setbacks, when added to the relative incoherence of the Interim Report and the inherent conservatism of the medical profession evident in a number of its proposals – hence Honigsbaum's 'deceptive radicalism' – help explain the SMA's rather muted response to the Report's publication. Murray, while acknowledging what he saw as its good points, also argued that the Report undoubtedly sought to 'leave loopholes in what is essentially a State, salaried service, so that a certain small number of doctors may continue to take large fees from the highest income groups'.

This was an explicit reference to the document's claim that 90 per cent of the population would be covered by its proposals, the implication being that the remainder would be served by private practice. Even more worryingly, Murray continued, was the failure to address democratic control of the service, both internally and by society as a whole. Overall, he concluded, a minority of MPC members, by which he obviously meant himself and his SMA colleagues, 'have yet to speak'. The majority, on the other hand, had failed to realise that 'the consumer of medical care, the British public, wants no half measures in this matter'.[24]

Differences over local authority control

This last, general, statement was certainly something with which all of the medical left would have agreed. But this did not mean that all socialist health workers – including some Association members – subscribed fully to the 'official' SMA line. In particular, the subject of local authority control, of hospitals, general practitioners, or both, was seen by some as highly problematical. The MPC provides a useful starting point from which to examine such internal disagreements in the early part of the war. In a number of documents considered by the Commission, Brook stressed that while in favour of a unified system with a 'considerable degree of local autonomy', ultimately a central body should directly control the whole service. This was to ensure 'optimum standardisation': in other words, that services be equally available throughout the country, irrespective of the local government area in which a patient or consumer lived. Brook was also anxious to ensure professional rights and representation in a socialised system, something which potentially conflicted with the idea of democratic control. In short, any new service should be 'a national one and not placed under the local authorities'.[25]

Brook clearly took a less optimistic view of the virtues of local government than did his friend, colleague, and fellow LCC member Hastings. His speech to the 1940 Association AGM was, he later noted, 'strongly criticised' for some of his proposals. It is reasonable to assume that his questioning of the efficacy of local control and more conciliatory attitude to general practitioners, almost certainly a consequence of his direct involvement with the MPU, upset SMA colleagues. For Brook argued that while previous schemes had assumed a central role for local bodies, he was of the opinion that not only would it be a 'grave mistake' to give these any direct control over GP services, but also that they should 'be deprived of the present functions of control of hospitals and medical services'. Brook here drew specifically on his LCC experiences and on his observation that local government health services varied enormously in terms of efficiency. These points were also made to the MPC.[26] Brook had a perfectly valid argument, one which had already been made by another left-wing doctor.

Stephen Taylor was attached to the Ministry of Information during the war, and in 1945 won the parliamentary seat of Barnet for the Labour Party, by which time he was apparently an SMA member as well as health correspondent for the *Daily Herald*. As will be seen, he was an important contributor to Labour's plans for a National Health Service. In 1939 Taylor devised 'A Plan for British Hospitals'. This pointed out that rich counties, such as Middlesex and Surrey, had developed good municipal hospital services, but that poorer counties had often had to put up with 'converted public-assistance institutions'. Hence the need, he suggested, for 'hospital finance on a national basis'. Furthermore, while groups of hospitals should be allowed 'as much local autonomy as possible', there should also be some form of national organisation. This, he continued, should be neither part of the Health Ministry nor connected with local authorities. Rather, there should be a 'statutory National Hospital Corporation, with a charter subject to a five-yearly review by Parliament'. This should be controlled by a 'board of governors, of whom at least a third should be medical men'. Taylor's interest in the organisational model of the British Broadcasting Corporation is evident here.[27] His hostility to local authority control derived, Taylor later recalled, from his 'bitter experience' of an LCC hospital. It was, he claimed, 'the worst run hospital' in which he ever worked, beset by bureaucracy and run by poor quality administrators. Councillors themselves were at best 'dull and inefficient', and at worst 'self-seeking, corrupt, and power lusting'. Taylor's view of the LCC was, therefore, somewhat at odds with that of its propagandists such as Hastings.[28]

This scepticism about the efficacy of local authorities was at least partially shared by another prominent SMA activist, R.A. Lyster. Asked by the Fabian Society to comment on early drafts of Hastings's *The Hospital Services*, noted above as an important Association document contemporary to the MPC's deliberations, Lyster suggested that among its defects was its apparent reliance on

> conditions in and around London. It blandly assumes that the Local Govt. Act 1929 has been carried out generally whereas a great proportion of the local authorities have defied the letter and the spirit of the Act.

Lewis Silkin, an LCC colleague of Hastings, was also asked to comment on the drafts of Hastings's pamphlets. While full of praise for his administrative experience and professional knowledge, Silkin was not entirely convinced by Hastings's arguments for the inclusion of GPs in a full-time salaried service. This, he suggested, was a matter which he and Hastings had discussed 'many times' in the past. Other criticisms of Hastings's draft text included the suggestion that he was not clear enough about hospital control, and that – rather surprisingly – he was too soft on the voluntary hospitals.[29] All this suggests the fluidity of socialist proposals for health care in the early years of the war, and the potential problems for the SMA in having all aspects of its plans accepted and implemented. And, as we shall see in the next chapter, the idea of local authority control of health services in particular remained highly contentious within the labour movement.

The impact of Beveridge

The mood of some leading Association members at the time of the Interim Report's publication is perhaps best captured by a meeting of June 1942. This was evocatively entitled 'The Frustration of Medicine', almost certainly a conscious echo of the phrase much employed by left-wing scientists in the 1930s, 'the frustration of science'. Here Murray suggested that the 'primary object' of medicine was defeated if any doctor, no matter how successful his record of curative work, had to deal with 'a single case of preventable disease'. Bourne similarly emphasised the environmental basis of much ill health, and thereby its preventable nature, citing as evidence data on army rejection rates and maternal morbidity. One consequence was the frustration of the medical profession, attributable to the 'lack of public responsibility for the preservation of health'. Pressing his point home, Bourne argued that society had for so long seen health as 'the absence of obvious disease' that many had never experienced 'that positive feeling of well-being which is health'.[30] This clearly relates to the point made above on Bourne's claim that the 'right to health' involved not only the provision of socialised services, but the attainment of an optimum of individual well-being; as well as to the more general emphasis the Association placed on health and health care as a total package, a vital constituent of society as a whole. The 'frustration' of Murray and Bourne therefore derived from the mixed progress of proposals for medical reconstruction, and possibly also the disagreements within the medical left itself over what course this should take.

These ruminations, and the debate over the MPC's findings, were, however, soon overshadowed by the publication of the Beveridge Report in December 1942. Although this said nothing specific about a future health service, its plans for post-war social insurance were

predicated on three 'Assumptions'. The second of these – Assumption B
– was the creation of 'a national health service for prevention and
comprehensive treatment available to all members of the community'.
As Webster notes, this was the

> first official source signifying that the Government was considering
> undertaking a full reconstruction of the health services, rather than
> merely sponsoring rationalisation of the hospital service.

It was on this strong implication of a unified and comprehensive medical service, something for which it had argued since its foundation, that
the SMA focused. Murray, ever the optimist and exponent of Association influence, even suggested at one point that Assumption B 'had
taken the Socialist Medical Association policy as its own'.[31]

The SMA did not itself give evidence to Beveridge's Committee, but
the London County Council did. Among its recommendations were that
services such as hospitals 'be administered by local authorities'. This is
not, of course, especially surprising in the sense that the LCC as a whole
was committed to the municipal socialist model, as is witnessed by the
comment of its Labour leader, Charles Latham, in 1941. Responding to
an initiative which might have sidelined local government, Latham
protested that 'the fifth columnists against democracy are preparing to
steal the people's municipal hospitals', part of a broader attack by
'reaction' on popularly elected local government. He counterposed a
comprehensive hospital system under local authority control. However,
it is worth noting that the LCC's evidence on hospitals to Beveridge
precisely mirrors the approach adopted in July 1942 at a special meeting of the Hospital Committee, whose SMA representation had been
further strengthened by the co-option of Murray.[32] As we saw in Chapter Five, the council's pride in and commitment to its municipal hospital
system was due largely to the initiative of Association members on the
Hospital Committee, and their own dedication to and propagandising
for local authority control.

The SMA clearly recognised from the outset the importance of
Beveridge's proposals, and their impact on both the medical community
and the general public. In other words, they realised that an historic
opportunity was being presented for a wholesale reform of British
social welfare. At an EC meeting on 10 December 1942 it was agreed
that Murray prepare a draft statement on Beveridge, with a view to this
ultimately appearing as a pamphlet. At the following meeting a resolution was passed approving the 'principle underlying the Beveridge
Report', and calling for the 'carrying out to the full the terms of Assumption B by means of Socialised Medical Services'. On Murray's
initiative, it was also agreed that Association members eligible to do so

should attend BMA meetings to oppose its stance on Beveridge.[33] This was an obvious indication that the relative, and recent, coincidence of views between the Association and the BMA which had characterised the MPC's Interim Report was now over. The respective attitudes of the two organisations towards Beveridge diverged sharply. Consequently the SMA was competing with the main professional body, ultimately without any real success, for the support of the mass of medical practitioners. The Association was, as we shall see, to become involved in an increasingly acrimonious relationship with the BMA, which it characterised as being led by a reactionary, and aged, clique.

The SMA nonetheless pressed on with its support for Beveridge. The *Bulletin* outlined the organisation's interim analysis and position. There was no doubt, it suggested, that the implementation of Beveridge's plan would profoundly affect the British people's health. But caution had to be exercised. While the Report aimed at the abolition of poverty, 'we are more than sceptical as to the power of any provisions of social insurance *under capitalism* (emphasis in original) to achieve such an object'. The need for a socialised health service, based on the now familiar components of teamwork; preventive medicine; and democratic control – a new health service should not be 'imposed from without or above'; was restated, as was hostility to any extension of the panel system. Such reservations notwithstanding, the article concluded on the upbeat note that the SMA now had a unique opportunity to put to 'people in all classes the ideas for which [it] has striven since its inception'.[34]

The Report certainly prompted a whole range of Association initiatives and activities, including the publication of two propaganda leaflets. Significantly, these eschewed the anti-capitalist rhetoric of the *Bulletin* to put as favourable a gloss as possible on Beveridge's proposals. Assumption B was 'an indication of a necessity of modern times', although it 'hints only at the method to be adopted to make the assumption a reality'. The SMA was, unsurprisingly, happy to elaborate on this method. Particular attention was paid to the alleged iniquities of the insurance system, and a warning given that sections of the medical profession – and especially the BMA – were prepared to fight for their 'vested interest in disease'. But the Association had no doubt that, essentially, 'Assumption B means a National Health Service'.[35]

Meetings with ministers

By 1943 the SMA clearly felt that positive change was a distinct possibility, and that it had itself an important part to play in promoting and advancing such change. The March edition of *Medicine Today and*

Tomorrow pointed out that proposals were 'piling up so fast that it is almost impossible to keep pace with them'. From this, it deduced that British society was quickly approaching 'that third stage in the history of all social advances, that at which all men, having previously condemned, now accept the new idea'. But this stage had not yet been reached. Parts of the profession still stood out against medical progress. This sense of a real possibility of change combined with the need to combat reactionary forces was continuously present throughout this period. The idea of a 'third stage' is, furthermore, strikingly similar to the idea being put forward contemporaneously by John Ryle, that 'social medicine' was the 'third epoch' of preventive medicine.[36]

One way in which the SMA sought to counter medical reaction, go beyond simply propagandising about Assumption B, and help force the pace of change was by direct discussions with government ministers. Two such meetings in 1943 are worth examining, for three reasons: first because they further illustrate the kind of demands the Association was making, in this case to important politicians, at a time when the future of the health services was under intense discussion; second, and related to the previous point, because they will ultimately contribute to an assessment of the Association's influence both within the labour movement and more generally; and third, because they reinforce the earlier suggestion that 1943 was a year of particular significance for the SMA.

Hastings first approached the Minister of Health, Ernest Brown, about a meeting in late February. In an internal memorandum a civil servant gave an interesting, if not necessarily flattering, view of the Association and its place in medical politics: 'I assume the M will have to see these people, even though they may not be one of the bodies representative of the profession with whom discussions will be carried on in detail.' The timing here is nonetheless crucial, for Brown was beginning the process ultimately resulting in the publication of the 1944 White Paper. This included discussions on a 'Comprehensive Medical Service' with various branches of local government, the voluntary hospitals, the BMA, and the Royal Colleges. One specific initiative by the Ministry was the appointment, in January 1943, of a sub-committee of the Medical Advisory Committee to look into health centres, an SMA preoccupation whose case had been successfully argued on the MPC.[37] Of course as the civil servant's comments attest, the Association was not, as an organisation, officially part of this process.

However Hastings, as a local authority representative, was. At one of a series of meetings at the Ministry from March onwards, at all of which Hastings was present, the LCC delegation stressed their hostility to the inclusion of any 'outside interests' – that is official delegates chosen exclusively by the medical profession – on local Health Authorities or any of their executive bodies. The reason for this was a principled objection to having such interests formally involved on bodies with revenue raising powers. This emphasis on democratic accountability and suspicion of the organised medical profession was shared by the SMA, whose members had raised such matters on, for example, the MPC. It is therefore not unreasonable to see the LCC's stance as at least in part dictated by Association ideas.[38] Moreover the SMA was also directly involved with labour movement campaigns for reformed health services. In February 1943, for instance, a conference on health took place in London, attended by around 500 delegates. Although primarily organised by trades unions, the Association played a significant administrative and supportive role. And while largely concerned with industrial health matters, the meeting did voice wider demands, including the adoption of Assumption B by the government.[39] Even more importantly, and as the following chapter shows, the SMA was at precisely this time playing an instrumental role in the preparation of what was soon to become the Labour Party's 1943 policy statement, *National Service for Health*. Its request for a meeting with Brown was therefore a conscious attempt to become involved in crucial discussions on future policy. This was a process with which Hastings as an individual was personally acquainted; and which in certain specific areas – such as health centres – was addressing issues of considerable concern to the Association. It was also a process in which the Labour Party, whose health policy was being shaped by the SMA, had a considerable interest.

This last point is borne out by official party support for the proposed delegation, civil service reservations notwithstanding. J.S. Middleton, Labour's General Secretary, wrote to the Health Minister pointing out that the Association was an affiliated organisation, and that 'Dr Hastings and his colleagues have been of great service to the Party in the years gone by in connection with medical matters'. Consequently, Association members met with Brown at the end of March.[40] By this time he and his civil servants would certainly have been aware of the labour movement's strong desire for health service reconstruction, and of the SMA's role in its formulation and advancement.

Prior to the meeting itself, Brown received a long memorandum from the Association welcoming the government's acceptance of Assumption B and the Minister's acceptance of 'the principle of group practice based on health centres'. On the latter, the document continued, it was undoubtedly the case that promotion by the SMA had led to their current acceptance. Furthermore, only the Association had a detailed plan for health centre organisation. To illustrate this, it was suggested that each centre should serve a population of 20 000 people, and be staffed by twelve GPs.[41] While there is obviously a certain amount of self-advancement going on here, it is also reasonable to assume that the Association genuinely felt it had made a significant breakthrough on health centres in the light of the MPC's Interim Report and the setting up of an official committee on the issue.

The rest of the memorandum made a range of familiar points, including the end of private practice, a salaried service, and local authority control. On the last point, local government required reorganisation so that elected authorities controlled not less than half a million people, and not more than two million. This was preferable to 'any form of "joint board"'. Interestingly, though, an implicit acknowledgement of the vexed question of doctors' rights – or at least, and rather more ambiguously, the rights of health workers – was made when it was argued that doctors should not be disbarred from local elections. Similarly, the 'health unit' – by which was presumably meant institutions within a given local authority area – 'should be operated by a committee of the whole health personnel'. The complexities, ambiguities, and qualifications here once again illustrate the problem of reconciling democracy with professional status in health service administration. On the more general question of the need for a national health service, however, the Association was more clear cut. It pointed out that it had a 'much more diverse membership' than other health organisations, and that it was in close touch with the general population's mood through its propaganda meetings. This led the SMA to firmly believe that 'the public is ready for this change'.[42] While not explicitly stated, the obvious contrast here was with what the Association saw as the medical profession's increasingly reactionary position, at least as expressed by the BMA.

At the meeting itself, the Association reiterated and expanded upon its proposals. Murray raised the question of health centres, and Brown pointed out that this was now under official consideration. Horace Joules stressed the need for a hospital service which was unified, not just coordinated. The Minister replied that this was not currently 'practical politics', and that the government had 'certain commitments to the voluntary hospitals which must be honoured'. The Chief Medical Officer asked what exactly was meant by a 'unified service'. Hastings responded that the Association had 'two things in mind: a single type of hospital – the distinction between voluntary and municipal being abolished – and also a close coordination of the preventive and curative sides of medicine'. The meeting concluded with Hastings promising to provide memoranda on various points raised during the discussion.[43]

The second meeting of 1943 worthy of examination was with a minister whom the Association could reasonably expect to be rather more sympathetic to their case than the National Liberal Brown, namely the leader of the Labour Party and Deputy Prime Minister, Clement Attlee. The idea for this came from John Wilmot, parliamentary private secretary to Hugh Dalton, President of the Board of Trade, in the course of a discussion on the SMA's role in London politics. The meeting duly took place in November 1943.[44] By this time Attlee would have been well aware of the Association's views through its role in Labour's health policy formation and through the initiative of Joules, who had written to Evan Durbin, Attlee's personal assistant, a few weeks earlier. Joules's letter made two main points: first, that the Ministry of Health was being successfully bluffed by 'a small minority of elderly, rich, reactionary specialists and medical politicians'; and, second, that now was the time for the introduction of a salaried service. Durbin was particularly impressed by the first point, remarking to Attlee that it was 'of the greatest importance in dealing with the unsatisfactory proposals that we fear the forthcoming Draft White Paper by the Minister of Health is likely to contain'. He suggested a meeting between Attlee and Joules, describing the latter as 'of our way of thought and a most remarkable and statesmanlike Doctor'.[45]

The official starting point for the discussion between Attlee and the SMA representatives was Assumption B, although by now this was really a pretext for a much wider ranging and more detailed expression of Association ideas. Hastings began by stressing his organisation's commitment to current Labour health policy; and by acknowledging the constraints on the party resulting from its participation in the coalition government. Even so, he continued, three particular issues should remain to the fore. There should be a unified service, covering the whole population; and there should likewise be a 'real partnership' between local authority and voluntary hospitals. The service should not, however, be built on the basis of an extended panel system. This was, Hastings claimed, disliked by those it was meant to benefit. Furthermore, it existed for 'the treatment of declared disease and not for the prevention of disease', another instance of the Association's belief that 'vested interests' – in this case general practitioners' economic interests – stood in the way of medical progress.

Questioned by Attlee on the difference between the SMA and the BMA positions, the delegation primarily stressed administrative concerns. The BMA envisaged a Medical Corporation as the principal governing device, whereas the Association advocated 'enlarged Local Authorities or Health Boards under the general control of the Ministry of Health'. The delegation also pointed to differences of opinion within the BMA itself, with (even among its older members) only about 20 per cent favouring a 'completely reactionary policy'.[46] This echoed the claim about the nature of the BMA leadership made by Joules to Durbin, which the latter had seen as being especially significant, and is also consistent with the Association's contention that the BMA was out of touch with medical opinion, especially among younger doctors and those in the armed forces.

The broader political context is important. By the time of his meeting with the SMA, Attlee was also a member of the government's Reconstruction Priorities Committee. As such, he had developed a critical stance on the government's developing health policy, for example over voluntary hospitals and health centres. Too many concessions were being made to the former, too little emphasis being placed on the latter. Similarly, Attlee was unhappy about the capitation system of paying doctors, preferring instead a salaried service. All of these points were Labour Party policy as formulated largely by the SMA, as the following chapter further substantiates, as well as being the kind of issues raised by both Joules and the Association delegation. Attlee's concern over the direction of official policy resulted in his sending a number of memoranda to the Ministry of Health, one significant instance of which came in December 1943, that is shortly after his discussions with SMA members. This document, described by Brooke as an 'exercise in Labour-SMA planning', was written by Stephen Taylor. While this may be something of an overstatement, given that Taylor was at this stage sceptical about at least some aspects of Association policy, it is also the case that he was coming closer to the organisation, as shall become evident in subsequent chapters. His 1943 memorandum rejected 'any combination of private and public practice and made strong arguments for a fully salaried service'.[47] Although this may have been commonplace among certain sections of the medical left by this stage, the SMA's role in articulating and pushing forward such ideas should not be underestimated.

The meetings with ministers, and the circumstances leading up to and surrounding them, show the Association building on its relative success on the MPC, which if nothing else had proved a useful propaganda platform; and responding to the proposals of, and the reaction to, the Beveridge Report. They also demonstrate the organisation seeking to influence, at the highest level, the discussions then taking place in government circles over the future of Britain's health services. This was significant not only because a Labour minister such as Attlee was, at this stage, clearly sympathetic to certain Association ideas, but also because even before these meetings it is evident that Health Ministry officials were fully aware of the SMA's views on medical reorganisation. Such an awareness was almost certainly heightened by the profile the organisation adopted in the first four years of the war. This in turn was important for the Association because of its belief, especially in the wake of the Beveridge Report, that the forces of medical reaction were now seeking in earnest to undermine any progressive proposals for a state medical service. It is in this context, of optimism tempered by the need for constant vigilance, that another crucial aspect of the SMA's activities in this period needs to be examined, namely the participation of leading members in the Labour Party's policy-making process. The results of this activity, the organisation's reaction to the 1944 White Paper, and its position as the war in Europe and the wartime coalition government both came to an end, are the subjects of the next chapter.

Notes

1. On the volume of Association literature, see Hilliard's comments in SMA, *The SMA and the Foundations of the National Health Service*, p. 3; Aleck Bourne, *Health of the Future*, Harmondsworth, Penguin, 1942; David Stark Murray, *The Future of Medicine*, Harmondsworth, Penguin, 1942; on the 'Penguin Specials' see Nicholas Joicey, 'A Paperback Guide to Progress: Penguin Books 1935–c. 1951', *Twentieth Century British History*, 4, 1, 1993.

2. DSM 5/1, cutting from *The Listener*, 11 February 1943; Somerville Hastings, 'The Development of the Health Services', *The Medical Officer*, 27 February 1943, pp. 69–71. The programme for the lecture series on 'Social Medicine and Public Health', inspired by a speech to the Association by John Ryle – Murray, *Why a National Health Service?*, p. 58 – can be found in DSH, File 57, 'Public Health'.

3. MSS.79/MPU/1/2/2, Minutes of Council Meetings 1937–48, Minutes of the Emergency Sub-Committee, 25 May, 26 July, 23 October 1940 and 28 January 1941, and Minutes of Council, 12 February 1941; SMA, *Bulletin*, March 1941, p. 1; MH 77/26, 'Office Committee on Post-War Hospital Policy: Salaried Medical Service', undated but presumably early 1942.

4. 'Whither Medicine', *MTT*, vol. 2, no. 4 (new series), December Quarter 1939, pp. 3–18 – this was later published as a pamphlet.

5. Parliamentary Debates, 5th series, vol. 365, col. 895ff.

6. *Lancet*, 1941, I, pp. 187–8.

7. Webster, *The Health Services since the War*, p. 25; Bartrip, *Themselves Writ Large*, pp. 227–32.

8. MPC Minutes 7 May 1941, p. 2, and 29 May, p. 2; Honigsbaum, *Health, Happiness and Security*, pp. 18, 74; *idem*, *Division in British Medicine*, p. 185; Webster notes the influence of Ryle in *The Health Services since the War*, p. 37, on whom see also Dorothy Porter, 'Changing Disciplines: John Ryle and the Making of Social Medicine in Britain in the 1940s', *History of Science*, XXX, 1992, pp. 137–64; and *idem*, 'John Ryle: Doctor of Revolution?', in Porter, Dorothy and Porter, Roy (eds), *Doctors, Politics and Society: Historical Essays*. The copy of Brook's *Making Medical History* in the library of the Wellcome Unit for the History of Medicine, Oxford, is dedicated by the author to Ryle.

9. MPC Minutes 7 May 1941, pp. 3–6; MPC, 'A Preliminary Survey of the More Important Reports and Opinions on the Development of Medical Services'.

10. 'Planning Medicine: Commission's Great Task', *MTT*, vol. 3, no. 1, March Quarter 1941, pp. 1–5; SMA, *Bulletin*, no. 29, February 1941, p. 1.
11. SMA, *Medicine Tomorrow*, SMA, rev. edn, 1941/42, p. 21.
12. Elizabeth Bunbury, *Health and the Medical Services*, SMA, 1941/42, pp. 3–5.
13. Somerville Hastings, *The Hospital Services: Research Series no. 59*, Fabian Society/Victor Gollancz, 1941, pp. 17–20.
14. *Lancet*, 1941, I, p. 527. On the various 'experiments' in South Wales, and the rather dubious nature of some of their conclusions, see A. Susan Williams, *Women and Childbirth in the Twentieth Century*, Stroud, Sutton Publishing, 1997: I am grateful to Charles Webster for this reference.
15. Bourne, *Health of the Future*, p. 115; SMA, *The Socialist Programme for Health*, p. 8.
16. MPC Minutes, 7 May 1941, p. 3.
17. MPC General Practice Committee, Minutes, 6 August 1941, p. 3; MPC Hospitals Committee, Minutes, 4 September 1941, p. 7; MPC Public Health Committee, memorandum 'The Health Centre Unit' submitted to the meeting of 11 December 1941, pp. 1, 2.
18. On 'regionalisation' see Webster, *The Health Services since the War*, p. 28ff; and Fox, *Health Policies, Health Politics*, Chs 2, 4, 6.
19. Murray, *The Future of Medicine*, p. 103ff.
20. Beach, 'The Labour Party and the Idea of Citizenship', p. 156ff.
21. SMA, *The Socialist Programme for Health*, SMA, 1942, pp. 2–5.
22. *BMJ*, 1942, I, 'Medical Planning Commission: Draft Interim Report', pp. 743–53, and p. 745 for the health centre proposals; Webster, *The Health Services since the War*, p. 25; Honigsbaum, *Division in British Medicine*, pp. 182–3; MPC General Practice Committee – Minutes of the Committee, 6 August and 18 September 1941.
23. MPC General Practice Committee – Minutes of the Committee, 8 October 1941.
24. DSM (2) 4, cutting from *Reynolds Illustrated News*, 21 June 1942, Dr Irwin Brown (David Stark Murray), 'A Revolution in Your Health'.
25. MPC, Minutes of the General Practice Committee, 2 July 1941, Document 3 Appendix I, Charles Brook, 'The Co-Ordination of a National Medical Service', p. 8; and MPC, 'A Preliminary Survey of the More Important Reports and Opinions on the Development of Medical Services', Appendix XV, Charles Brook, 'Problems of the Post-War Practitioner', p. 11.
26. Brook, *Making Medical History*, p. 12; *idem*, 'Problems of the Post-War Practitioner', *MTT*, vol. 2, no. 6 (new series), June Quarter 1940, p. 7 – this was the basis of one submission to the MPC by Brook. See also Honigsbaum, *Division in British Medicine*, p. 258.
27. Special Commissioner (Stephen Taylor), 'A Plan for British Hospitals', *Lancet*, 1939, II, pp. 946, 951.
28. Stephen Taylor (Lord Taylor of Harlow), *A Natural History of Everyday Life: a Biographical Guide for Would-Be Doctors of Society*, The Memoir Club, 1988, pp. 293, 253. I am grateful to Charles Webster for drawing my attention to this work.
29. Fabian Society Papers, K10/4, R.A. Lyster to John Parker, 19 April 1941; Lewis Silkin to John Parker, 18 April 1941; and general comments on the

draft. Lyster was also involved with the MPU, which almost certainly contributed to his scepticism about local authority control.

30. *Lancet*, 1942, I, p. 713.
31. Webster, *The Health Services since the War*, p. 35; DSM 4/2, 'Report of the Health Workers' Convention, May 16th 1943'.
32. Social Insurance and Allied Services: Report by Sir William Beveridge – Appendix G, Memoranda from Organisations, Parliamentary Papers 1942–43, vol. VI, p. 218; quoted in Rivett, *The Development of the London Hospital System*, p. 244; LCC/MIN/2219, 6 July 1942; Minutes of the London County Council, 30 June 1942.
33. DSM 1/6, EC Minutes, 10 December 1942, and 10 February 1943.
34. SMA, *Bulletin*, no. 51, January 1943, pp. 3–4.
35. SMA, *SMA Leaflet no. 1: The Beveridge Report and the Health Services*, London, SMA, n.d., but 1943; and *SMA Leaflet no. 2: Assumption B or the 'Panel'*, London, SMA, n.d., but probably 1943.
36. *MTT*, vol. 4, no. 1, March 1943, p. 1; Porter, 'Changing Disciplines', p. 146.
37. MH 77/63, Hastings to Brown, 27 February 1943; and internal memorandum, 1 March 1943; MH 71/103, Medical Advisory Committee: Sub-Committee on Health Centres; for the context, see Webster, *The Health Services since the War*, p. 44ff.
38. See MH 80/25 and 26, and MH 77/26 for the meetings between the Ministry and local authority representatives. The meeting referred to is in MH 80/25, 'Second Meeting between Representative of Local Authorities and Officers of the Ministry of Health, March 29th, 1943'.
39. SMA, *Health: What Needs to Be Done*, SMA, 1943.
40. MH 77/63, Middleton to Brown, 5 March 1943.
41. MH 77/63, memorandum from the SMA to Brown, March 1943.
42. MH 77/63, memorandum from the SMA to Brown, March 1943.
43. MH 77/63, notes of the meeting of 26 March 1943.
44. DSM 1/6, EC Minutes, 7 October 1943.
45. Piercy Papers, 8/20, memorandum from E.F.M. Durbin to Attlee, 30 September 1943.
46. MH 77/63, Notes of a Deputation from the Socialist Medical Association which attended the Lord President, 11 November 1943.
47. Brooke, *Labour's War*, pp. 204–5; see also Webster, *The Health Services since the War*, pp. 51–4.

CHAPTER EIGHT

'The Battle for Health'

To examine SMA activities within Labour's policy making structures, it is necessary to go back to early 1941 when, yet again, the Public Health Advisory Committee was reconstituted. This first met in March, and the timing here is important for, as we have seen, the MPC was shortly to begin its deliberations. Post-war medical reconstruction was a matter of mounting concern, and the Labour Party anxious to be involved in the public debate. Of the committee's 15 members, around half belonged, or were close to, the Association. The most important of these were Murray, Lyster, and, in the key position of chairman, Hastings. In a letter to the committee, the party secretary defined its purpose as twofold: an examination of wartime health problems and the formulation of a long-term health policy. A document was produced on the PHAC's behalf by Hastings – 'A Scheme for a War Time National Medical Service' – which, as its title suggests, was concerned primarily with short-term arrangements.[1] Over the next three years, however, the PHAC, now integrated into the party's policy structure as part of the Central Committee on Reconstruction, increasingly concentrated on proposals for the post-war period. As Brooke suggests, it was 'among the most active of the party's policy bodies, producing a considerable corpus of memoranda on a range of health-related subjects'.[2] It is worth stressing that the committee's output was largely the work of its SMA members, with Hastings and Murray playing a particularly prominent role.

The PHAC's deliberations produced their first significant outcomes in late 1942 and 1943. In September 1942 the Central Committee acknowledged that the creation of a 'state medical service' was one of its five post-war aims, an important shift in emphasis from the relative neglect of health matters in the inter-war period.[3] This was followed by a special weekend meeting of the Central Committee in December – coincident with the publication of the Beveridge Report – at which various aspects of reform were discussed. Here Hastings introduced, on the basis of eight pre-existing and largely SMA-authored documents, the PHAC proposals. He urged the party to produce a health policy statement, and it is notable here that his committee had recently complained that the Central Committee was ignoring its work, and that other organisations were producing policies 'while the Labour Party has failed to do so in spite of the basic documents having been prepared eleven months ago'.[4] This was an interesting comment – a reflection of, on the one hand, the zeal of the SMA and, on the other, of the classic social democratic dilemma we have now encountered on a number of occasions, namely whether to prioritise social or economic policy. Also of importance here is Brooke's observation that the Beveridge Report had a contradictory impact on Labour policy-making. It undoubtedly made social reconstruction a 'central issue in wartime politics'. But, as far as Labour was concerned, it also initiated a shift from 'active to passive, from making policy to evaluating it'. The first of these was to work, at least in the short term, in the SMA's favour. On the other hand the latter was, for a body so much concerned with the creation of radical policy initiatives, clearly more problematical.[5]

It is thus significant that at the December meeting Hastings was rather cautious in his approach. This was perhaps because of his own misgivings about the possible pace of change, but more probably because of his perception that the party's policy makers were anxious not to be seen to be too far ahead of public or professional opinion. He argued, for example, that the hospitals 'should be brought under State control eventually, but it was better to do it in stages'. An important factor here was the current strength of the voluntary institutions, and Hastings suggested that it would be better to take these over when they were, as they had been in the 1930s, in a more difficult financial position. This was something with which the ever-cautious Morrison appeared to agree. Similarly, Hastings took a relatively moderate line on the question of all doctors being salaried state employees; and argued once again, when asked about the economic implications of a state scheme, that it should be brought in step by step. It was therefore decided that a financial estimate should be produced for, at present, internal purposes only. Nonetheless, the meeting concurred with the PHAC's general strategy, an essentially SMA strategy, subject to minor modifications and clarifications.[6]

The second major outcome of the committee's activities in this period had its origins in late November 1942 when Harold Laski, secretary of the Central Committee, suggested that the PHAC produce a health policy pamphlet. A draft was prepared by Murray – and apparently circulated to the Central Committee at the weekend meeting – which, after further consultation and drafting, was published as *National Service for Health*. This in turn was the basis of an NEC resolution agreed by party conference in June 1943, which Brooke suggests represented the 'dominance of SMA influence'.[7] The PHAC was clearly pleased with its work, noting with approval conference's decision and the production of *National Service for Health*. By July 1943 the first edition of the pamphlet had nearly sold out, a second edition was to be drafted, and press reports had been favourable. Nearly 30 years later Murray was to see this document as a 'complete vindication' of the Association's 'years of effort', a process which had begun with its success at party conference in 1934. A copy was sent to every SMA member, and the text itself was 'very largely' an echo of the memorandum presented earlier in the year to Ernest Brown, discussed in the previous chapter.[8]

Clearly the Association felt that 1943 was a year when much was going its way. In April, for instance, Murray claimed that the SMA was preparing a scheme which would 'answer the needs of a Social Security Service within the capitalist state as visualised by Sir William'. But this scheme, based on the experience both of Britain and of other countries, especially the Soviet Union, would also 'be capable of expansion into a completely socialised system of medicine'.[9] As we shall see later, what Murray subsequently identified as the paradox of a service created with socialist intentions but within a capitalist framework was to come back to haunt him. But in the early 1940s he was certainly making ambitious claims for his organisation, and it must be recognised that after years of relentless propagandising and, more recently, assiduous and committed work on Labour Party bodies, its efforts seemed to be paying off. The experience of war had helped focus and refine its proposals, a process further enhanced by participation on the MPC and the organisation's response to Beveridge. The outcome of these various factors was *National Service for Health*, worth examining as a specific and important example of official Labour policy predominantly shaped by the SMA.

National Service for Health

The pamphlet was broken into three 'chapters': the first asked what medical services were needed, and why; the second described the current system; and the third showed how the criteria adopted in the first could be met only by a state medical service. The underlying aim of any scheme, it was argued, must be the maximum mental and physical fitness of every citizen. Full health was an individual's greatest asset, and a nation's greatest asset was a healthy population. A properly-functioning service should be planned; preventive as well as curative; comprehensive and open to all; efficient and modern; and easily accessible. It should also retain confidence between doctor and patient while ensuring that medical workers were not exploited; and allow for the medical profession's fuller participation in national affairs. The last was an indication of the high status accorded to science and medicine by many socialists at this time, and justified on the grounds that increasingly 'in planning policy about food, education, industry, etc., the nation will need the guidance of medical science'.[10] It is also a further instance of the potential tension between professional status and democratic control, as we have already seen a recurring problem for the medical left.

Unsurprisingly, the current system did not fulfil the stated aspirations. This was true whether analysed in respect of control, the patient, the doctor, the hospital service, the system of funding, the maternity and child welfare service, or the school medical service. Equally unsurprising, therefore, was the conclusion that the nation required a state medical service. Proposals were then made as to how this would work in the various sectors of the health care system. Similarly, health centres were promoted, as was the need for doctors to be remunerated by salary. The latter would ensure that the practitioner would thereby be 'free to do his best work in the wide field of preventive, as well as curative, medicine'. Although for a short time it might be necessary to allow the continuance of private practice, for the Association the epitome of 'capitalist medicine', the service should be so efficient and complete that 'no patient could desire a better and every doctor will wish to serve in it'.[11] Such statements were typical of the SMA belief that even if private practice were not immediately abolished (although this was the ideal), then under a properly socialised system it would soon wither away, a consequence of consumer choice and producer altruism.

National Service for Health was, however, rather more cautious on the issue of hospitals. It certainly sought a unified system, and suggested that each local authority be required to put forward a 'coherent but adaptable plan, each plan covering a large area – a "Region"'. But the voluntary sector was not to be abolished outright; rather it was to be absorbed into the system gradually, perhaps through the mechanism of local authority subsidies. This was surprising when compared with the attitude of Hastings and the LCC in the 1930s, and Elizabeth Bunbury's cry of 'no taxation without representation'; rather less so when placed in the context of Hastings's December 1942 speech. The document was clearly anxious that voluntary hospitals were seen to be treated fairly, 'on terms which will satisfy the nation's sense of equity'.[12]

On administration, *National Service for Health* made a valiant attempt to be all things to all people. Ultimately, control was to reside in the Ministry of Health, reconstructed to take over responsibility for matters such as school meals and industrial health. Indeed the Ministry was of central importance, for no other body had its 'accumulated knowledge' of health conditions, nor its nation-wide authority. Given that health was a national concern, then it was 'Parliament, representing the whole nation, which must have ultimate control'. So just as the War Ministry directed 'the strategic placing of the Home Forces for defence against invasion', so should the Health Ministry be able to plan 'the strategic disposition of the nation's defences against ill-health'. Such military metaphors were a long-standing characteristic of left-wing proposals for health reform and were, understandably, particularly common during the Second World War when questions of national health were about more than simply the achievement of social justice. Hastings, supporting the health service resolution at 1943 party conference, suggested that one reason for a socialised service was the changes which had taken place in medicine itself, for 'medical science and the medical services, like the army, have been mechanised'. *National Service for Health* was itself suffused with military and technocratic vocabulary.[13]

On the other hand, it was recognised the Ministry could not do everything: 'That would mean certain breakdown.' Rather, another administrative layer would be required – yet another variant of 'regionalism' – and this would be provided by reformed local government, democratically controlled. Hence the need to leave wide powers with the local authorities, which must be responsible for the 'detailed administration of the service'. It would require, however, a 'National Health Service' to grant local government the powers, and the 'necessary democratic control', to carry out these responsibilities.[14] If *National Service for Health* was not entirely coherent about the respective responsibilities of centre and locality, it did nonetheless make it clear that democratic accountability was important, and that here local government had a crucial role to play. This is a further instance of how the document was strongly shaped by SMA preoccupations, perhaps moderated or modified either to accommodate the centralising tendencies in the party; or, more probably, as a result of the labour movement debates over the future of local government and 'regionalism' noted in the last chapter.

In respect of the funding of a future socialised service, revenue was to be derived partly from general taxation, partly from local taxation. As to the crucial question, 'Can We Afford It?', costing estimates were derived from PEP, Beveridge, the SMA, and David Stark Murray. Murray's *The Future of Medicine*, although not explicitly acknowledged, was extensively drawn upon, not surprisingly given his part in the pamphlet's creation. The answer to the question was, of course, that apart from any other consideration, a comprehensive service *had* to be afforded. It was 'literally a "vital" need', but in any case the cost of ill-health also had to be taken into account, as did the inefficient use of resources in an uncoordinated system. Money spent on health was not wasted: rather, it was productive, since it bought 'not only release from the frustration and pain of ill-health, but also fullness of life, new strength for new endeavour'. Summing up, *National Service for Health* claimed that:

> In the interests of the nation's health, vigour and happiness; in the interests of true economy; in the interests of the medical profession as well as the interests of the sick, the Labour Party appeals to every citizen to support this great reform – the organisation of a National Service for Health.[15]

As suggested, SMA members felt a considerable sense of achievement over the publication of *National Service for Health* and the passing of the associated conference resolution. Hastings reminded delegates that some ten years previously the same assembly had endorsed an Association motion on a state medical service. Now an 'excellent' health policy statement had been published, and the psychological moment had arrived for the working class movement to press for a scheme providing 'a health service such as people like myself ... have dreamed of for many years, but which we, perhaps, never hoped to see'. This gaining of the psychological initiative, especially given the rallying of medical reaction, was also stressed by H.B. Morgan. It was important, he argued, to pass the resolution unanimously as 'our opponents are gathering their battalions to undermine the Beveridge Report by concentrating their opposition on the medical service and trying to prevent its adoption'. Edith Summerskill, demanding the abolition of the profit motive in medicine and the institution of a salaried service, went on to urge Labour members of the coalition government to 'reject a Conservative interpretation of Assumption B'.[16]

The sense of an impending fight against socialised medicine's actual and potential opponents was also evident in a party guide to *National Service for Health*, which devoted considerable attention to arguments which might be used against a state system, and how they could be countered. Similarly *MTT*, in an editorial welcoming the policy statement, denounced the 'hysteria of BMA meetings' whipped up against 'ideas which neither the Ministry of Health, the Socialist Medical Association, nor the Labour Party have suggested'. The piece continued that the 'true basis of the struggle will become increasingly clear' as the introduction of legislation drew closer.[17] The need to keep pressing the case for its vision of a socialised service is further exemplified by an Association delegation in November 1943 to the body on which it already exerted considerable influence, the PHAC. The delegation expressed full support for *National Service for Health*, but sought to emphasise three points as requiring particular attention: first, the need for a unified system of control; second, the danger of extending the panel system; and, third, the need to abolish the dual hospital system. As we saw in the previous chapter, the Association was to make these same points to Attlee three days later, and they also formed the basis of an SMA memorandum to the parliamentary Labour Party in January

1944. The delegation further expressed the view that 'the Government's programme was unlikely to provide a *full* national health service'. However no 'temporary expedients' should be adopted which might 'prejudice the later achievement of a full service'.[18]

The 1944 White Paper

By late 1943 the SMA was in a mood of anticipation and optimism, tempered by an awareness that the battle was not yet won. While the Labour Party appeared to have been largely converted to its ideas, nonetheless it was only part of a coalition government. Outside the party, furthermore, the forces of medical and political 'reaction' were preparing for a fight. The Association's position was summarised early in 1944, that is on the eve of the publication of the government's White Paper, by its next policy statement, *A Socialised Health Service*. Once again, questions of administration and of professional control received considerable emphasis. It was acknowledged, for example, that local government reorganisation was badly needed, and that 'regionalisation' might provide a way round existing problems. It was also suggested that the 'administration of a nationwide medical service requires at least three levels of control'. These were the national, where strategic planning would take place; the local, where the national plan could be modified in the light of local conditions, and which would be democratically controlled; and (confusingly) an administrative layer which would leave doctors 'to a large extent in control of the services as they affect the individual patient'. These possible complications notwithstanding, the service should be unified and subject to a national plan, comprehensive, and open to all.[19]

This document was, in turn, based on a memorandum submitted to the Ministry of Health late in 1943 which had acknowledged that the 'delegation of powers' within a socialised system was 'probably democracy's greatest difficulty', something of an understatement. The doctor's position had to be established from the outset, albeit within 'the normal democratic framework of this country'. Such a structure was, crucially, clearly distinguishable from

> the corporate body of the Fascist state with its professional supremacy; the totalitarian with all power in the hands of the Nazified 'State'; and the bureaucratic in which control is in the hands of a special class.

Full democracy was to be exerted especially at the regional level. At the most local level, that of the 'health unit', and here only, 'professional and vocational control are essential'. Even so, it was envisaged that lay bodies would emerge to 'advise the technical and professional staffs'. Such a development should, however, be spontaneous rather than imposed by statute, and derive from the 'people's educated desire for health'. Most important of all was that 'administration should be a vital and living thing; and that all trace of bureaucracy, red-tape and lack of freedom should be rigidly excluded'.[20] As we saw in the last chapter, this organic analogy was also used by Murray in *The Future of Medicine*, and was integral to the Association's view of an activist citizenry in a participatory democracy.

This was one of the SMA's bravest and most sustained efforts to reconcile professional status and democratic control, although as a comparison between the memorandum and its later published version clearly shows, even here its efforts remained, ultimately, highly problematic. The memorandum is also significant in its clear attempt to distance itself from bureaucratic forms of state medicine. The 'strong' version of this was the medical corporations of fascist Italy, the 'weaker' version the claim made, most notably by the BMA and the Conservative Party, that schemes such as those of the SMA would reduce doctors to civil servants. This was a point of some concern to the SMA throughout the war. Bourne claimed in October 1941 that state medicine was neither good nor bad in itself. What would determine its worth was the use to which it was put, and it was undeniably present in Nazi Germany just as it was, more positively, in the Soviet Union. State medicine's value, therefore, 'depends essentially on the political system within which it operates'. What was needed in Britain were fundamental changes in every aspect of social and political life.[21] Once again, we can see here how the wartime experience focused and refined Association ideas.

Some of the SMA's fears, as expressed in policy documents and in various committees and meetings, appeared to be borne out with the publication in February 1944 of the government's long-awaited White Paper on the future of the health services. This had already been the subject of considerable criticism by Labour members on the government's own Reconstruction Committee – we noted in Chapter Seven the reservations in Attlee's office at the time of his meeting with an Association delegation – and the final version was seen as a rather unsatisfactory compromise.[22] SMA members too were acutely aware of what they saw as the document's shortcomings. In a memorandum prepared for the PHAC, Hastings argued that its proposals were 'better than nothing', and should not be opposed by the Labour Party. On the other hand, there should be no weakening of 'the present compromise'. Hastings predicted that the White Paper would be attacked by the voluntary hospitals, the BMA, 'and the Tories generally', all of whom would attempt to further subvert the suggested scheme. As to the existing proposals, Hastings pointed out that they failed to press for the unification of services. If implemented as it stood, the White Paper would result in 'the general practitioners under Whitehall, hospitals and consultants under the Joint Board, and clinics and preventive services under the major local authority'. There would be a tripartite system of administration, and so the SMA aim of integrating services would not be achieved. A not dissimilar administrative structure was to be set up by the 1946 Act and, as we shall see, was one cause of Association disillusionment with Bevan's scheme. Murray too was prepared to acknowledge the White Paper's significance while pointing out its drawbacks. At a meeting in October 1944 he argued that the document envisaged 'the finest possible service for all', but also suggested the continuance of private practice. 'What', he rhetorically demanded, 'would they say if the police or the fire service were run on these lines?'. It is clear from other parts of his speech that Murray here detected (and he was right to do so) a concession to the BMA.[23]

Nonetheless the Association was, like most of the rest of the labour movement, ultimately determined to put as positive a gloss as possible on the White Paper and to counter the arguments of its opponents. Indeed, the civil servant John Pater later contrasted the radicalism of *National Service for Health* with the Association's willingness to accept the more equivocal official document. The *Bulletin* claimed that the White Paper's publication was a 'pivotal point in the history of British medicine'. Consequently it was the duty of all SMA members to make themselves conversant with its proposals, and its relationship to *A National Service for Health* and *A Socialised Health Service*. As well as this, members should use such comparisons to put forward suitable resolutions at professional, trade union, and Labour Party meetings, and letters should be sent to both the medical and the lay press. All this was to combat the vested interests, 'both professional and general financial', which would seek to maintain the current position. *Medicine Today and Tomorrow* also welcomed the White Paper, albeit with considerable reservations. It also noted, without any obvious irony, that nowhere did the official text acknowledge that 'it has clearly drawn on material that first appeared in these pages'.[24]

All this suggests, quite correctly, that from the outset the Association was quick to realise the White Paper's significance. Within three hours of its publication, Hastings called a press conference attended by 11 journalists at which a statement was issued on the organisation's position. At the EC meeting at which this was announced and endorsed it was also agreed to produce a leaflet and speakers' notes for SMA members, and to draft a motion for Labour Party conference. The leaflet attributed the White Paper's weaknesses to the need for compromise 'inherent in Coalition government', and reiterated the concerns expressed by Hastings to the PHAC, including that on hospital unification. This last point was also picked up by Summerskill, Haden-Guest, and Morgan, MPs as well as SMA members, in the Commons. Nonetheless there was much to welcome. The extension of health insurance had been rejected, and the principle of universal provision of care accepted. All this was a 'great step forward'. Assuming the government meant what it said, and was concerned to pursue the Atlantic Charter's call for 'freedom from want', then 'we may yet build up a system in which health is possible for all and medical care is sufficient to maintain it'.[25]

The EC resolution for party conference was, with one minor modification, proposed by Murray on the SMA's behalf. This too welcomed the White Paper, with reservations, and urged the labour movement to press for changes to bring it in line with *National Service for Health*. Talking to his motion, Murray argued that failure to support the official document would allow opponents to erode its proposals, so making it unworkable. Opposition from the medical profession was 'reaction at its very worst', with 'Harley St.' developing a new definition of democracy – 'Government of the people, for the doctors, by the doctors'. BMA conference, he continued, had attacked local government 'in a way reminiscent of Mussolini'. Rhetorically stimulating as this was, Murray's characteristic abrasiveness was hardly likely to win over vacillating professional colleagues, and was in contrast to the tone adopted in *National Service for Health*. Nonetheless, on the NEC's behalf Barbara Ayrton Gould accepted the SMA motion, which was subsequently carried unanimously, adding that Murray, although he had not himself mentioned it, 'had a great deal to do with the drafting' of Labour's health policy.[26]

The SMA and medical 'reaction'

We have already noted Brooke's view that it was in 1943 that the SMA reached the peak of its influence. Clearly, however, and as the 1944 conference attests, the Association continued to play a crucial role in the formation of Labour health policy.[27] This is therefore an appropriate point at which to begin to assess the SMA as the war drew to a close, and as plans for post-war reconstruction were increasingly part of the national political agenda. In 1944 membership was officially recorded as 1200, nearly double the figure of the previous year and making the Association Labour's second largest affiliated organisation after the Fabian Society. This was the beginning of a membership expansion which was to peak at 2000 during the passing and implementation of the 1946 NHS Act, before declining thereafter. As Murray later recalled, in 1944 over 29 branches and groups were active, with propaganda literature being produced both locally and nationally.[28] The organisation was, therefore, vigorous, and participating in labour movement politics in a variety of situations, from local meetings to national policy making bodies.

But by 1944, as closer and closer detail became essential in the articulation of plans for a future health service, it was evident that having the Association's vision of a socialised service fully accepted was not going to be a straightforward task. This operated on a number of levels. For one thing, and as Murray's conference comments suggest, any radicalism which the BMA may have exhibited in the MPC Interim Report was now long since forgotten. The BMA was resolutely hostile to the White Paper, despite the evidence of its own survey that certain sections of the medical profession were a good deal more sympathetic than the official line.[29] This point was pursued relentlessly by the SMA, and we noted in the last chapter Joules's claim that the BMA leadership was, essentially, an ageing and reactionary clique.

However true this might have been, the BMA was not going to take matters lying down, and part of its response involved attacks on the SMA. This was presumably unsurprising to the Association, given its repeated warnings about the forces of medical reaction and the kind of language individuals such as Murray were prepared to use about professional colleagues. The debates around the White Paper clearly illustrate the antagonism between the two organisations. Early in 1944, for instance, Murray and Charles Hill of the BMA took part in a heated radio discussion broadcast to no doubt bemused United States service personnel. Murray's opening statement outlined the SMA position, concluding that he strongly believed in a salaried service. Hill, in reply, accused Murray of not understanding the doctor-patient relationship, as he was a pathologist. This not especially enlightening remark was countered by one equally irrelevant from Murray, that Hill was a bureaucrat who did not see patients either.[30] Fatuous as all this was, it does show the feelings now being aroused by the prospect of some form of state health service. Hill's willingness to publicly discuss health service issues with overtly socialist individuals such as Murray (and we encountered Hill in the last chapter in a radio debate with Bourne) certainly suggests that the BMA took the Association 'threat' seriously. This in turn led, according to Harry Eckstein, to its making a particularly bizarre allegation.

In the wake of the White Paper's publication the BMA leadership sought to establish its members' views by means of a 'Questionary'.

This survey's result, as Webster points out, supported the leadership line in general, but was 'scarcely a gesture of unrestrained approval'. The SMA analysis was even more sceptical. As Murray put it, to count on the

> political ignorance and conservatism of any group of citizens in times of great social disturbance, such as war, may be to produce a set of answers which are diametrically opposed to those the questioner expects.

Such, he continued, was the BMA Council's fate. The government, however, had been given a 'clear signal' by the profession that it could 'safely proceed with its National Health Service'. This was grossly over-optimistic. The BMA leadership was certainly given an unexpected shock by the results. Equally, however, Murray's claim that the answers on the principles involved in a socialised service had been so favourably received that 'not even the most violent reactionaries within the BMA can have any hope left of influencing national policy' was somewhat wide of the mark.[31] Even assuming the BMA leadership was prepared to abdicate, which it was not, there is little evidence that the mass of GPs in particular sought the kind of service put forward by Murray and his colleagues. The point made earlier about an expanding membership notwithstanding, Murray's comments may reflect his organisation's metropolitan bias, rather than the mood among the medical profession nationwide.

This incident is cited by Honigsbaum as a key instance of Murray's misreading of medical opinion in the 1940s, and will be one more factor in our ultimate assessment of the SMA. For present purposes, however, what is important is the response of the BMA leadership to the survey's results. According to Eckstein, this involved the suggestion that its members had not fully understood the White Paper's implications, and that the SMA had 'stuffed the ballot boxes'.[32] It is difficult to substantiate Eckstein's claim, but it is both plausible and illuminating in the context of the libel action brought by the BMA against Association members over alleged ballot-rigging, discussed in the next chapter.

A further instance of the medical establishment's approach came in October 1944, when the *BMJ* launched an attack on so-called 'dissident doctors'. Noting the SMA's activities, and accepting that its members' views, although those of a 'vociferous minority', were sincerely held, the journal nonetheless went on to make a number of critical points. A large number of doctors, it suggested, were equally convinced that 'the introduction of doctrinaire politics into medicine is doing untold harm to a profession which has never held it to be its duty to act as political proselytizers'. Moreover Association members, while 'parading the fact that they are members of the BMA', were not content to work within the latter organisation in a democratic manner. The article also found it 'disquieting' that at a time of an acute shortage of doctors, some were 'prepared to spend time, money, and paper in fomenting political activity and indeed in directing it'. Not surprisingly, given its staggering hypocrisy, this prompted a flurry of correspondence. Much of this was from SMA members disputing the points raised, but it is also notable that non-members criticised the double standards the *BMJ* appeared to be operating.[33] What is clear, though, is that the medical profession's more conservative members were taking the SMA seriously, almost certainly because of its influence on Labour Party thinking. They were thus prepared to attack the Association at any opportunity, and willing to raise the political temperature in their efforts to forestall a state medical service.

Differences on the Left over health policy

It has been argued in this and the previous chapter that the Association had important successes in the first five years of the war. It has been further suggested that, partly as a result of these achievements, its relationship with one of the main professional bodies was increasingly acrimonious. But it is also the case that there were differences within the labour movement – and indeed within the Association itself – over health service reorganisation; and that the Labour leadership, as the war drew to an end and a general election became imminent, took over more and more health policy formulation at the expense of the influence which the SMA had previously been able to exert. A small but telling instance of this came in the summer of 1944, when Hastings reported to his EC that Labour was soon to bring out a document on the proposed national health service 'very much on the lines of SMA policy'. He was going to seek the leadership's agreement, he continued, that this be a joint Labour Party/SMA publication. Although the way in which this decision was reached is not entirely clear, the EC noted a few months later that after discussion with the party 'our representatives had agreed that the pamphlet should be published by the Labour Party only'.[34]

It is necessary, therefore, to look at some of the less positive aspects of the Association's position in the post-Beveridge era, beginning with the fourteenth Nuffield College Reconstruction Conference. Held in late March 1944, this dealt specifically with the reorganisation of the health services.[35] It was attended by just under 100 people representing a broad spectrum of opinion and including prominent SMA members

Hastings, Churchill, Joules, Murray, and Sayle. The Nuffield gatherings were not open to the public, and the Health Conference chairman John Ryle stressed that everyone could speak freely. The contributions of Association members were for the most part along familiar lines. A particularly optimistic approach was taken by Murray, who suggested that the White Paper would make medicine 'a social science', and that while it did not 'usher in a millennium ... it was possible to plan for a millennium, and to do so was necessary for its achievement'.

But although SMA members generally pursued similar approaches, there were differences of emphasis both as compared with previous pronouncements and between individuals. Hastings, discussing the ever-vexing matter of administrative control, claimed that the Ministry of Health was capable of supervision 'but not of direct administration'. So in a unified service, the only possible options were 'the new Joint Board or the existing local authority, and he felt the former was much to be preferred'. Of course Hastings had for some time acknowledged the need for local government reorganisation, probably through regionalisation – hence, presumably, his lack of enthusiasm for the idea of the '*existing* local authority' (my emphasis). Nonetheless, his apparent favouring of a 'Joint Board', something which his organisation had previously been not at all keen upon, comes as something of a surprise.

Stella Churchill too seemed to want the best of both administrative worlds. Pointing out that she had been both an employer and an employee on local authorities – specifically the LCC – she concluded that there was in such bodies a considerable wastage of time: consequently a 'democratic system was necessary, giving medical representation on local authorities and on the Central Advisory Board. Far more professional representatives were needed in the new health service'. To this rather curious view of democracy was counterposed the 'purer' version of Joules, who argued that on many issues 'the layman had a broader vision ... than the doctor'. It was therefore necessary to proceed to the 'democratic organisation of the whole of the health services', and those involved should 'consider themselves as an integral part of a team'. Joules also felt that the problems over local authority boundaries had been exaggerated, and that these would disappear with the introduction of a 'universal and enforceable optimum'.[36]

The point here is not to ridicule the inconsistencies in Association pronouncements, or the differences between its various activists. Rather, it is to recognise that on the political left, as elsewhere, envisaging a new health service was no easy task, and one subject to disagreements, debates, and the vagaries of personal experience. This, as we have already seen, came into the open in forums such as the MPC and in the sometimes confused documents and statements of the Association and its individual members. An important area of contention was, as has become evident, local authority control, among whose Association critics were Brook and Stephen Taylor, and it is here appropriate to say something more about the latter.

Taylor was involved not only with the Labour Party, which he appears to have formally joined only in 1943, but also with a group of young, radical members of the medical profession, Medical Planning Research, which produced an 'Interim Report' late in 1942. Stressing its 'scientific' basis, this challenged the efficacy of democratic control, local or national, of any future reformed health service. Rather, it recommended 'a statutorily appointed public corporation, subject to periodical parliamentary review, with its governors directly elected by ministers of the Crown', a proposal strikingly similar to that of Taylor himself in 1939 and discussed in the preceding chapter. Significantly, the bibliography appended to this Report cited health analyses by bodies such as PEP, but not the SMA. Taylor was clearly well thought of by the Labour leadership. We noted in the last chapter his authorship of a memorandum for Attlee for the Reconstruction Priorities Committee, and archival evidence makes it clear that he was in close contact with Evan Durbin, the Deputy Prime Minister's assistant and one of his principal admirers.[37]

Taylor expanded on his views in his book of 1944, *The Battle for Health*, published after the White Paper and a work whose title was later adopted by the SMA for its travelling exhibition on the NHS. As is suggested by the title, this work again made extensive use of military metaphor. Taylor stressed that 'we in Britain believe in individual freedom, in government by consent, and in the democratic process'. Nonetheless he was not at pains to extend this to health service administration. He remarked that, at present, most health functions were carried out through local authorities, 'some big, some small; some efficient, some inefficient'. But in any future service, planning was essential, and the medium through which this was to be done was 'area health planning', such areas of necessity being larger than most existing local authorities – another version of regionalisation. In this, and in the accompanying diagram, there was no sense that the resulting administrative bodies were to be democratically controlled. Finally Taylor, rather disingenuously, claimed that the question of whether 'doctors should be employed by a Corporation, a medical board, local authorities, or universities' was irrelevant.[38] It was not 'irrelevant' to, for example, the SMA or the BMA.

In September 1944 a document, 'The Health Services White Paper: The Labour Party's Policy', was presented to the PHAC. The authorship of this text is not clear, but as will become evident its arguments corresponded closely to those of Taylor. The unsuitability of existing local government boundaries for a future health service was stressed, and in their place 'new large health areas' were advocated. It was agreed that public money should be spent only by publicly accountable bodies, but this did not necessarily mean that 'the elected representatives themselves must directly control all such bodies'. What was important was that control should not be in the hands of 'vested interests'. The BBC and the universities were cited approvingly as models of public administration, although at other points more direct democratic control was also proposed.[39] Whoever the author, and Taylor must be a strong candidate, what is important here is the further example of diversity of opinion on the political left over future medical reorganisation.

Taylor was, of course, only one individual, albeit an increasingly influential one. How, then, did other interests within the labour movement see the future of health policy by this stage of the war? The SMA was highly conscious of the need to organise against what it saw as the forces of medical reaction. But it was also aware of the need to monitor the pronouncements of fellow socialists. In May 1943, for example, the EC noted that the journal *New Statesman and Nation* was taking a 'very reactionary attitude on medical organisation', and that its arguments were being quoted in the Commons by 'reactionary speakers'. The journal's editor was approached with a view to receiving an SMA delegation, an offer he declined, certainly once and possibly twice. However an article by Hastings – 'The Doctors and the Beveridge Report' – appeared the following September, optimistically asserting that 'doctors will certainly make many protests, but, in my opinion, if the conditions offered them are fair and reasonable the majority will be ready to accept service'.[40] It is significant, however, that the SMA felt obliged to question the journal's stance in the first place.

More crucial, though, was the approach of one of the labour movement's most powerful institutions, the TUC. Historically more concerned with industrial workers' wages and conditions than with social reform, nonetheless the TUC had previously become involved in health policy through, for example, its discussions from the late 1930s onwards with the BMA. It was also a constituent part of bodies such as the Joint Medical Sub-Committee, composed of representatives of the Labour Party and the Cooperative Party, as well as of the TUC itself. In the wake of the MPC and Beveridge this committee, whose party representatives included Murray and Hastings, held an intense debate over the form of any future health service, much of this revolving around MPU policy statements.

The principle area of disagreement was over the question of administration, with the MPU adamantly opposed to any form of local authority

control. In one particularly revealing exchange of letters, the MPU's
Alfred Welply suggested that so long as

> the TUC insists (if it does insist) upon the Labour Party view that
> democracy requires that elected councils should have supreme and
> undisputed authority in all matters with which they have to deal, it
> is little use trying to reach a working agreement.

In reply, the Secretary of the TUC's Social Insurance Department, J.L.
Smyth, assured Welply that 'the General Council have not made up
their minds as between your view and that of the Labour Party'. Even
though the MPU did eventually somewhat modify its stance, correspondence between the Labour Party and the TUC in October 1943
shows Hastings still unable to accept the MPU position.[41]

At precisely this time, the TUC submitted a memorandum to the
Ministry of Health. This stressed the need for a unified national health
service, comprehensive and freely available to all, and for a shift towards preventive medicine. But no mention was made of a salaried
service. Similarly, although it was suggested that, in respect of administrative structures, there should be powers of delegation to regional and
'further to local representative bodies', the document also sought central administration and coordination 'through a Government Department
– the Ministry of Health – responsible to Parliament'. Overall, therefore, the service should be 'uniform in all parts of the country'. In turn,
this reflected the TUC's decision in 1942 in favour of a centrally run
hospital system.[42] The principal issue here is that while the TUC undoubtedly desired a state medical service, and while its position was in
general terms compatible with current Labour Party policy, nonetheless
the administrative details were of less importance to it than the actual
provision of services themselves. The possibility remained, and was
implicitly favoured, of a national rather than a devolved system. As we
shall see below, this also put the TUC in a position to be much more
sensitive to the demands of the majority of the medical profession than
the SMA.

In response to the White Paper the TUC created a small sub-committee, which produced its initial findings in early March 1944. Like the
rest of the labour movement, the sub-committee saw the government's
proposals as both flawed and a great step forward. On the crucial
question of control, however, little was said other than to note that the
proposed Central Medical Board would be primarily composed of doctors. The reasons behind this were appreciated, but it was suggested
that 'similar arrangements should be made for other workers'. Nothing
was said, in other words, about democratic control at either local or
regional level.[43] Later the same month the Labour Party's Policy

Committee noted a suggestion from the TUC that a joint committee consisting of representatives of itself, the Cooperative movement, and the party be set up to examine the White Paper's policy implications. The party's nominees to this body were Hastings, Murray, Barbara Ayrton Gould, Percy Collick, and Morgan Phillips. The first two were prominent SMA members. But the others were not, so that even in terms of the party's representation Association members were in a minority. This was even more the case on the committee as a whole. Although SMA strength was enhanced by H.B. Morgan, the TUC's medical advisor, he was in an ambiguous position, and overall those attached to the Association constituted at most one-third of the body.[44]

Of course one way of interpreting this would be to argue that the very fact of having representation at all was testimony to the SMA's role in Labour's health policy formation. Nor were the Association's plans for a socialised service rejected wholesale. On the contrary, the text produced by the joint committee, and unanimously agreed by its members, emphasised a number of points central to the Association case. The White Paper's recognition of the need for health centres, for example, was praised, just as that document's failure to recommend a unified hospital system was deprecated. On matters such as private practice and administration the sub-committee was, nonetheless, more equivocal. While stating the usual aim of medical care as a wholly public service, it also allowed the right of individuals to opt for, and doctors to provide, private treatment. Regarding hospitals, it suggested these be integrated on the basis of 'natural hospital regions', whose boundaries 'should not be co-terminus with the boundaries of existing local authorities'. Overall, the service as a whole should be 'subject to proper democratic control', although precisely what this meant was not made especially clear. The proposal for a Central Medical Board primarily representing medical interests was noted but not remarked upon; and, similarly, little comment was made regarding the suggested Statutory Central Health Services Council, to be set up to advise the Minister of Health, save that it should consult with all professional interests involved.[45]

This document was clearly designed as a broad labour movement response to the White Paper and as such might be seen as understandably preoccupied with general principles rather than particular detail. But its significance for this study is that although the SMA certainly had a presence on the body which produced it, the Association did not hold a dominant position such as it had on the PHAC. This should be further placed in the context of the point made earlier, that the Labour leadership was more and more concerned to centralise policy formation; and that powerful forces within the labour movement, most notably the

TUC, were beginning to play an increasingly important role in these deliberations. So from an Association point of view, statements such as that on the White Paper issued at the annual Congress meeting in 1944 would have caused considerable anxiety. While again agreeing the necessity of a national health service, this also argued that for the scheme to be successful it should have the 'goodwill of the profession'. To this end, the 'circumstances peculiar to the profession' should be recognised, and there should be 'full consultation' with it on all relevant matters.[46] Given the TUC's ongoing relationship with the BMA, this must have seemed to the Association an unwarranted acknowledgement of the status of the leading reactionary 'vested interest' against which it was itself waging war.

It is abundantly evident from the records that the TUC's views on medical reorganisation were shaped not only by Labour Party policy and its own concerns – for example on industrial health – but also by wider influences. These included bodies such as the BMA and even the MPU, at the expense of the SMA. It was certainly prepared to look outside the labour movement. In May 1944 the General Secretary of the Fire Brigades Union suggested to the TUC that 'a conference could be organised, similar to that on Education, and the support of the Socialist Medical Association could be enlisted'. In reply, it was noted that while the TUC was discussing the White Paper with the Labour Party, 'to which the Socialist Medical Association is affiliated', and the Cooperative movement, it was also involved with the BMA through 'the Joint Committee which has been in existence for some years'.[47]

This coolness on the part of the TUC towards the SMA is more explicitly exemplified by the former's response to an invitation for a General Council representative to attend the Association conference on the national health service held in April 1945. The Social Insurance Committee felt that

> the invitation should not be accepted in view of the fact that the General Council were acting on behalf of all its affiliated organisations in this matter and would, if necessary, convene conferences to deal with it.[48]

As we shall see in the next chapter, this was not the last occasion on which the TUC declined support for an SMA-sponsored gathering. In short, therefore, the Association clearly had much greater problems in its relationship with the TUC than with, at least up until 1945, the Labour Party. The TUC, while committed to some form of state medical service, did not appear especially interested in the question of devolved democratic control in the way so characteristic of the SMA. One of its constituent organisations, the MPU, was hostile to any such form of administration. Rather more importantly, so too was the BMA, with whom the TUC had a long-standing if somewhat difficult and controversial working arrangement, and which was also opposed to any form of salaried service. The TUC was thus surprisingly accommodating to contemporary medical opinion, in a way that the SMA certainly was not. Given the TUC's position within the labour movement and the Labour Party, its attitude was clearly a large obstacle in the Association's path.

Another body with views on health service reorganisation was the influential Fabian Society. At the very beginning of the war R.B. Thomas, a prominent figure in Fabian social reform circles, suggested that recent plans for health service reform, 'drawn up by the Socialist Medical Association and others, have all been urban in conception and have taken little account of rural areas'. Furthermore, he continued, it was time that 'Socialist thought escaped from the metropolis and from the view that local government is a synonym for the LCC'.[49] This was a view not dissimilar to that we have already seen expressed by Lyster in his critique for the Fabian Society of a pamphlet by Hastings. There was, certainly, no hard and fast boundary between the two organisations – Murray, for example, was a member of the Fabian Medical Services Group. Dr Brian Thompson, another member of this body, put forward proposals for medical reorganisation in 1942, the vast majority of which would have been easily acceptable to the Association. These included a comprehensive and free service, with an end to the panel system; health centres; and a salaried service. On the question of control, Thompson recognised that with the war had come 'breakdowns of local government administration and their chaotic finances, with the irresistible trend towards regionalisation'. But in a future socialised service doctors would have to get used to a new type of discipline. The GPs' boss would be a 'Superintendent of Clinics', in turn responsible to a committee composed not only of medical practitioners, 'but also, and indeed predominantly, of lay members'. Although doctors were instinctively suspicious of lay control, they would come to recognise the justice of this arrangement whereby 'the public, as consumer of the service you give, has a voice in the provision of that service'. Municipal services had operated in this way for some time and had, when sensitive to appropriate medical advice, 'shown themselves to be good masters'.[50]

There were, however, powerful currents within the Fabian Society much more cautious about the way in which a socialised service should be implemented, exemplified by the document 'Principles of a Comprehensive Health Service', produced sometime in late 1943. Stressing that medicine was largely an 'art' (cf. Murray's comments to the Nuffield Conference cited above), and having warned against a sudden, wholesale takeover of hospitals and of medical staff, the key point was then made that since health was a national concern, so should it be dealt with nationally. The only 'rational' way in which this could be done was by central government assuming direct responsibility. Local interests must undoubtedly be acknowledged, but given the financial demands on a socialised service local authorities could at best be 'only ... Government Agents'. These bodies were, the document continued, 'fond of sneering at the insolvency and revenue raising methods of Voluntary Hospitals but their own position does not appear really any better'.

But it was not only financial problems which counted against local government administration of health services. The present behaviour of many local authorities was 'often petty, arrogant, vain, disrespectful when they should not be animated by a vulgar love of power'. Such was the power-hungry attitude of, for example, the recent speech by LCC leader Lord Latham, that many 'true socialists must have felt ashamed' on hearing it. Hence to hand over

> important national services too completely at the present time to local authorities is to hand them over to bodies that are in many instances at best described as Bourgeois and at worst are almost Fascist in their methods – and with petty corruption by no means always distant.

We have seen that SMA members such as Murray used anti-fascist and anti-corporatist arguments when advocating decentralised control. Here was a similar argument being used against just such an administrative structure, an argument with strong similarities to Taylor's comments on the potential for local government corruption. Lest it be thought that here was a prime instance of Fabian central planning, the document also urged that individual hospitals, although under Regional Health Councils, should be self-governing through 'lay and medical committees' in accordance with 'democratic principles as defined by G.D.H. Cole'. Health centres and GP teamwork too were to be encouraged, although the final goal of a salaried service should not be introduced immediately. Rather, if private practice was to die, it should do so 'gradually in a truly Fabian manner'.[51]

Once again, we can see that there were differences within the labour movement over the direction and content of any future health policy. It is consequently not surprising to find these being played out at the upper levels of the party. In 1943 discussions on the embryonic White Paper took place in the War Cabinet Committee on Reconstruction Priorities. At one of these the Labour minister Ernest Bevin, a powerful voice within the movement, suggested that *if* government proposals came down in favour of a health care system administered by local authorities, then certainly there should be democratic control. What should not happen was that any health service plans be delayed by local government reorganisation. At a previous meeting, when Morrison argued strongly for local authority control while stressing the potential dangers to local government of instituting large regional bodies, Bevin suggested that consideration might be given to the possibility of health service administration 'on a national basis, local interests being represented by means of advisory committees'.[52] The fluidity of views over medical reconstruction therefore found expression in the highest reaches of the Labour Party. The Reconstruction Committee deliberations also suggest that for some in the Labour leadership – as in the TUC, and these were of course overlapping groups – the actual creation of a service providing its consumers with comprehensive and free medical care was seen as more important than what might be considered relatively unimportant, or endlessly complicated, or potentially obstructive, administrative details.

The tensions between the somewhat pragmatic approach of important elements within the party leadership and the SMA's more 'purist' line can be seen in the conference between Thomas Johnston, Secretary of State for Scotland and Labour MP, and a delegation from the Association's Scottish section. This meeting took place at almost exactly the same time as that between Attlee and the SMA, discussed in the last chapter. It was, however, marked by a much greater degree of recorded disagreement, despite common ground on a large number of issues. The Secretary of State suggested, for example, that it might take time to provide health centres, given potential shortages of staff and materials. By contrast Dr Lipetz, SMA Scottish secretary, argued that health centres were vital and that 'after the war buildings and equipment would become readily available'. Johnston stressed that he was concerned not to coerce doctors into a full-time salaried service, and that he 'wished to develop the present services and so make the comprehensive service practicable'. Lipetz, on the other hand, emphasised his opposition to capitation fees for doctors employed at health centres, as this would lead to competition between them. Johnston thought this 'not wholly true', and that a limited system of capitation payments might be possible. The Scottish Association members also showed the over-optimism to which the Association was prone, with the Scottish section chairman, Dr Dunlop, claiming that 90 per cent of medical practitioners would accept a salaried service if the salary was sufficient.[53]

The SMA at the end of the war

Health care reform was, therefore, a highly contested field, both in general and within the labour movement. There is no doubt that the SMA was aware of this, and of the need for vigilance if its plans were to be in any way realised. The difficulty of the task facing the Association in having its proposals fully accepted had certainly become all too apparent. One further problem was that the Labour Party body over which it had exerted considerable influence, the PHAC, appears to have effectively ceased to exist by the end of 1944 – more evidence that policy-making was being centralised in the party. Medical reaction too was fighting back, and of particular concern was the revelation that the Conservative Minister of Health, Henry Willink, had been conducting secret negotiations with the BMA and apparently making fundamental concessions on matters such as the sale of practices.[54] These negotiations were the subject of extensive comment in *MTT*. In December 1944 the journal noted that early in the war, its most stressful period, the BMA had initiated the Medical Planning Commission and that the 'Conservative-dominated coalition proposed a complete nation-wide service controlled by the representatives of the people'. Now that the war was going Britain's way, however, the Conservatives were reverting to plans for insurance – 'a possible let-out for capitalism and private enterprise' – while the medical profession had revealed itself as adhering to 'a form of Fascist-Individualism which is the negation of democracy and a denial of the centuries-old ethics of medicine'.[55] As we have had cause to comment before, such language could hardly have endeared the Association to many of the doctors whom it was trying to win over. It is also in marked contrast to the conciliatory approach of the TUC.

The next edition of *MTT* nonetheless continued to pursue a confrontational course. No doubt with the *BMJ*'s 'dissident doctors' revelations in mind, it remarked that certain sections of the medical profession had previously deemed politics 'a dirty business'. Now, however, some of the strongest advocates of this argument were 'indulging in political activity which if not shady is at least sharp'. The principal culprit here was

> that great non-political organisation, the British Medical Association, trying by secret political negotiations to dictate the fate of our democracy and the whole timetable of medical advance.

Here, then, was the principal 'vested interest' conducting negotiations, apparently successfully, with a member of the party to which it was politically most closely aligned, the Conservatives. In such circumstances, progressive and democratic forces had to be vigilant and to fight back –

failure to do so might result in the 'altering of the whole basis of democracy as we have known it'. One further consequence of these negotiations was, an Association internal memorandum claimed, that they had precipitated a Tory attack on local government 'in an effort to delay and prevent all social advance which threatens privilege'.[56]

The Association itself was not prepared to let any of this happen without a fight. At a meeting organised by the SMA and held on 15 April 1945 – the meeting to which, as we have seen, the TUC declined to send an official delegate – a resolution was unanimously passed calling for the White Paper's immediate implementation. The government, still at this point the wartime coalition, was urged to resist those blocking social progress 'because they are not prepared to give up their positions of privilege'. This was a clear reference to the BMA, as was the objection made to the Health Minister negotiating with 'an interested organisation on which the public are not represented, on principles already approved of by the House of Commons'. In this period, Kevin Jefferys argues, health policy became for the first time during the war a 'source of political controversy', with the Minister of Reconstruction later recalling the very considerable differences there would have been between a Conservative national health service and that actually introduced by Labour.[57] This is an important argument, and certainly an indication of the rising political temperature of the time. But it is worth stressing the SMA's repeated warnings, especially post-Beveridge, over the strategy of socialised medicine's opponents.

The following month the Association raised the negotiations issue at party conference. Murray, the SMA delegate, proposed a long motion with seven basic points: public accountability for public expenditure; local authority control over municipal hospitals and medical services; an end to the 'panel'; local authority control over health centres; abolition of the sale of practices; medical education to be free to all suitable candidates, irrespective of sex; and integration of the NHS with other welfare reforms. Hence the government, that is the caretaker Conservative government, should immediately implement 'nothing less than the proposals of the White Paper as a basis for a comprehensive health service'. Regret was expressed that the Health Minister was considering 'radical alterations in the scheme violating democratic principles and sacrificing the health of the people to the vested interests of the medical profession', another instance of the SMA's repeated hostility to what it considered the anti-democratic agenda of medical reaction.[58]

Murray's speech provoked no dissent and, indeed, little discussion. The only other major contribution came from fellow Association member Summerskill, replying on behalf of the NEC. Like Murray, she objected to the secret negotiations between Willink and the BMA as well as refuting medical and Conservative claims that Labour sought to deny professional freedom. On the contrary, clinical freedom would be enhanced by the kind of system Labour supported, another longstanding SMA assertion. Summerskill also paid a warm tribute to the Association's activities. It seemed only a few years ago, she reminisced, that 'half a dozen of us used to sit in a very small room at a time when a Socialist doctor was looked upon as an eccentric and an untouchable'. In particular she praised the April meeting, which had attracted 600 delegates. Murray's motion was duly carried.[59]

This party conference success must have been something of a boost for the SMA. While its grip on party health policy was not what it had been two years earlier, it was clearly still able to command support for its plans for a socialised service, and the 1945 resolution can be seen as a further official endorsement of these. There was still, apparently, everything to play for during the coming election and, hopefully, a consequent Labour administration. *Medicine Today and Tomorrow* captured this mood when it suggested that the summer of 1945 'may well mark the turning point in the history of this country and, if this is so, in the history of the whole world'. Whatever way the election went, it would have repercussions in all areas, and perhaps especially in health since 'the medical service is one which comes so close to the people'.[60]

Differences within the labour movement notwithstanding, the SMA retained the advantages of having a relatively coherent plan; the professional and administrative experience to speak authoritatively on medical matters; and, most importantly, a number of years of close involvement in party policy making. It had also received at least some measure of official recognition, as a Ministry of Health memorandum of February 1944 illustrates. This document listed the organisations and institutions with whom negotiations would take place over a future health service. As in 1943, these were primarily the BMA, the local authorities, the Royal Colleges, and so on. However a further category – organisations which would 'have to be heard', but not through 'continuous "negotiation"' – included the TUC, the MPU, and the SMA.[61] In all these circumstances, how did the Association's aspirations fare under the post-war Labour government?

Notes

1. Public Health Advisory Committee (Unclassified), File 2, Minutes of the Public Health Advisory Committee, 27 March and 13 May 1941.
2. The committee's change in status is noted in Labour Party Central Committee on Reconstruction (Unclassified), Minutes of the Second Meeting

of the Special Sub-Committee of the Central Committee, 10 September 1941; Brooke, *Labour's War*, p. 139.

3. Public Health Advisory Committee (Unclassified), File 3, Minutes of the Public Health Sub-Committee, 14 November, 4 December, 10 December 1941; and File 2, Minutes of the Public Health Advisory Committee 24 June 1941; Labour Party Central Committee on Reconstruction (Unclassified), Minutes of the Central Committee on Reconstruction Problems, 16 September 1942.

4. Labour Party Central Committee on Reconstruction (Unclassified), Minutes of the Thirteenth Meeting of the Labour Party Central Committee on Reconstruction Problems, 19 and 20 December 1942; Public Health Advisory Committee (Unclassified), File 3, Minutes of the Public Health Sub-Committee, 24 November 1942.

5. Brooke, *Labour's War*, p. 167.

6. Labour Party Central Committee on Reconstruction (Unclassified), Minutes of the Thirteenth Meeting of the Labour Party Central Committee on Reconstruction Problems, 19 and 20 December 1942.

7. Public Health Advisory Committee (Unclassified), File 3, Minutes of the Public Health Sub-Committee, 24 November 1942 and 15 January 1943; Labour Party, *National Service for Health*, Labour Party, 1943; Labour Party, *Report of the Forty-Second Annual Conference*, Labour Party, 1943, p. 146; Brooke, *Labour's War*, p. 143.

8. Public Health Advisory Committee (Unclassified), File 3, Minutes of the Public Health Sub-Committee, 8 July 1943; Murray, *Why a National Health Service?*, p. 61.

9. DSM (2) 4, David Stark Murray, 'Beveridge and Health', *Labour Monthly*, April 1943.

10. Labour Party, *National Service for Health*, pp. 2–4.

11. Ibid., pp. 4–12, 16–22.

12. Ibid., pp. 15–16.

13. Ibid., pp. 15, 12; Labour Party, *Report of the Forty-Second Annual Conference*, Labour Party, 1943, p. 145.

14. Labour Party, *National Service for Health*, pp. 15, 12.

15. Ibid., pp. 23–4; on Murray's estimates, see *The Future of Medicine*, Ch. 9.

16. Labour Party, *Report of the Forty-Second Annual Conference*, Labour Party, 1943, pp. 144–5.

17. Labour Party, *Notes for Discussion Groups on National Service for Health*, Labour Party, 1943, pp. 9–12; *MTT*, vol. 4, no. 2, June 1943, p. 1.

18. Public Health Advisory Committee (Unclassified), File 2, Minutes of the Public Health Advisory Committee, 8 November 1943; DSM 1/30, SMA, 'The Essentials for Health: a Statement to the Parliamentary Labour Party, January 1944'.

19. SMA, *A Socialised Health Service*, SMA, 1944, pp. 3–4.

20. DSM 4/2, 'Administration of the Health Services: A Memorandum prepared by the Socialist Medical Association for presentation to the Minister of Health, October 1943'; see also 'Administration of the Health Services', *MTT*, vol. 4, no. 4, December 1943, pp. 3–14.

21. SMA, *Bulletin*, no. 37, October 1941, pp. 1–2.

22. Brooke, *Labour's War*, pp. 206–9; Webster, *The Health Services since the War*, pp. 52–3. For a review of the issues, see Martin Powell, 'The Forgotten Anniversary? An Examination of the 1944 White Paper, "A

National Health Service"', *Social Policy and Administration*, 28, 4, 1994, pp. 333–44.

23. Public Health Advisory Committee (Unclassified), File 2, Minutes of the Public Health Advisory Committee, 28 February 1944, with appended document 'Notes on the White Paper on the Health Services', by Somerville Hastings; DSM 2 (4), cutting from the *Berkshire Chronicle*, 27 October 1944.

24. Pater, *The Making of the National Health Service*, pp. 105–6; SMA, *Bulletin*, March/April 1944, pp. 1–2; MTT, vol. 4, no. 5, March Quarter 1944, p. 1; for the response of the rest of the labour movement, see Brooke, *Labour's War*, pp. 208–11.

25. DSM 1/6, EC Minutes 17 February 1944; SMA, *A National Health Service: the White Paper Examined: SMA Leaflet no. 3*, SMA, n.d., but 1944; Murray, *Why a National Health Service?*, p. 67.

26. Labour Party, *Report of the Forty-Third Annual Conference*, Labour Party, 1944, pp. 154–6.

27. Although see also Earwicker, thesis, p. 347 where he suggests that another aspect of the 1944 conference was the party's willingness to 'abandon the objective of a whole-time salaried service for the embrace of Willink's White Paper'. This is a valid point, but it is also the case that such a system remained official party policy.

28. For membership figures, see Labour Party Annual Reports for the appropriate years; Murray, *Why a National Health Service?*, pp. 65–6.

29. Webster, *Health Services since the War*, p. 57ff.

30. DSM 5/1, cutting from *London Calling*, no. 240, no date but early 1944.

31. Webster, *The Health Services since the War*, p. 61; MTT, vol. 4, no. 7, September Quarter 1944, pp. 3–4.

32. Honigsbaum, *Division in British Medicine*, pp. 285–6; Eckstein, *The English Health Service*, pp. 150–51.

33. *BMJ*, 1944, II, pp. 506–7, 540–41, 576–7, 608–10.

34. DSM 1/6, EC Minutes, 26 July and 4 October 1944. Nor is it entirely clear if this proposed pamphlet was ever actually published.

35. The background to these conferences can be found in Daniel Ritschel, 'The Making of Consensus: the Nuffield College Conferences during the Second World War', *Twentieth Century British History*, vol. 6, no. 3, 1995.

36. Fabian Papers, G59/7, Fourteenth Nuffield College Social Reconstruction Conference, 25–26 March 1944: Reorganisation of the Health Services in Great Britain, pp. 19, 36, 38, 39, 11.

37. Webster, *The Health Services since the War*, pp. 26–7; 'Medical Planning Research: Interim General Report', *Lancet*, 1942, II, p. 610; Piercy Papers, 8/20.

38. Stephen Taylor, *Battle for Health: A Primer of Social Medicine*, Nicholson and Watson, 1944, pp. 9, 113, 121, Chart XIII on 104–5, 121–2.

39. MSS/292/847/3.

40. DSM 1/6, EC Minutes, 6 May and 3 June 1943; DSH, File 11, 'Health/NHS', leaflet reprinted from *The New Statesman and Nation*, 4 September 1943.

41. MSS 292/847/2.

42. MH 77/73, 'Trades Union Congress: National Medical Service', 20 October 1943; Earwicker, thesis, p. 264.

43. Trades Union Congress, 'Report of Sub-Committee Appointed on 1 March to Examine the Government's White Paper on "A National Health Service"', in Public Health Advisory Committee (Unclassified), File 2.

44. Public Health Advisory Committee (Unclassified), File 2, Minutes of the Public Health Advisory Committee, 29 March 1944; Joint Committee of the TUC, the Labour Party and the Co-operative Congress on the Government White Paper 'A National Health Service', 5 September and 3 October 1944.

45. Public Health Advisory Committee (Unclassified), File 2, Joint Sub-Committee of the TUC, the Labour Party and the Co-operative Congress on the Government White Paper 'A National Health Service', pp. 2–4.

46. 'Trades Union Congress, Blackpool 1944: Government White Papers on Social Insurance: Government White Paper on A National Health Service', p. 9 – copy in MH 77/73.

47. MSS/292/847/2.

48. MSS/292/847/3.

49. R.B. Thomas, *The Health Services*, Fabian Society: Research Series No. 49, 1940, p. 3.

50. Brian Thompson, *A Letter to a Doctor*, Fabian Society: Fabian Letter No. 6, 1942, pp. 19, 12, and *passim*.

51. Fabian Papers, K10/5, 'Principles of a Comprehensive Health Service', pp. 1, 3–4, 7, 9–10, and *passim*.

52. MH 80/26, War Cabinet Committee on Reconstruction Priorities: Conclusions of a Meeting of the Committee held on 8 September 1943, and of a Meeting of the Committee held on 30 July 1943.

53. MH 80/26, 'Note of meeting with representatives of the Scottish Section of the Socialist Medical Association at St. Andrew's House on 17 September, 1943'.

54. Webster, *The Health Services since the War*, p. 71ff; for labour movement reaction, Brooke, *Labour's War*, p. 213.

55. *MTT*, vol. 4, no. 8, December 1944, p. 1.

56. *MTT*, vol. 5, no. 1, March 1945; DSM 4/2, Socialist Medical Association, 'BMA and Ministry of Health "new proposals"', 10 April 1945.

57. *Lancet*, 1945, I, p. 605; Kevin Jefferys, 'British Politics and Social Policy During the Second World War', *Historical Journal*, 30, 1, 1987, pp. 135, 136.

58. Labour Party, *Report of the Forty-Fourth Annual Conference*, Labour Party, 1945, p. 138.

59. Ibid., pp. 139–40.

60. *MTT*, vol. 5, no. 2, June 1945, p. 1.

61. MH 80/27, memorandum 'Negotiations outside the office', February 1944.

CHAPTER NINE

'We Thought of It First': The SMA and the National Health Service

With victory in Europe came the end of the wartime coalition government, and Labour's subsequent landslide election victory in July 1945 at which 12 SMA members were returned to the Commons. Significantly, economic rather than social policy was emphasised during Labour's election campaign, yet another example of the social democratic dilemma over whether to prioritise economic change or social welfare aimed at ameliorating existing conditions.[1] The Labour governments of 1945 to 1951, led by Clement Attlee, were nonetheless to create some of the central institutions of the 'welfare state', including the NHS. This chapter's purpose is not to examine in detail the complicated negotiations between the Minister of Health, Bevan, and, in particular, the BMA over the shape of the NHS; nor Bevan's Cabinet battles with, most notably, Morrison. These have been more than adequately analysed and described elsewhere.[2] Rather, it examines the Association's activities in the post-war period, with particular emphasis on its critique of Bevan's scheme, enacted in 1946 and brought into operation on the so-called 'Appointed Day' in July 1948.

The basis of these doubts will become apparent as this chapter progresses but a sense of what these involved, in both the immediate and the longer term, is worth noting here. The SMA's press release on the day of the 1946 Bill's publication welcomed the proposed health service as 'far in advance of anything yet available in this country'. But it also claimed that Bevan had gone further than necessary in giving way to 'existing interests and institutions'. The Association pledged to support the Minister in resisting any further concessions, while expressing particular concern over doctors' remuneration and the proposed administrative structure.[3] This sense of unnecessary compromise, particularly with the BMA, remained, often expressing itself as regret for opportunities lost. In 1969, for example, MacWilliam wrote to Murray of 'the efforts we made to establish an efficient Health Service and the way we were reduced to impotence by Charles Hill and the Harley St. Consultants'. Murray himself, in a 1972 interview, suggested that it was 'time for Nye's compromise to be redeemed'. He had no doubt that Bevan 'allowed private practice within the NHS as a bribe', and that the Minister had openly and cynically spelt this out to Murray himself. But, he continued, this was clearly wrong in principle. Rather touchingly, in view of subsequent events, Murray suggested that one objection to private medical practice was that it employed 'public resources for private gain' in a way that nobody would think of applying to the railways or the Post Office.[4]

Bevan's National Health Service

However in order to contextualise the Association's critique, it is necessary to briefly examine the form the NHS took; and the organisation's relationship with Bevan, the politician commonly credited with the service's creation. Bevan's appointment as Health Minister was, at least outside the higher ranks of the Labour Party, unexpected. Civil servants had speculated on Ellen Wilkinson and Association member Edith Summerskill as prospective candidates. At the 1945 election Murray stood for parliament in the Richmond constituency. Commenting on his adoption, a local newspaper claimed that 'many regard him as a "probable" for the office of Minister of Health in a future Labour Government'. Even had Murray been elected, which he was not, the chances of him receiving any ministerial appointment were, to say the least, remote if only because it appears that Attlee was firmly convinced that Bevan, in recognition of his dynamism and commitment, should become Health Minister. But for the SMA, this appointment was problematical. As Webster points out, Bevan was to maintain a distance between himself and Labour's health experts, including the Association. And while he was to receive much advice – in public and through personal communication – from the SMA, ultimately 'his relations with this group were not particularly close'. Webster further argues that by 1945 the Association was 'no longer a force to be reckoned with', and that 'there is no evidence that its wisdom exercised any particular charm for Bevan'.[5]

Other historians have reached broadly similar conclusions. Honigsbaum describes at length what he sees as the 'defeat' of SMA policies in the 1940s. Kenneth Morgan suggests that Bevan was 'fully acquainted' with the Association's arguments, and then demonstrates how the Minister ignored most of them. He also, rather curiously, suggests that the SMA had 'succeeded in forcing' its ideas on Labour Party conference in 1934; and makes the interesting remark that Bevan's own experiences had made him deeply sceptical of 'the vested interests of middle-class pressure groups such as the medical profession'.[6] While it is clearly the BMA Morgan has in mind, it is worth speculating on how the working-class Bevan responded to advice – often unsolicited – given by the predominantly middle-class SMA.

Bevan's biographers, and that of his wife Jennie Lee, also help throw light on his relationship with the Association. Lee later recalled her partner's problems in persuading both parliament and his Labour colleagues of the merits of his health service plans. These problems were in part due, she claimed, to the public attacks by 'hot-heads, led by the Socialist Medical Association'. Bevan's private response was to see the demands of 'Dr Stark Murray and his Socialist Medical Association colleagues' as 'pure but impotent', a revealing comment from a politician at once highly principled and highly pragmatic. John Campbell suggests that Murray in particular 'never forgave' the Labour Health Minister for his neglect of a key Association demand, health centres. Michael Foot, a great admirer of Bevan, has little to say directly about his relationship with the SMA, although he does claim that the Association's 1945 conference resolution was directed more against the actions of Conservative government ministers than it was to 'the kind of service which a Labour government should consider'. This, it might be argued, tells us as much about Foot's desire to let Bevan off the hook for ignoring established Labour policy as it does about the SMA.[7]

Finally, Patricia Hollis, in her biography of Lee, sees Bevan as situated between the demands of the SMA, 'which had drawn up Labour's health policies'; and those of the BMA. In the end, she continues, Bevan was probably right in his judgement that 'most of these issues did not matter greatly', a telling remark on the importance of internal democracy in the Labour Party. Nonetheless Hollis also notes that Bevan's scheme had 'heavy costs', for example in its administrative structures, but concludes that the

> strain on Nye, and on Jennie, as he was denounced by the Socialist Medical Association for selling out, by the BMA for his despotic tendencies, by the Tories ... , and by his Cabinet colleagues for incurring the wrath of all of them, was immense.[8]

In fact, the SMA well understood that any Health Minister faced in the BMA a powerful and politically well-connected pressure group. It had devoted considerable energy, especially post-Beveridge, to attacking what it saw as the main professional body's reactionary attitude, and this continued after the Labour government's election. An Association internal memorandum acknowledged that Bevan faced difficulties in dealing with 'vested interests', and that this had been made worse by Willink's secret negotiations with the BMA. The White Paper was therefore no longer the basis on which to proceed, raising the possibility that Bevan would have to seek Cabinet agreement to new proposals 'cutting right through all the previous discussions and difficulties'. In consequence this might force the SMA to decide whether it could support a system not controlled by local authorities; in which doctors were remunerated using a capitation system; and in which private practice was allowed to continue.[9] Given Bevan's plan, this was a prescient analysis of the dilemma the Association was soon to confront.

The main point, however, is that on taking up his ministerial post Bevan did not feel obliged to take particular heed of the SMA, despite its important contribution to Labour Party health policy up until 1945; and that this was something which, unsurprisingly, the Association increasingly saw as a flaw in the Minister's strategy. The National Health Service as set up by Bevan provided comprehensive and universal medical care, free at the point of consumption. The sale of GP practices was abolished; the hospitals were effectively 'nationalised', thereby both circumventing and doing away with the voluntary/municipal divide; and the system was financed out of general taxation rather than through an extended version of health insurance. All this was, by any standards, a huge and radical step forward in social welfare, and achieved by extremely demanding negotiations between Bevan and the medical profession right down to the Appointed Day. Bevan's political skill in these trying circumstances, particularly as he was also responsible for the housing programme, cannot be overstated.

On the other hand, the health services were not unified. A tripartite system was created, consisting of the hospital service (with the teaching hospitals having their own special status); general practice; and remaining local authority health functions. Unification and integration through democratically controlled local authorities was hence rejected. Within this complex system, private practice remained and salaried status for doctors abandoned in favour of remuneration by capitation. The majority of practitioners therefore continued as independent contractors. Furthermore, the medical profession (although not other health workers) exerted considerable power over the NHS, in terms of both administration and policy. This was at the expense of democratic control within the service and, arguably, by society as a whole.

The handing over of power to the medical profession had, for its critics, a further unwelcome consequence. During the Act's passage much was made of the need to move from curative to preventive medicine, a longstanding Association aspiration. This proved, however, highly problematic. In part this was because one early outcome of free health care was a huge consumer demand which meant that resources had to be allocated to curative medicine. But the professional power of doctors also contributed to this inasmuch as they had, so those such as the SMA argued, a 'vested interest' in ill-health. Hence the jibe increasingly voiced by its members that a national 'sickness', rather than a national 'health', service had been created. This was reactive rather than proactive, thereby failing to address the fundamental causes of poor health; and was the product of welfare capitalism rather than full-blown socialism, despite Bevan's own undoubted socialist credentials.

A further problem with the NHS was slower to make itself apparent, but was no less important for that. Health centres, one of the key institutions for which local authorities were envisaged as having re-sponsibility and seen by their supporters as essential to engendering teamwork in the new service, were promised by the 1946 Act. But in reality they were painfully slow to get off the ground. This was partly because building materials were being diverted to domestic housing, understandably given the condition of the post-war housing stock. How-ever it was also of significance that the BMA leadership used the health centre issue as part of its campaign against Bevan's proposals, and that this in turn led the Minister to severely curtail the original health centre plans. As will be apparent from previous chapters, Bevan's concessions involved matters of considerable concern to the SMA. The Association viewed issues such as a salaried service, democratic control, and health centres as not only important in themselves, but also because a fully integrated and socialised medical service was crucial in the transition to a democratic socialist society. Such a service was not only to meet the nation's health needs, but in organisation and ethos was to provide a model for socialism.

SMA support for the National Health Service

A more detailed analysis of the SMA's critique is given below. But first it is important to establish that in the immediate post-war period the organisation did not simply carp about Bevan and his scheme. On the contrary, the Association found much to celebrate in the Minister's plan, as well as being quick to claim credit for what it saw as its positive aspects, an attitude succinctly summed up in a 1946 article by Murray entitled 'We Thought of it First'. A variety of means were employed to put forward the various themes of the SMA message. Hastings and Murray both participated in radio broadcasts, for example in May 1947 when Hastings spoke on the BBC's Far Eastern Service on the implications of the NHS for hospitals. The previous year, Murray took part in another radio debate with the BMA's Charles Hill. When Hill accused Murray of wanting to turn doctors into civil servants – a standard BMA debating ploy – the latter replied that the state in Britain was not a 'bogey man'; rather, it was 'the people', hence the need for Hill to clearly distinguish 'between a fascist state' and that now being planned. We can see here the kind of point Bourne was making during the war, that state medicine was in itself neither good nor bad, but rather existed in a broader political context.[10]

One crucial component of this was highlighted in the *Scottish Co-Operator* on the Bill's publication, once again by Murray whom the journal described as the 'brain behind' the new measure. For the ordinary citizen, he explained, it could not be stressed enough that services would be provided '*as a right of citizenship*' (emphasis in the original), irrespective of individual economic status. At least one aspect of the 'right to health', discussed in Chapter Seven, was therefore being fulfilled. In turn, this also implied that Labour's election would see the full achievement of previously only partly-realised citizens' rights. One way in which the public could be informed of these was through the travelling exhibition – 'The Battle for Health', named after Taylor's book – set up in 1946. This stressed a number of themes, including the need for teamwork and, especially, the centrality of health centres. The exhibition made extensive use of illustrative material, and was used not only by SMA branches, but also by local Labour Parties, Cooperative Political Committees, and Fabian Societies. Its aim was, as *MTT* put it, to 'crystallise public opinion in favour of the new service'. According to Murray, requests for BMA representatives to debate with Association members at exhibition meetings rarely came to anything since the 'BMA was exceedingly reluctant to put up speakers as their case was really too weak to be exposed in public'.[11]

Nor was the importance of enlightening professional colleagues as to the true nature of Labour's plans ignored. In a letter to the *Lancet* in autumn 1945, Hastings, Murray, and Joules claimed that many doctors had inadequate knowledge of Labour's plans, and suggested that those interested obtain a copy of *National Service for Health* direct from the SMA. Similarly, *MTT* warned its readers of the 'flood' of leaflets being circulated to both the public and the profession by the BMA. In some of these, it claimed, '[t]ruth and accuracy are the only things missing'. The medical profession's sensibilities were nonetheless also recognised, and as the Appointed Day approached the EC agreed not to be 'too outspoken as a body but work individually in as many spheres as possible to influence doctors'.[12]

This did not, however, stop four prominent Association members having a libel action brought against them. Bevan had expressed doubts about the procedures involved in the BMA's referendum of its members on the 1946 Act. This allegation was repeated by SMA members – and MPs – Hastings, Jeger, Morgan, and Louis Comyns in letters to the press, and the BMA sued. The end result was that the four apologised to the BMA in open court, met its legal costs, and donated £1000 to a medical charity. It is notable, although understandable, that the Labour

Party felt itself unable to take any responsibility, financial or otherwise, for Hastings and his colleagues during these proceedings.[13] The incident again illustrates the acrimonious relations between the Association and the main professional body.

This episode notwithstanding, Association MPs also sought to pursue a positive approach, and one which would not unduly antagonise Bevan, during the Bill's parliamentary passage. The eight SMA members on the NHS Select Committee kept a low profile, their only significant intervention being an abortive attempt by Hastings to amend, in such a way as to involve greater local authority participation, clauses relating to London. In an important sense, this was a battle already lost. A defence of voluntarism and a positive role for local government were put forward in Cabinet by Hastings's old LCC ally Morrison, who at this time was, according to Taylor, inclined to criticise Bevan's 'left-wing speeches and right-wing policy'. Morrison argued, quite correctly, that hospital nationalisation was not existing party policy and that voluntary and municipal hospitals should continue under local control; and that it would be disastrous were local government allowed to languish through the erosion of its 'most constructive and interesting functions'. Bevan's position, however, was that while a few local authorities ran a good hospital service, the vast majority were unsuited to this purpose, and had a record of inefficiency and poor service. He also rejected the idea of specially created local government bodies for health service administration as this would simply add to the already complicated local authority functions, and would in any case be 'unlikely to attract polling interest'. Bevan's arguments won the support of the majority of his Cabinet colleagues.[14]

This helps explain Hastings's speech during the Bill's Second Reading. Here he stressed the importance of the LCC experience and of 'local interest' and 'local patriotism'. Surprisingly, given his previous attitude but pursuing a similar line to Morrison, he also suggested that however good public provision was, there would always be 'opportunity for voluntary effort and for experiment in social service'. Nonetheless, Hastings conceded that Bevan's ministerial team had clearly shown the impossibility of handing over a new hospital service to either existing sector. Overall, he concluded in a contemporaneous journal piece, the NHS Bill was a 'masterpiece of political strategy' which had 'called the bluff of the BMA'.[15] As we shall see, Hastings was on other occasions highly critical of the emerging structure of the NHS. But he also tried both to support the government where at all possible and to take the wider view, as an article published in May 1948 – that is just before the Appointed Day – clearly shows.

Hastings began by claiming that 'since time began' never had so much been done 'for the people' in such a short period as by the current administration. He himself had recently visited a number of European countries, and nowhere were conditions as good as in Britain. For this reason alone criticism of the government should cease. The domestic context is significant here, for the 1947 economic crisis had severely shaken Labour's confidence. But there was an even more important reason why the current government should remain in power, namely that 'its existence is the most important factor in world peace today'. The world was dividing into two camps, one led by the United States, with its high degree of individual and political freedom, but also its 'economic anarchy'; the other by the Soviet Union, with its planned economy – 'which all socialists must admire' – but diminishing personal freedom. Britain, standing between these two, needed the sort of 'planned socialist economy' which only Labour could deliver. Had the Tories won in 1945 Britain would have become a client state of the US, 'with what international result we dare hardly contemplate'.[16] There are two crucial points being made here: first, that it was essential to avoid, whenever possible, any unwarranted criticism of the Labour administration. Second, however, there was also a positive sense that Britain was entering a transformative era. We have already noted this as implicit in Murray's remarks on citizenship, and Hastings explicitly spelt this out in another, slightly earlier, article when he suggested that the English (*sic*) were living through perhaps the greatest period in their history. An 'evolutionary process' had been started by the war and continued by the post-war government, a situation which would have been very different had the Tories won in 1945.[17] The emphasis on both Labour's election victory and the changes brought about by the war is noteworthy, as is the clear sense that the potential existed for genuine social transformation which had implications not only for Britain, but also for the whole world. Such broader concerns are also evident in the SMA's attempt to promote medical internationalism, discussed further below. More specifically on medical politics, Hastings's attitude here suggests that while the creation of the NHS certainly had its problems, nonetheless it should be recognised as at least a step in the right direction.

The more positive side of the Association's analysis was also reflected in aspects of its relationship with Bevan. In the run up to the inauguration of the NHS, the SMA held a celebratory dinner with the Health Minister as principal guest. The toast to the Appointed Day was moved by Hastings, who also reminded Bevan of the role of the Association, as well as that of the Minister himself, in the new service's creation. Bevan's reply, according to Murray, showed full appreciation of the debt owed by himself, and the new service, to the SMA and its president, Hastings. While the Bill was still being drafted, a deputation met with the Minister who, in a subsequent letter, expressed his gratitude

that the general view of the Association's representatives was 'favourable to the proposals I outlined'. There followed a friendly
correspondence on a number of administrative points raised by Murray,
and Bevan also agreed to let the Association know in advance the Bill's
main points, so that it could best deal with press enquiries. All in all,
therefore, it is clearly not the case that the SMA was always and on
every occasion critical of Bevan. On the contrary, the Association frequently showed its support, publicly and privately, for some of his
scheme's general principles. However as Webster points out, simultaneously with the relatively friendly correspondence just cited, the
Association was also beginning to adopt a more critical line, expressing
unhappiness at the Labour minister's 'departure from some of Labour's
favoured policies'.[18]

The SMA's critique of Bevan's scheme

This is therefore an appropriate point to examine in more detail the
Association's critique of Bevan's NHS, and we use as a starting point a
1946 pamphlet written by Stephen Taylor. As we have seen, Taylor had
not always pursued the same line as the Association, although by the
post-war period he was not only an MP but an SMA member as well.
He was also soon to become Morrison's parliamentary private secretary
in which capacity, Beach suggests, he was responsible for impressing on
the LCC veteran ideas about participatory citizenship in a democratic
socialist society, very much the Association's approach.[19]

Taylor's pamphlet was published in a discussion series which carried
the rider that the Labour Party did not necessarily endorse all the points
made. The document itself was largely descriptive, although a rationale
for the health service's creation was also given. Taylor exercised caution
in certain areas – anxious, perhaps, not to unduly antagonise the medical profession nor to compromise the party leadership. He argued, for
instance, that it was necessary that both patients and doctors join the
service willingly and of their own accord; and that ultimately private
practice would 'die a natural death'. Although Taylor acknowledged
that this was a compromise, and was clearly opposed in principle to
private medicine, he also felt that such a policy was, in the long run,
better than 'compulsory strangulation'. This was an argument similar
to that used in the 1943 Fabian Society document discussed in the last
chapter, and rather at odds with the long-standing support for private
practice claimed in his memoirs.[20] In such respects, therefore, Taylor's
analysis and description was moderate; relatively unthreatening, even to
the medical profession; and clearly supportive of Bevan's scheme.

Interestingly, however, he also ventured into potentially more problematic areas. The current Bill, he suggested, was extremely important. But it was 'neither the beginning nor the end of the job of building a real national health service for Britain'. This strongly implied that in the near future the proposed service would require further amendment and expansion; and that the creation of a socialist health service was an ongoing, rather than a once and for all, process. Taylor also stressed the need for a measure of democratic control over the NHS, which was to be 'made and moulded by public opinion'. It was necessary to 'make our say in the running of the service a big one' so as to forestall the possibility of the new service becoming 'bureaucratic and managed from above'; and the danger that the 'high measure of freedom granted to the doctors may degenerate into license'. He also emphasised the 'revolutionary' nature of the proposal for health centres, based on teamwork; and acknowledged that the 'administrative link-up' between hospitals, GPs, and local authority clinic services was 'one of the points in the plan which can be criticised'. Taylor concluded with five suggested points for discussion, including the next stage of health service development, and to facilitate this provided a reading list which included both *National Service for Health* and the SMA's *The Socialist Programme for Health*.[21]

These more controversial points indicate some of the potential areas of criticism of the NHS Act; suggest a need for a flexible and dynamic vision of a state medical service; and thus can also be seen as part of an ongoing Labour Party debate about the meaning of 'socialism' in post-war Britain. On the last point the Labour intellectual Margaret Cole, for instance, noted that while the party had come to power with a 'definite programme for the social services', nonetheless this did not purport to be a 'programme of "full Socialism"', even in this particular field. Such a plan would, she continued, for many on the left include 'the turning of the medical service into a salaried profession'. Cole also acknowledged that the 1946 Act was a compromise, and that although there were currently good reasons for delays in implementing the health centre scheme, nonetheless it was unlikely that they would be put off for very long because 'teamwork is on the way, in medicine as everywhere else'.[22] The SMA's critique of Bevan must therefore be seen in this broader ideological context. In the following discussion it is organised under issues raised or implied by Taylor, namely: the unification of all health services; democratic control; doctors' remuneration and private practice; the shift from preventive to curative medicine; and teamwork and health centres.

A central theme in the Association's critique of the pre-war health services was their lack of planning and coordination. This, it was argued, led to muddle and inefficiency, and a poor delivery of health care. SMA literature often used illustrative diagrams to show just how complex the system was, and how different members of the same family could find themselves having to seek out different forms of care depending on, for example, their age or economic status.[23] We have also seen how Hastings had noted the difficulties of coordinating services provided by the LCC and by the metropolitan boroughs. It was therefore envisaged that post-war medical reconstruction would fully address these problems. As Murray put it around the time of the 1946 Bill:

> If we are to establish a system of health care, if we are to provide a single route to the whole medical service, if the people are to play a part in its development and running, we must plan the service as a single integrated whole. Fundamental changes must be made if chaos is to give place to order.

Planning, as in other aspects of post-war life, was therefore essential, and unification the foundation on which a socialised service would be built.[24]

This issue was raised in the March 1946 press release, which expressed unhappiness with the proposed administrative arrangements 'chiefly because general practice is not integrated with the rest of the service'. As we have seen, it was assumed by the SMA that health service integration would be carried out by local authority bodies, but that the Association had also long recognised the stumbling block of existing local government boundaries. In an essay published early in 1948, Hastings agreed that the most serious objection to the 1946 Act was that in any given locality health services would be 'under the charge of three separate committees' – that is the tripartite system which Bevan had introduced. But as matters stood, there were no local authorities covering a population large enough to guarantee economic and medical efficiency.[25]

However, this conciliatory tone was to be replaced by what Hastings clearly saw as a return to the basic principles of socialised medicine. He told the 1953 Association AGM that 'time and experience' were clearly showing that Bevan's error was in 'failing to take the advice we offered him' over the framing of the Act. This was especially so in two areas – a salaried service and 'the complete unification of the different branches of preventive and curative medicine'. The tripartite system was, he continued, 'manifestly absurd'. One solution was a two-tier administrative structure. In England and Wales, this would consist of ten to fifteen large units – yet another version of regionalisation, as well as a possibly unconscious echo of the wartime EMS – responsible only for planning. Beneath these would be smaller units, each covering a population of around 250 000 people. Although Hastings acknowledged that all this would require a 'radical change in the present structure of local government', his general opposition to the existing arrangements was clear enough.[26]

While concerned in the first instance with the service's rationalisation through unification, underlying this was another important constituent of the SMA's vision of a socialised service – local government, and thereby democratic, control. Historically, the SMA had laid great emphasis on the need for popular participation in a truly socialised health service, particularly since its experiences on the inter-war LCC. It was certainly the case that 'planning' was essential to medical reconstruction. But it was emphasised, particularly during and after the war, that this was not a matter of non-accountable bureaucracy, such as had characterised the fascist states. Democratic participation was to be a bulwark against those 'vested interests' deemed to be concerned more with sickness than with health, especially the reactionary elements in the medical profession. Furthermore, we have seen that the Association's conception of the 'right to health' involved not simply the passive receipt of health care, but also the duty both to maintain individual health and to be actively involved in service administration. The Association had, in short, an activist view of citizenship combined with the belief that socialism and democracy were virtually synonymous terms.

Unsurprisingly, therefore, the administrative structures of the NHS caused concern. Lack of unification was one aspect of this, not least since it meant that the medical profession had successfully avoided any form of local authority – and thereby directly democratically accountable – control. Indeed, the medical profession had succeeded in gaining considerable power within the new system at the expense of both its fellow health workers and the population at large, another form of the corporatism against which the Association had long campaigned. In the first instance the SMA devoted less attention to the absence of devolved accountability in Bevan's plan, recognising the genuine case for local government reform and that in the meantime it might be possible to place sympathetic personnel on the various boards and committees set up by the Act. Furthermore, we have seen that the Association had long had problems in reconciling professional rights with what it saw as citizens' democratic rights.

Although this tension remained, and remained unresolved, in the post-war period, nonetheless the SMA became increasingly preoccupied with the introduction of democratic control within, and of, the service. A survey carried out by the Sheffield branch in February 1949 identified as a serious problem 'the undemocratic and often reactionary professional membership of the authorities under the Act'. The local medical committee and the medical representation on the local executive council

– the latter the body which administered general practitioner services under the NHS, the former one its professional sub-committees and usually composed of local BMA leaders – consisted almost entirely, it was claimed, of doctors who had opposed the service's introduction. Even an authority composed of the 'progressively minded' could find itself 'entirely dependent for advice in professional and technical matters' on doctors unsympathetic to the state service.[27] Apart from any other consideration, this suggested that seeking to place individuals favourably disposed to a full-blown socialised service on the many existing NHS committees might achieve at best only limited success.

The answer therefore lay elsewhere. Published in the late 1940s, the policy statement *A Socialist Health Service* asserted unequivocally that the NHS did not have 'the democratic structure and outlook that it should have and which is a fundamental objective of the Labour Movement'. Consequently, the introduction of democratic principles was an 'urgent necessity'. Much of the criticism levelled at hospital administration in particular – both in terms of membership and its 'tendency to bureaucratic action' – would be met if the various boards and committees were formed by the 'well-tried democratic method of election'. Local government reorganisation was undoubtedly necessary. But even prior to this Regional Boards, for example, could be made directly electable. Within hospitals themselves, democracy had made 'slow progress'. Staff committees, in hospitals and in future health centres, ought to be truly representative, and should have the right of delegation to management committees. The medical profession was currently well served, but it was equally important that other occupational groups have a say in management. This process of hospital democratisation was to be completed by the creation of local 'Hospital Associations' consisting of the 'widest representation of all the people who regard the hospital as their own', and these too should have the right of membership of management committees.[28]

One Association sub-committee even went so far as to suggest that the service's large-scale administrative structures were a 'grave danger to democratic government'; and that unless devolution of control, involving popular and staff participation, occurred, 'more will have been lost than gained by reorganisation'. But while some (extremely limited) progress had been made by 1951, even after six years of Labour government it could not be remotely suggested that the health service was run on anything approaching democratic lines. The issue was raised in the summer of that year at a special SMA conference, 'The Next Five Years in Health'. Dr Ian Gilliland, for example, welcomed the introduction of the NHS, but argued that Labour 'must go on to build a Socialist service to fit into the Socialist Society in which we are going to live'.

This would involve organising the NHS in a 'new democratic way so that those using it and those working in it play their part in running it'.[29] The democratic rights of both producers and consumers had, therefore, yet to be fully realised. To do so would move towards a truly socialist health service, in itself a significant contribution to the achievement of a socialist society.

A further problem with Bevan's scheme, and a consequence of his ceding power to the medical profession, lay in the method of doctors' remuneration. Murray, reviewing the NHS in 1951, declared the capitation system of GP payment 'a failure' which had even 'more faults than were prophesied'. It benefited only those out to 'grab every penny he can' at the expense of the quality of service delivered. Certain types of doctor – for example those in rural areas, and the conscientious – were penalised, and this was exacerbated by regional differences in living costs. The only solution, Murray concluded, was 'a salaried service coupled with collective responsibility for the health of the nation'. The same year an *MTT* editorial, almost certainly also written by Murray, suggested that the 'problems of general practice will never be solved until we have a whole-time salaried service'. A salaried service had, of course, been an SMA demand from the outset. One of the reservations expressed in its press release on the Bill's publication was that the proposed payment system went against its own, and the Labour Party's, established policy.[30]

The Association therefore took this matter extremely seriously, and an internal memorandum of the late 1940s spelled out exactly why. The SMA, it claimed, approached the whole issue of remuneration differently from other medical organisations. It recognised that satisfactory conditions were essential to a good service. But it was also important to set this in the framework of total NHS costs. The service's quality and content should be fixed first, and doctors' payment discussed in that context. Furthermore the SMA, because it recruited not only medical practitioners but also other health workers and because of its political philosophy, believed that doctors' income had to be viewed in relation to that of other NHS personnel. All health workers, including medical practitioners, should therefore be salaried employees.[31] What was being argued for was a structured, and unified, service in which everyone, including doctors, were integrated into the system and rewarded according to their ascribed place in it rather than by their ability to exert political pressure. This would, in turn, end private entrepreneurialism and encourage teamwork. Teamwork is dealt with more fully below. However it is worth noting here that Hastings saw the capitation system as potentially subversive of health centres and the ability of doctors to work in 'true partnership', a crucial issue if medicine were to provide the model for a socialist society. How, Hastings demanded, could there possibly be cooperation among medical staff if a doctor's first consideration was 'the increase of names on his list'? The continuance of 'capitalist medicine' was to be deprecated, and could have no more than 'sentimental value' once the sale of practices was abolished. Once again showing optimism touching on naivety, Hastings predicted that with the ending of the sale of practices 'doctors will be as keen to be remunerated by salary as they now are for payment by capitation'.[32]

But persuading the government to implement what was undoubtedly part of Labour's official health policy proved more problematical. An SMA resolution on a salaried service was not reached at party conference in 1949, and party secretary Morgan Phillips wrote to Elizabeth Bunbury explaining the NEC's position. Phillips agreed that such a system would have certain advantages. There was, however, strong opposition from doctors, and for any employing agency there would also be issues of discipline and supervision. Consequently it was the government's view that it was 'neither politic nor practicable' to force on any profession a remuneration system to which it was opposed. The Health Minister's position, Phillips concluded, was to 'let the situation develop naturally in the light of further experience', hardly the most dynamic of attitudes. In fact Bevan had long since conceded that a salaried service would not be introduced, and this was legislatively enshrined in the 1949 National Health Service (Amendment) Act.[33] This can be seen as yet another example of Bevan's willingness to ignore established party policy; of his distance from the SMA; and his apparent belief that it was, from a consumer's point of view, more important to have the service introduced than to worry about the precise nature of its administrative arrangements.

A salaried service, a cornerstone of the Association's proposals, was therefore not achieved. Nor was the ending of private practice. In the immediate post-war period the main thrust of the SMA's argument was the need for a full-time salaried service, which carried with it the implication of an ultimate end to private practice, rather than on the continuance of 'capitalist medicine' itself. But the issue was not forgotten. In an Association publication celebrating (rather critically) Bevan's life, one of the next generation of activists, David Kerr, found it 'no accident' that private sector medicine was 'aided and abetted by both the organised medical profession and through the big insurance companies'. These were each looking after their members' concerns 'in a competitive capitalist society'. Both remained, however, 'in no way accountable to the public – the electorate – the consumer – the patient – call the poor mortal what you like'.[34] This problem clearly had its historic roots in the compromises made by Bevan.

The failure to implement a salaried service, and the associated failure to bring the medical profession under democratic control, was thus a triumph for the 'vested interests' of which the Association had long warned. One implication of this was that those who had a stake in sickness – doctors, with their emphasis on curative medicine – had won out over those seeking a significant shift to preventive medicine. Hastings agreed in 1948 that if 'we want to prevent we must treat'. Equally, however, if 'we want to treat intelligently and efficiently' then it was necessary to provide for 'the recognition of disease at its earliest beginning'.[35] This in turn involved the acknowledgement that ill-health was as much a socio-economic as an individual problem; that the solution to this was socialism; and that a truly socialised health service would be instrumental in affecting the transition from one social system to another.

An Association committee set up under Dr Duncan Leys to investigate child health concluded that working class children were still dying unnecessarily, and that this was a problem of environment rather than heredity. Making the 'average standard of health' equal to the best was therefore primarily an economic issue, hence the need for a 'social revolution', of which socialised health services formed a part. The promotion of good health ought to be a fundamental concern of the entire labour movement, and should include demands for adequate nutritional standards and better quality housing. Of course everyone had, as we have seen, considerable responsibility for their own health. As Murray put it, the 'preservation of that degree of ... health is something in which the individual must play his or her part'. But this had also to be placed in a broader context. Health protection had become one of the state's 'primary duties', and the state's actions in the entire socio-economic sphere were crucial in determining the individual's working and living environment. This was clearly a radically different view of health from that offered by, say, the BMA. Its strong implication was that full health could only be achieved under socialism, and in a fully socialised medical service. Preventive medicine was a matter of both individual and collective action, and was not, as yet, fully understood or implemented.[36]

Preventive medicine was crucial to a fully integrated health service, and one of the key institutions in its promotion was to be the health centre. The creation of health centres had always featured strongly in Association plans and was promised by the 1946 Act. Their significance to the SMA was made clear by Murray at 1947 party conference when he claimed they would become 'the symbol to the whole of the people of this country of what a Socialist Medical Health Service really means'.[37] Health centres were consequently not just bricks and mortar, or even aggregations of general practitioners. They were also crucial to preventive medicine, to the integration of health care in the widest sense, and in providing the opportunity for the realisation of that template for socialist society, medical teamwork. The concept of teamwork had, as we have seen, a number of dimensions for the Association. Medical science's increasing complexity made it impossible for any one practitioner to embrace it fully. Teamwork was therefore essential 'if the great technical developments of modern medicine are to be of benefit to patients'. The isolation – and implicitly (and occasionally explicitly) in Association literature, the medical ignorance – of GPs in particular would therefore disappear, and all doctors thus enjoy the 'fine sense of team spirit which they learn as students and junior hospital officers'.[38] The primary role of medicine – the optimum in both curative and preventive care – would therefore be fulfilled.

The health centre was particularly important here, for it was to be the location of primary care practitioners and other medical and associated personnel; was to be closely linked to hospitals, so that specialist care would be readily accessible; and would bring under one roof the 'two great branches of medicine' – the preventive and the curative – leaving them 'no longer isolated from each other'. As a report produced by SMA dentists claimed, local authority health centres should be 'the primary instrument of health'. There the dentist would join 'the health centre team, which will include every other type of health worker'. Consequently dentists too would lose their existing feeling of isolation. Medicine would gain by the combating of diseases in which 'disorders of the mouth' played a part, while dentistry would gain by the new contact with GPs in particular, but also with the consultant and specialist services available at the centres.[39]

It was certainly recognised that creating a comprehensive system of health centres was problematic at a time of building material shortages and the need for new homes, a point explicitly acknowledged in Murray's 1947 conference speech.[40] However, even before the Appointed Day SMA members had considerable reservations about the government's commitment to health centres. MacWilliam suggested in March 1948 that not all of the blame for the 'present situation' – the tense build-up to the Appointed Day – was attributable to the BMA. Bevan could be criticised on a number of grounds, but undoubtedly his greatest error was in failing to appreciate the importance of health centres. Their neglect had made the NHS 'very much inferior to what it might have been' as well as destroying its attractiveness to many doctors. In addition to its combative approach to Bevan, this piece is another example of SMA optimism – or naivety – about medical opinion, given that the BMA's attitude to health centres was, at best, one of indifference. But it also needs to be placed in the context of the recent issuing of two Ministry of Health circulars, of which MacWilliam was undoubtedly aware, curtailing previous plans for health centre development. Hence, as a 1951 Association pamphlet put it, health centres 'faded into the background'. But the NHS would fail, no matter how much money was spent on it, if they were not provided. For health centres alone could create the circumstances whereby health personnel, 'combining as a team, can give the highest standard of satisfying work, and the only way of providing a focal point for the health and healthful activities of a community'.[41]

This neatly sums up the main characteristics for the Association of the ideal health centre. But once again, as MacWilliam anticipated and the 1951 pamphlet claimed, Bevan proved a disappointment. An official committee, on which the BMA but not the SMA was represented, was set up subsequent to the circulars to which MacWilliam had reacted with such annoyance. This deliberated for two years, but its delayed report of early 1951 did not move matters any further forward. Ironically, the most comprehensive health centre built in the post-war period – Woodberry Down, set up by the LCC in Stoke Newington – was officially opened by Hastings in 1952, almost certainly a recognition of his services to the council. Commenting on the occasion, *MTT* suggested that after a 'life of fighting for health centres' it was right that Hastings should have been 'publicly acknowledged in this way'. Woodberry Down's expense, however, was to be used as one excuse for not continuing with a health centre programme. Overall, therefore, the demise of this programme was attributable to, as Webster puts it, 'medico-political tensions' and 'resource constraints'.[42]

It is possible to get a synoptic sense of what the SMA wanted in the late 1940s by way of two speeches and a report. Hastings in May 1949 was brief and to the point. The good parts of the NHS were attributable to the SMA; its drawbacks to Bevan's failure to take SMA advice. The existing service involved the 'bulk purchase of the services of capitalist medicine for the mass of the people'. What the Association wanted was a 'unified service for preventative medicine by means of team work'. Only the SMA, on whom the service's future depended, could fully argue this case. The underlying political philosophy was explained in the report of the previously referred to child health sub-committee. The Association sought to 'achieve, in health, the purpose of socialism'. Means were as important as ends, and the socialist means were democratic and aimed at 'implementing in every possible way the direct power of the consumer and producer to determine the structure of social service'.[43]

Also in philosophical vein, Association member Dr J.H.F. Brotherston – later Chief Medical Officer, Scotland, and Honorary Physician to the

Queen – addressed the 1948 International Conference (discussed further below) on 'social medicine', a topic widely debated in the 1940s and defined by him as the 'application of medicine to man in his environment'. This was a necessary counter to the increasingly scientific nature of medicine which isolated the disease from the patient, and meant that the doctor in 'applying the facts of science overlooked the social facts of his practice'. The war, however, had re-emphasised the importance of social factors, and it was now realised that 'science could not be fully applied if social science was neglected'. Social medicine therefore involved doctors working alongside other scientists, social scientists, and social workers. This in turn depended on the provision of health centres wherein 'scientific and social medicine would be one'.[44] In a rather rarefied way, this was an assertion of the need for not only health centres, but also preventive medicine and teamwork across professional boundaries.

The SMA and the post-war labour movement

Clearly, then, the SMA had a detailed critique of Bevan's service and a not always easy relationship with the Minister himself. This was certainly not helped by the Association's criticisms, although this also should be put in the context of the point made above about the support which the organisation offered its ministerial colleague. But of course its place in left-wing medical politics was not simply a matter of its dealings with one individual. What success, if any, did the Association have in the post-war period on Labour Party committees, at party conference, and within the labour movement generally?

Previous chapters argued the importance of the SMA's wartime role shaping Labour's health policy, particularly through its influence on the Public Health Advisory Committee. As we have seen, however, by the end of the war this had apparently been allowed to lapse. A discussion on this took place on the Association's EC in August 1945, and the idea mooted of attempting to establish a joint SMA/Labour Party health committee. This got nowhere. However in 1948 the PHAC was revived as the direct result of an Association conference resolution arguing for the committee's re-establishment on the basis that while Bevan was to be congratulated on the steps he had taken, nonetheless there was also a need for 'further developments and extensions'. As we shall see, this sense of uncompleted business was an important dimension of the SMA's post-war position. Despite the implicitly critical tone, the NEC agreed to the creation of a new health forum.[45]

The re-established PHAC was a sub-committee of the Policy and Publicity Committee (one of whose members was Bevan) and, like other similar bodies set up at the same time, charged with coming up with proposals for the next edition of the Labour Party programme. It had 11 members: the chair, Edith Summerskill; four NEC nominees; and six co-opted individuals, of whom four – Hastings, Murray, Taylor, and Fred Messer – belonged to the SMA, as did Summerskill.[46] This was a strong, although hardly commanding, Association presence. Moreover Summerskill was beginning to hold increasingly senior party and governmental positions, and while undoubtedly fully committed to the NHS, she also had demands for loyalty other than to the SMA placed upon her. Indeed, Hastings's replacement as chair by Summerskill must also be seen as a loss of status for the SMA president, given his previous long tenure of that position, and a signal by the NEC that its own members were to be in key positions on subordinate committees. Taylor too, as we have seen, now had official responsibilities, and although his approach was at this point in many respects in close accordance with that of the Association, he was a rather ambiguous member of what he later called 'a tiny body with ... extreme left wing tendencies'.[47]

The PHAC was not, therefore, the SMA power base it had once been; it was more closely under the supervision of the party leadership than its wartime predecessor; and it now had to work within established parameters – Bevan's NHS – rather than the more fluid situation of the first half of the 1940s. All this gave less opportunity for radical policy innovations, and is reflected in the mostly uncontroversial issues – for example patent medicines – which the SMA Executive decided to have its members present to the PHAC. The committee's first report, in December 1948, was uncontentious, although it did reflect a number of Association concerns. It was suggested, for example, that preventive medicine was entering the stage where individuals should do more to look after themselves, the aim being to 'produce a new attitude to life and new habits of mind and body'. The PHAC also gave the occasional opportunity for the more direct propagation of SMA ideas. In November 1949 Hastings, in a memorandum for the committee, denounced current Labour policy on medical education as 'most reactionary'. More state funding was required and, echoing the 1948 report, he claimed that in future doctors would have to appreciate 'the shift that is taking place from curative to preventive medicine'. Hence, once again, the need for medical students to be drawn from all parts of society.[48]

Essentially, though, the PHAC had ceased to be of any real significance as a platform from which the SMA could influence Labour's policy making. This was paralleled in the parliamentary Labour Party, despite increased Association representation. Following the 1945 election a number of groups, consisting entirely of backbench MPs, were set up to liaise with ministers. Among these were the 'Health Group' (later the Health and Social Insurance Group, and later still the Social Services Group), initially chaired by Hastings. Between May 1947 and May 1948, however, he was replaced by Percy Daines, an individual with no especially obvious qualifications for the post. It is difficult to see from the records why this occurred. However Hastings had found himself in trouble in this period through being one of the 13 signatories of the so-called 'second German telegram', a message of support from left-wing MPs to a German political body which the party leadership considered a communist front.[49] It was also at this time that Hastings was passed over as chair of the revived PHAC; and when he and three colleagues were involved in the previously noted BMA libel action. Hastings, it is reasonable to assume, was not the Labour leadership's favourite comrade in 1948.

The Association's inability to penetrate the post-war labour movement is also shown in other ways. At 1948 party conference Murray failed miserably in his attempt to be elected from the constituency section to the NEC, gaining only 64 000 votes. To put this in perspective Bevan, who came top of the same ballot, attracted over 700 000 votes. This poll took place just weeks before the Appointed Day when the Association might have expected, given its self-assessment as the intellectual source of the NHS, to gain significant support. That it did not, while Bevan remained a party favourite, is an important indicator of the SMA's failure to put down deep roots in the wider labour movement, irrespective of whether its claims about itself were actually true.[50] Similarly, Association members now found it much more difficult than previously to make an impact on party conferences. Murray's resolution in 1946, seeking greater democracy in a future, enhanced health service was not even responded to by Bevan, and no vote appears to have been taken. The language of his speech, particularly given that the NHS Bill had only recently been published and that Bevan was fending off criticism from all sides, is notable. Murray warned that the Association would be watching 'exceedingly carefully' for any abuse of the 'compromise' made by the Health Minister. This can have done little to endear him to his ministerial colleague. The following year Murray again proposed the Association resolution, this time on the necessity of pushing ahead with health centres. On this occasion Bevan did respond, displaying the political skills for which he was justly renowned. He welcomed Murray's statement, but suggested that it was inappropriate, and indeed not conference's place, to go into too much detail on policy matters. The SMA had, Bevan suggested, 'all kinds of ways of getting at the Executive as well as through the conference itself'. He therefore asked Murray to withdraw his resolution, which the latter duly did.[51]

Bevan was being more than a shade disingenuous when he implied that the Association had easy access to the Labour leadership. Furthermore, the failure to take votes on its resolutions meant that the Minister's negotiating strategy was not in any way compromised by conference decisions although Bevan was, as we have seen, in any case perfectly capable of ignoring established party policy on health. Putting a brave face on the matter, the Association Council noted in June 1947 that the conference had given Murray the 'opportunity ... to put our point of view'. Significantly, though, Murray also suggested that there was a 'widespread feeling' that the party's annual meeting had to be reorganised, given the number of resolutions which failed to be reached.[52] This may, of course, have been wishful thinking, or a subconscious recognition of the SMA's weakening position. More generally it is striking just how little conference time was devoted to the NHS, the Association's efforts notwithstanding.

The problems the SMA increasingly faced in having its message accepted were, furthermore, not confined simply to the Labour Party. In autumn 1947 it began organising a conference of health workers to discuss the NHS. This soon, however, ran into trouble, first through the Transport and General Workers Union and the MPU retracting initial support. A letter to Bunbury showed that the TUC had recommended the transport workers' withdrawal on the grounds that the 1946 Act was under 'detailed and continuous consideration' by its General Council, and that concern had been expressed that at the proposed conference support might be given to 'policies not in accordance with those laid down by Congress'. It was also made clear that the TUC considered the proper forum for discussion of 'broad points of policy' to be with Labour's NEC. Further withdrawals and complications followed. Letters from Hastings to H.B. Morgan, TUC medical advisor and SMA member, appear to have got nowhere, and the conference was eventually postponed.[53]

The TUC's stance raises two important points about the Association's post-war situation. First, it was suggested in the previous chapter that the TUC was, during the war, careful to keep a distance between itself and the SMA over medical reconstruction. This attitude, of indifference bordering on hostility, clearly continued after 1945. Given the union movement's influence on the Labour Party, this did not work to the Association's advantage. Second, this episode also suggests that the Association was already known for publicly criticising aspects of Bevan's proposals, and that this further alienated an important section of the labour movement. The SMA was, therefore, progressively marginalised within the post-war labour movement, and this manifested itself in increasingly uncompromising criticism of Bevan's scheme. The Appointed Day in July 1948 was certainly welcomed as a huge step forward in health care provision, and one for which the Association claimed considerable credit. But the period 1947–1948 in particular saw significant setbacks for the organisation in its attempt to retain a foothold in Labour Party policy formation.

Medical internationalism

Much of the SMA's time after 1945 was devoted – understandably – to the NHS. However it also found the collective energy to engage in other activities, and a brief examination of these is required before moving on to the concluding chapter. The Association had a long-standing concern over tuberculosis which in the post-war era resulted in a number of conferences aimed at not only socialist health workers, but at the whole labour movement. At a meeting jointly organised with the London Trades Council in early 1951 Hastings once again claimed that 'all which is best' in the NHS derived from the SMA, and that anything wrong in the 1946 Act resulted from the government not doing 'the things we told them to'. More specifically on tuberculosis, he argued that the increasing concern and interest in its prevention and treatment also had a great deal to do with the Association initiatives. Given the SMA's preoccupation with preventive medicine, it is therefore not surprising to find that emphasis was laid on improvements in environmental conditions, such as food and housing; and on vaccination against, and early detection of, the disease. This approach had earlier led Association member Richard Doll to demonstrate the relationship between infant mortality, tuberculosis, and poor housing conditions, and in consequence to call for the government to build 400 000 houses per year.[54]

Nor did the SMA neglect its international commitments. Even before 1945, considerable concern had been expressed over the nature of any post-war settlement and two members – Marrack and Bourne – contributed to a Fabian Society volume proposing a humane policy of European reconstruction so as to avoid the miseries and upheavals subsequent upon World War I. Similarly Hastings, whom as we have seen had a lifelong interest in child welfare, suggested in 1947 that in seeking to avoid a further conflict an important consideration was the instruction of German children in the 'principles of truth and honesty, and conditions of normal life in a democratic country'. With rising concern over the international situation in the early 1950s, Doll, Joules, Gilliland, and Leys were among the signatories of a letter to the *Lancet* appealing to their fellow doctors to think more positively than simply in terms of treating casualties in the event of war. Rather, the medical profession should come together – 'in the spirit of our chosen profession of healing' – in an attempt to end war preparations and contribute to the cause of world disarmament.[55]

One practical way in which the Association's internationalism operated in this period was its continuing involvement with medical refugees. In autumn 1945 *MTT* noted that Nazism was a 'many-headed monster' whose 'racial theories will die very slowly'. Contemporary attempts to stir up prejudice against refugee doctors, and here the allusion was almost certainly to the MPU, were deprecated. It was simply wrong, the piece continued, to imagine that if every refugee medical practitioner left the temporary register established in 1940 then every British doctor would automatically find employment. It was to be hoped, therefore, that the government would recognise that 'the new health service can easily absorb the small number of our continental friends who would prefer to remain with us'. The official situation nonetheless appeared satisfactory, almost certainly because the temporary register remained in force.[56] However this expired in 1947, and from 1948 the SMA again found itself concerned with the fate of medical refugees. The MPU was once more playing the anti-semitic card, albeit briefly, and seeking the expulsion of foreign health personnel. The Association's response was to demand the admission of refugee doctors to the medical register, not least because of the 'good service' given to the Royal Army Medical Corps by non-British practitioners. Correspondence with Bevan and Morrison followed, with the response of the former being clearly felt as inadequate. The outcome of all this is unclear, but particular Association interventions could have positive results. In early 1948 Drs Grunberg and Herschan, both refugee doctors but now British subjects, were nonetheless dismissed from their posts at Birkenhead Municipal Hospital. The two were subsequently reinstated, and wrote to thank the Association for its part in this. Ultimately, refugee doctors gained permanent status and British citizenship.[57]

While not the issue it had been in the 1930s and early 1940s, the SMA nonetheless retained its commitment to medical refugees. Its belief in socialist and medical internationalism – a controversial issue at a time of intensifying Cold War – is also evident in other ways. Hastings, for example, was chairman of the Medical Supplies Committee for Germany and Austria, an organisation providing hospitality for German doctors brought over to Britain by the Foreign Office in 1948 in an attempt to re-establish relations between the medical professions of the two nations. The nature of this belief in internationalism was eloquently, if optimistically, spelled out by Murray when he suggested in 1948 that the 'problem of our time' was international cooperation. In medicine, with its single set of aims no matter where practised, there should be no barriers to the setting up of transnational mechanisms whereby all doctors would 'co-operate, not only to solve the remaining problems of medicine, but also to protect, to preserve, and to promote the health of the citizens of the world'.[58] Its internationalist beliefs were thus not simply an appendage to the Association's socialist vision, but central to it.

This is further witnessed in the revival of the International Socialist Medical Association, first agreed to at an EC meeting in October 1946. After protracted negotiations and a number of setbacks, a conference eventually came together in June 1948, particularly propitious timing given the imminence of the Appointed Day. In addition to SMA members, it was attended by delegates from nine nations, and observers from Hungary and the USA. Messages of support were received from Bevan and Foreign Secretary Ernest Bevin, as well as from other countries, including the Soviet Union. In essence, however, this was a meeting of socialist doctors from the democratic states of western and northern Europe, an unwitting example of emerging Cold War divisions. The international body was formally constituted, under the supervision of the British organisation, with Murray as chairman and Bunbury as secretary of its provisional committee. Its aims – international cooperation to help maximise health and health services throughout the world – were agreed, and *MTT* assigned the task of acting as clearing house for international news and information. Conference also heard speeches from both British and foreign delegates, including a further claim by Hastings that the NHS was 'in most ways a direct outcome of SMA policy'. The message for socialist health personnel from other countries was obvious.[59]

Reporting to the next EC, Hastings described the meeting as a 'phenomenal success', and the formation of the international organisation as especially important. But the conference scheduled for Sweden in 1949 does not appear to have happened, and while some sort of International SMA congress seems to have taken place in Berlin the same year, no Association member was able to attend because of late notification.[60] Overall, there is virtually no further mention in the SMA's records of international activities of the kind originally envisaged. Like other aspects of the Association's post-war programme, therefore, considerable energy was devoted to projects only partially achieved, if at all. There can be no doubt that the SMA's vision, domestic and international, was inspired by socialist and medical idealism. But the political situation, at home and abroad, placed limits on what could be achieved. The International Socialist Medical Association got off the ground at SMA instigation. But apparently it got little further. The NHS was brought into being, and this too owed its creation to the Association, at least as far as the organisation itself was concerned. But while the new service was celebrated, it was also incomplete, and thereby unable to fulfil its historic role in the transition to socialism. Consequently we now need to assess the Association's position by 1951, when the Labour government was replaced by another Churchill administration; and then evaluate its role in the creation of the NHS and its contribution to socialist analyses of health care.

Notes

1. Brooke, *Labour's War*, p. 325; the Association MPs were Hastings, Haden-Guest, Summerskill, Morgan, Santo Jeger, Taylor, Louis Comyns, Barnet Stross, Samuel Segal, Richard Clitherow, John Baird, and Will Griffiths. All of these were medical doctors of one kind or another, with the exception of the last three who were, respectively, a medical student; a dentist; and an ophthalmic optician, *MTT*, vol. 5, no. 3, September 1945, pp. 4–6.

2. The standard and best account of the creation of the NHS is Webster, *The Health Services since the War*, especially Ch. 4; the debates within the Labour government are covered in Kenneth O. Morgan, *Labour in Power 1945–51*, Oxford, Oxford University Press, 1984, pp. 151–63. See also Peter Hennessy, *Never Again*, Jonathan Cape, 1992, pp. 135–44.

3. DSM 4/2, Socialist Medical Association, 'Message to Press on publication of Health Service Bill', 21 March 1946.

4. DSM (2) 7, H.H. MacWilliam to David Stark Murray, 14 January 1969; Naseem Khan, 'Out of the Market Place', the *Guardian*, Thursday 16 March 1972, p. 11.

5. Webster, *The Health Services since the War*, p. 76; see also Pater, *The Making of the National Health Service*, p. 106; DSM (2) 9, cutting from the *Surrey and Middlesex Clarion*, April 1945; Webster, 'Labour and the Origins of the National Health Service', p. 197.

6. Honigsbaum, *Division in British Medicine*, part 7; Morgan, *Labour in Power*, p. 152.

7. Lee, *My Life with Nye*, p. 177; John Campbell, *Nye Bevan*, Hodder and Stoughton, 1987, p. 179; Michael Foot, *Aneurin Bevan 1945–1960*, Granada, 1975, p. 112. See also Stewart, 'The "back-room boys of state medicine"', p. 230.

8. Patricia Hollis, *Jennie Lee: A Life*, Oxford, Oxford University Press, 1997, pp. 129–31.

9. DSM 4/2, D. Stark Murray, 'New Views on the Health Service', n.d., but mid-1945.

10. Irwin Brown (David Stark Murray), 'We Thought of It First', *MTT*, vol. 5, no. 6, June 1946, pp. 9–10; DSH, File 44 'Radio and Other Talks', script of 'The Public Hospital' for the BBC Far Eastern Service, 6 May 1947; DSM (2) 4, cutting from *The Listener*, 24 January 1946.

11. DSM (2) 4, cutting from the *Scottish Co-Operator* 13 April 1946; for the themes and organisational details of the exhibition see DSM 6/43 and DSM 1/36; *MTT*, vol. 5, no. 7, September 1946, p. 5; and Murray, *Why a National Health Service?*, pp. 83–4.

12. *Lancet*, 1945, II, p. 479; *MTT*, vol. 5, no. 6, June 1946, p. 2; DSM 1/2, EC Minutes, 28 January 1948, p. 2.
13. Bartrip, *Themselves Writ Large*, pp. 259–60; Minutes of the Labour Party Liaison Committee, 9 March 1948.
14. Parliamentary Papers 1945–46, vol. VII, Standing Committee C: Minutes of the Proceedings on the National Health Service Bill; Morgan, *Labour in Power*, p. 155; Hennessy, *Never Again*, p. 139; and MH 80/29, Aneurin Bevan, 'Draft Cabinet Paper – National Health Service: the Future of the Hospital Services', August 1945, pp. 4, 5; Taylor, *A Natural History of Everyday Life*, p. 286.
15. Parliamentary Debates, 5th series, vol. 422, cols. 275–8; Somerville Hastings, 'Those Sixty-six Million Pounds', *MTT*, vol. 5, no. 6, June 1946, p. 4.
16. Somerville Hastings, 'Rifle Shots at Night', *London News*, no. 259, May 1948, p. 3.
17. Somerville Hastings, 'Common Man is All that Really Matters', *London News*, no. 253, July/August 1947, p. 1.
18. Murray, *Why a National Health Service?*, pp. 86–7; DSM (2) 7, Bevan to Murray, 11 February 1946, Murray to Bevan, 21 February 1946, and Bevan to Murray, 11 March 1946; Webster, *The Health Services since the War*, p. 89.
19. Beach, 'The Labour Party and the Idea of Citizenship', p. 161.
20. Stephen Taylor, *National Health Service: Labour Party Discussion Series no. 6*, Labour Party, 1946, pp. 1, 2, and *passim*; *idem*, *A Natural History of Everday Life*, p. 251 and *passim*.
21. Taylor, *National Health Service*, pp. 1, 10, 14, 16–17.
22. Margaret Cole, 'Social Services and Personal Life', in Munro, Donald (ed.), *Socialism: The British Way*, Essential Books, 1948, pp. 117, 100–102.
23. See, for example, Murray, *The Future of Medicine*, p. 77.
24. David Stark Murray, *Your Health, Mr. Smith*, Today and Tomorrow Publications, n.d., but 1946(?); for a discussion of 'planning', particularly in the economic context, see Jim Tomlinson, 'Planning: Debate and Policy in the 1940s', *Twentieth Century British History*, 3, 2, 1992.
25. DSM 4/2, Socialist Medical Association, 'Message to Press on Publication of Health Service Bill', 21 March 1946; Somerville Hastings, 'Public Health' in Tracey, Herbert (ed.), *The British Labour Party – vol. 2*, Caxton Publishing, 1948, p. 141.
26. Somerville Hastings, 'New Ideas for Health Administration', *MTT*, vol. 9, no. 4, July–August 1953, pp. 4–7.
27. DSM 4/2, Sheffield Branch of the SMA, 'How is the National Health Service Working?', February 1949; for a brief description of the role of the Executive Councils and the Local Medical Committees, see Eckstein, *The English National Health Service*, p. 193ff.
28. SMA, *A Socialist Health Service*, SMA, 1949, pp. 2–3; for subsequent, usually abortive, attempts by Labour governments to introduce some measure of democracy into the NHS, see Charles Webster, *The National Health Service: A Political History*, Oxford, Oxford University Press, 1998.
29. SMA, *Child Health: a Survey and Proposals*, Today and Tomorrow Publications, n.d. but probably 1948, p. 6; *MTT*, vol. 8, no. 2, summer 1951, p. 4.

30. David Stark Murray, *Good Health, Mr. Brown*, SMA, n.d., 1951(?), p. 24; *MTT*, vol. 8, no. 1, spring 1951, p. 2; DSM 4/2, Socialist Medical Association, 'Message to Press on publication of Health Service Bill'.

31. DSM 4/2, Socialist Medical Association, 'The Financial and Contractual Aspects of the National Health Service', undated internal memorandum, probably summer 1948.

32. Somerville Hastings, 'Those Sixty-six Million Pounds', *MTT*, vol. 5, no. 6, June 1946, pp. 4–5.

33. DSM 4/2, Morgan Phillips to Elizabeth Bunbury, 29 July 1949; Webster, *The Health Services since the War*, pp. 116–21, 129–32.

34. David Kerr, 'Politics and the National Health Service', in SMA (ed.), *Aneurin Bevan: an Appreciation of his Services to the Health of the People*, SMA, 1960, pp. 3–4.

35. Hastings, 'Public Health', p. 134.

36. SMA, *Child Health: a Survey and Proposals*, p. 3; SMA, *A Socialist Health Service*, pp. 6–8; David Stark Murray, *The Search for Health*, Watts and Co., 1948, p. 148.

37. Labour Party, *Report of the Forty-Sixth Annual Conference*, Labour Party, 1947, p. 196.

38. SMA, *A Socialist Health Service*, p. 4.

39. Ibid.; for a description of just how comprehensive the health centre was intended to be, see SMA, *Get the Health Centres Going NOW*, SMA, 1951, pp. 2–3; SMA, *A Socialised Dental Service: a Report produced by the Dental Group of the Socialist Medical Association*, SMA, 1948, p. 3.

40. Labour Party, *Report of the Forty-Sixth Annual Conference*, Labour Party, 1947, p. 196.

41. H.H. MacWilliam, 'For the Record', *MTT*, vol. 6, no. 5, March 1948, p. 8; Webster, *The Health Services since the War*, p. 383 – I am grateful to Charles Webster for drawing my attention to the exact timing of these events; SMA, *Get the Health Centres Going NOW*, pp. 1–2.

42. MH 133/63 and 133/64; *MTT*, vol. 8, no. 9, November–December 1952, p. 4; Webster, *The Health Services since the War*, pp. 383–6; *idem, The National Health Service: A Political History*, p. 50.

43. SMA, *Bulletin*, no. 109, June–July 1949, p. 3; SMA, *Child Health: a Survey and Proposals*, p. 4.

44. 'International Socialist Medical Association: Report of First Annual Conference', *MTT*, vol. 6, no. 7, Autumn 1948, p. 10.

45. DSM 1/6, EC Minutes, 8 August 1945; DSM 1/2, EC Minutes, 11 February and 28 July 1948.

46. Minutes of the Policy and Publicity Committee, 7 July 1948, p. 1; and 19 July 1948, p. 2.

47. Taylor, *A Natural History of Everday Life*, p. 296.

48. DSM 1/2, EC Minutes, 28 July 1948; Labour Party Research Department, RD/232 December 1948 'Draft Report of the Public Health Advisory Committee', pp. 2, 7; and RD/327 November 1949, memorandum by Somerville Hastings 'Medical Education in the New Programme', p. 1.

49. See the respective reports of the Labour Party Annual Conferences for 1946 to 1948, pp. 56 (1946); 64 (1947); and 73 (1948); Minutes of a Meeting of the Parliamentary Labour Party, 10 December 1947; for the 'German telegram' episode in more detail, see Jonathan Schneer, *Labour's Conscience: the Labour Left 1945–1951*, Unwin Hyman, 1988, p. 107.

50. Minutes of the National Executive Committee, 19 May 1948.
51. Labour Party, *Report of the Forty-Fifth Annual Conference*, Labour Party, 1946, pp. 132–4; Labour Party, *Report of the Forty-Sixth Annual Conference*, Labour Party, 1947, pp. 196–7.
52. DSM 1/2, Minutes of Council, 15 June 1947.
53. DSM 1/2, EC Minutes, 3 September and 8 October 1947, and Minutes of Council, 21 September and 30 November 1947.
54. For a history of tuberculosis in twentieth-century Britain, and a reference to an SMA intervention on the issue, see Linda Bryder, *Below the Magic Mountain*, Oxford, Oxford University Press, 1988, p. 231; for the first Association conference, see *MTT*, vol. 7, no. 6, summer 1950, p. 3ff; London Trades Council and the Socialist Medical Association, *TB: Report of Conference*, SMA, p. 4 and *passim*; SMA, *Bulletin*, 117, June-July 1950, p. 1.
55. Julian Huxley et al., *When Hostilities Cease: Papers on Relief and Reconstruction prepared for the Fabian Society*, Victor Gollancz, 1943; Parliamentary Debates, 5th series, vol. 433, col. 2492; *Lancet*, 1951, I, p. 170.
56. *MTT*, vol. 5, no. 3, September Quarter 1945, p. 3.
57. Honigsbaum, *Division in British Medicine*, pp. 312–13; DSM 1/2, EC Minutes, 28 April 1948, 30 June 1948; 10 March 1948, 5 May 1948.
58. *Lancet*, 1948, I, p. 729; Murray, *The Search for Health*, p. 156.
59. DSM 1/2, EC Minutes, 9 October 1946, and EC Minutes, 26 May 1948; 'International Socialist Medical Association: Report of First Annual Conference', *MTT*, vol. 6, no. 7, Autumn 1948, pp. 3–10.
60. DSM 1/2, EC Minutes, 30 June 1948; DSM 1/3, EC Minutes, 13 July 1949.

CHAPTER TEN

'Pure but Impotent'?

At the end of the Second World War the SMA was undoubtedly aware of the powerful opposition which existed to radical reform of the health services. Nonetheless it could also look forward to its vision of a socialised medical service being realised, in whole or in significant part. The Association had made much of the running in Labour's health policy and had a membership which, if not huge, was nonetheless expanding. Six years later it found itself in a very different situation. Although social reform had come a long way, the Labour government was suffering from terminal exhaustion and was soon to be replaced by another Churchill administration. Even before this Bevan left the Ministry of Health and then the government itself, in protest against the introduction of health service charges. These were also opposed by the SMA, but this did not mean that it immediately forgave the former Health Minister for his concessions to the medical profession. We saw in the last chapter that this sense of resentment lingered well into the 1960s, and it was further manifested by Hastings's apparent decision to vote for Morrison rather than Bevan in the 1955 leadership election.[1]

By the fall of the second Attlee government the Association itself was facing serious difficulties. It had been increasingly marginalised within the labour movement while becoming more and more unhappy about key aspects of Bevan's scheme. The resignation of Hastings as Association president in 1951 after 21 years in the post, although almost certainly due to his wider political commitments and his age, nonetheless symbolises the end of a particular phase in the organisation's history.[2] During this period it had rising hopes of playing a significant part in the formation of a socialised medical service, but saw these only partially realised, despite Labour's 1945 election victory. We now examine further the problems the Association faced in the post-war era and its responses to such circumstances, and use these as a platform from which to assess the SMA's role in medical politics from its foundation down to 1951. This in turn leads to a concluding discussion on the possible continuing pertinence of certain of the organisation's central ideas.

Problems of direction and membership

The post-war Labour administrations felt obliged to restrict public expenditure, including on the NHS, and impose health service charges. This resulted from the general economic situation, the belief that some patients were abusing the service through demands for unnecessary medicines and treatments, and concern that NHS costs were spiralling out of control. Jim Tomlinson argues that Labour created an 'austere' welfare state with, for example, no health centres or hospitals being built in the 1940s, hardly what radical reformers such as the SMA had in mind. One political consequence of such frugality was Bevan's move to the Ministry of Labour late in 1950, his resignation shortly thereafter from the Cabinet over charges for dental and ophthalmic work, and his subsequent vociferous campaign from the backbenches. These aspects of the government's economic strategy were deeply worrying to the SMA and even before the Appointed Day it expressed concern at the 'possible effects on the National Health Service of the recent announcements of cuts in capital expenditure'. More specifically on health policy, the clause in the 1949 NHS (Amendment) Bill allowing for the introduction of prescription charges was opposed by both Jeger and Hastings during its parliamentary passage. Hastings argued that the doctors making the greatest claims about widespread abuse of the service were precisely those who had opposed its introduction in the first place, and urged Bevan to ensure his place in history by rejecting the clause.[3]

Writing on the same issue, Murray claimed that it illustrated two particular points which had 'not been sufficiently emphasised and in Labour circles are too readily forgotten'. The first was that the party had not yet 'officially dropped' its policy of a full-time salaried service, although as we saw in the last chapter this was, in fact, a further dimension of the 1949 Act. Second, the service could only work efficiently and economically if doctors were concerned not with chasing after fees, but rather with devoting their entire energies to the functioning of the NHS. No single patient could abuse the system; rather, the onus was on those who actually did the prescribing. In a rather barbed manner, Murray suggested that the Health Minister 'may have made this point to his Cabinet colleagues but if so he failed to make them understand'. There was, in short, a clear relationship between the government's capitulation over a salaried service and its opening up of the possibility of charging fees. An SMA press statement the same month – partly drawn up by Murray – took a rather more conciliatory approach to Bevan, agreeing that if he had been fighting against charges in Cabinet then 'he deserves the thanks of the public'. But charges were, the statement continued, 'a complete denial of the basic principle of the

NHS for which the SMA fought and the Labour Party stood, namely, that it should be free at the time of use'.[4]

A letter to the press from a group of London Association members early in 1950 took the matter further. It noted that the prescription charges clause had been fully supported by the Conservative opposition. Any resulting costs would, the letter continued, fall most heavily on those in greatest need, for example mothers of large families. This would lead to 'unnecessary delay in sending for the doctor, and prevent the early diagnosis of disease while there is still time to effect a cure'.[5] The government's behaviour was thus, so the argument went, politically reprehensible and medically counterproductive, since fees would constitute the sort of economic barrier to health characteristic of the pre-war system. When placed in the context of the critique of Bevan's scheme dealt with in the last chapter, the question of expenditure and charges clearly added to the Association's worries over the direction in which the NHS was heading.

But the response of one SMA stalwart to these matters provides a way into an important dimension of the organisation's post-war problems. During the 1951 election campaign Edith Summerskill, now Minister of National Insurance, claimed that she and other Association founder members had been 'responsible for planning the National Health Service 20 years ago'. Bevan was not, she continued, the architect of the health service, only its midwife. Consequently, she and her SMA colleagues strongly resented 'any individual or group asserting for their own private political purposes that they are the sole defenders of the National Health Service', a clear reference to the former Health Minister and his well-publicised objections to the imposition of fees. Summerskill repeated her claim about the SMA a few days later at a May Day meeting where she was 'constantly heckled' on the charges issue. But, she urged her audience, their introduction was 'not a big breach of principle, so forget it. Close your ranks. Remember the real enemies are the Tories'.[6] On one level this graphically illustrates the SMA's strong sense of its own place in health service history, as well as personal antipathy to the now increasingly isolated Bevan. Nonetheless, the Association leadership was quick to distance itself from Summerskill's comments, issuing a press statement – a copy of which was sent to the errant member herself – reiterating its opposition to charges. Of course Summerskill was now bound by collective Cabinet responsibility. But as the records make clear, she was not the only individual to go against official SMA policy. During the Commons debate on the charges clause in the 1949 Bill, three Association members spoke. We have seen that Hastings and Jeger opposed fees. Sam Segal, while less adamant on the matter than the other two, suggested that its deferment might be appropriate at this stage, at least until further evidence became available. But when it came to the division he, along with Summerskill, actually supported the government. Hastings and Jeger do not appear to have voted, nor does any other Association MP, a curious stance on an apparently fundamental point of principle. Understandably, this led to concern inside the organisation over the Commons voting record of its members.[7] The essential point is, therefore, that while the SMA as a whole might pursue a particular line, this was not always adhered to by everyone in all circumstances.

Nor was such dissension confined to Cabinet Ministers or backbench MPs. Charles Brook, long sceptical of local government's role in health service administration, further argued in 1946 that health centres should not be under local authority control because of the different standards which prevailed across the country. Rather, they should be the responsibility of Regional Hospital Boards. Association member J.A. Scott wrote to the *BMJ* early in 1948 (that is during the tense run-up to the 'Appointed Day') to voice another kind of criticism of official SMA policy. Many in the profession, he claimed, had failed to appreciate Bevan's 'Machiavellian cunning'. The Minister was attempting to force the NHS on doctors, who should respond by taking strike action – precisely the sort of thing done in the past by Bevan himself. Scott further claimed that he was 'whole-heartedly opposed to the Act in its present form' and that this was a view shared by many others in the Association, despite the fact that 'Bevan relies to some extent on the SMA to help him push the Act upon us'.[8]

These divergences from the official Association strategy strongly suggest differences within the organisation over its role and purpose, particularly after the passing of the 1946 Act. This is now discussed in the context of a closely related matter, its problems in recruiting and retaining members. As recorded in Labour Party annual conference reports, SMA membership peaked at 2000 in the period 1946 to 1949, and the enthusiasm and idealism of some of the recruits of the 1940s has been captured by Anne Digby. After 1949 membership began to decline, but concerns were being expressed even in the immediate aftermath of the Appointed Day. Following an EC intervention by Hastings, an Association meeting was held at the Commons in November 1948. Statistical analysis showed the peak recruiting periods as the 1945 election, the publication of the 1946 Bill, and its Second Reading. The current decline in new members was noted and it was suggested that this might be due to a feeling that the organisation's work was now complete.[9] If this last point was true it implies that the official SMA line was not always agreed to, or perhaps even understood, by all who belonged to the organisation. It also reminds us of Elizabeth Bunbury's pre-war concern, referred to in Chapter Three, about the level of political awareness of Association members.

A further dimension to the membership issue was revealed by EC member and honorary treasurer, the surgeon Harry Barst, in early 1950. Following speaking engagements in support of Labour election candidates he had, he reported, spoken with 'many health workers who had not ever heard of the SMA'. At the subsequent AGM Barst, in addition to noting the ongoing financial deficit, stressed the need to make the Association known in all parts of the labour movement, in all parts of the country. It is undoubtedly significant that his contacts with these unenlightened medical personnel were in the provincial towns of Warwick and Goole.[10] This again illustrates the difficulties the SMA faced in putting down roots in the broader labour movement, particularly outside London. We have seen that this was no new phenomenon, and undoubtedly contributed to Murray's poor showing in the 1948 NEC elections discussed in the previous chapter.

The membership issue was clearly one of vital importance for the Association and was further taken up by Ian Gilliland, EC chair, at a Council meeting in March 1949. His statement was then discussed at the 1949 AGM and published, with amendments, in *MTT*; and with further amendments as the policy statement *A Socialist Health Service*. One immediately obvious organisational outcome of this flurry of activity was the reconstitution of the Association's Policy Committee, chaired by Murray and with Gilliland as secretary, in July 1949. Large sections of all three versions of Gilliland's statement sought to reassert what constituted a socialist health policy, ideas discussed in Chapter Nine.[11]

But Gilliland also gives an insight into matters more concerned with the very nature and purpose of the SMA. At the Council meeting he argued that now was the time for the organisation to 'put its house in order'. Despite its 'glorious history', enrolment since the Appointed Day had been slow. Indeed there had been more resignations and lapses of membership than new recruits. The Association had been content, he continued, to 'be the watch-dog of the new Service, following behind public demand and no longer putting forward a socialist policy'. Varying explanations were offered for this. In his Council speech, Gilliland claimed that since 1946 SMA strategy had shifted away from a 'fighting policy' to a preoccupation with the NHS Act's implementation. The *MTT* version omitted the point about the former 'fighting policy' but again stressed the significance of a shift in 1946, adding that since then many of 'our best and most active workers have found themselves endlessly involved with the day-to-day administration of the Act'. But the SMA had 'ceased to lead the fight'. It had become an advisory body, and although this was 'an important part of our work, it can only be a part'.[12]

This analysis raises, wittingly or otherwise, two crucial issues. First, Gilliland's point about the shift in 1946 away from a 'fighting policy' might be seen as something of an exaggeration given that from the NHS Bill's publication the Association, at least in its official statements, was sceptical about important constituents of Bevan's scheme. But it also reveals a greater truth. Like many such bodies, the SMA was stronger when it was battling against particular ideas or institutions and this adversarial stance clearly gave it a strong sense of identity and purpose. Of course there had been differences of opinion within the Association since its creation, and on occasions these could be embarrassing or troublesome. However between 1930 and 1945 the organisation went through a process whereby it refined and adapted its vision of a social-ised medical service. Despite differences, Association members were united in their desire for *some* form of socialised service, as well as being acutely aware of the need to combat medical 'reaction'. In such circumstances varying approaches could to a large extent be submerged in the common cause.

With the arrival of the NHS, however, internal differences took on a new importance. All Association members had welcomed central as-pects of the 1946 Act, particularly the provision of universal, free, and comprehensive services. The question now was what, if anything, to do next. For some, further important changes still had to be made. Murray, commenting on Bevan's departure from the Ministry of Health, claimed that the new Minister must address major policy issues if previous mistakes were to be rectified and new ones avoided. Above all, he continued, Bevan's replacement 'must act on the principle that the National Health Service cannot stand still. If it does not develop it will deteriorate ... '.[13] But as Summerskill's comments and the analyses of Gilliland and of the 1948 Commons meeting each in their own way show, for some in the SMA the creation of the health service was an end in itself. Although it might need tinkering with, the delivery of more or less free health care was the essential core of what was needed.

Many in the Association would have agreed with Bevan when he famously claimed that a 'free health service is pure Socialism and as such it is opposed to the hedonism of capitalist society'. It was possible for SMA members to hold such a view while being personally suspi-cious of Bevan, as in Summerskill's case; or a close friend, such as Will Griffiths MP, soon to be Bevan's parliamentary private secretary. Strate-gic differences posed the very real question of what purpose, if any, the SMA now served. For activists such as Murray and Gilliland there was much which remained to be done. For others, more pragmatic or more limited in their ambitions, what was required was consolidation of an essentially sound foundation. It was almost certainly from this group, as the Commons meeting suggested, that loss of membership primarily occurred. According to Martin Francis, this sense of completion was widely held in the labour movement itself, where Bevan's concessions were accepted as necessary for the achievement of what was nonetheless a socialist service. The feeling, at least among the majority in the Labour Party, that the NHS had resolved the major issues of health policy may account for the relative neglect of the issue in its election manifestos in 1950 and 1951.[14]

Nonetheless the disagreements within the Association clearly mirrored the acrimonious debates in the wider labour movement over what Brooke describes as the 'means and ends of socialism', debates which were to come to the surface and plague the Labour Party into the 1950s and beyond. A further reflection of this can be found at an SMA conference in 1955, when the present worrying state of the NHS was attributed in part to 'divergence of opinion in the Labour movement' over the service's future development. The complex relationship between the SMA and the rest of the labour movement is returned to below. Finally, while Klein rather overstates the case when he argues that the NHS became 'depoliticised' after 1948, his comment is illuminating in view of both Gilliland's claim that many Association members became absorbed in administrative work at the expense of fighting for further change in the system and Labour's apparent sense of closure on health policy.[15]

The second point arising from the Gilliland's analysis follows on from this. As we have seen, he claimed that some Association members were heavily committed to the 1946 Act's operation. It was certainly the case that, for example, Hastings and Joules belonged to bodies such as the Medical Advisory Committee of the Central Health Services Council, while Murray was now chairman of the Blood Transfusion Service of the South West Metropolitan Region.[16] This was, of course, in addition to other medical and political responsibilities. But again, as is often the case with such organisations, these burdens were not evenly shared. Hastings, congratulating Murray in 1949 for his efforts with *MTT*, went on to point out, quite correctly, that Murray himself had often been its sole contributor of articles. This had, in fact, been the case since the journal was founded. The trouble with the SMA, Hastings continued, was that 'the responsibility was left to the few'.[17] This places the membership expansion of the 1940s in a rather less positive light.

The amount of work falling on a handful of leading activists was clearly a serious concern, and another characteristic of the organisation during the period under consideration in this study. In view of this and other membership-related problems, and the course the health service had taken since its inception in 1948, it is therefore unsurprising to find

Murray stressing in June 1951 that the SMA had now more work to do than before the introduction of the NHS. There was, he argued, a need for detail rather than the previous general principles, and for the organisation to respond to others getting ahead of them in the production of health policy documents.[18]

Of course the SMA did not passively accept the difficulties which it faced in the post-war era. It worked extremely hard to ensure the passage of the 1946 Act and to continue to press for its own vision of a socialised service. Moreover it sought in one very specific way to deal with its increasing labour movement isolation, and its own membership problems, by attempting to improve its relationship with the Medical Practitioners' Union. As well as being affiliated to the TUC, the MPU had more than twice as many members as the Association, and indeed its numbers were rising in the wake of the 1946 Act.[19] Although the two organisations had been at odds in the past, by the late 1940s the MPU was, at least in some areas, pursuing policies similar to those of the Association. In October 1948, for example, MPU Council stressed its support for a system of health centres, with SMA member R.A. Lyster arguing that this should be a 'plank in our platform'. The same meeting noted the TUC's request for the withdrawal of an MPU conference resolution on health centres on the grounds that it 'implied criticism of the government'. As we saw in the last chapter, one year earlier the TUC had, for similar reasons, exerted pressure on potential participants, including the MPU, in an SMA-organised conference. Nonetheless the SMA was moved to congratulate both the MPU and the TUC on their health centre stance in autumn 1949. As Lyster's involvement also suggests, some individuals were active in both organisations, and indeed had been so for some time. Lyster and Brook are obvious examples here, to which can be added TUC medical advisor H.B. Morgan and Richard Clitherow, elected to parliament in 1945 and the following year appointed MPU Parliamentary Secretary.[20]

No doubt encouraged by the October 1948 meeting, the following month Hastings approached the MPU Executive with a proposal for cooperation, to which it duly agreed. It is worth emphasising that this came at exactly the same time as the SMA's discussion at the Commons of its membership problems. Hastings's plea for joint work must therefore be viewed as an attempt by the Association to gain direct access to MPU members in the hope of converting at least some of them to its policies. Unfortunately for the Association, MPU Council reversed the agreement to cooperate, almost certainly on the (rather disingenuous) grounds that the Union was 'non-political'. An SMA invitation a year later to co-organise a meeting on prescription charges was likewise turned down.[21] At a formal level the two therefore maintained their distance, and this avenue for an Association revival was effectively closed off.

Communists

The Association's post-war structural problems – some new, but also in large part inherent in the nature of the organisation itself – undoubtedly weakened its position, and can have done little for its credibility with the Labour leadership, even had the latter been inclined by this stage to adopt the whole SMA programme. Just as important here was the Association's political stance relative to the rest of the labour movement. It had always tended to the left and, at least at leadership level, this continued after 1945 and thus during the onset of the Cold War. We have already noted that Hastings was a signatory of the 'second German telegram', and other manifestations of this leftist inclination included a resolution condemning the Greek government's treatment of members of the medical profession. It was, this concluded, 'unbelievable' that the regime was being supported by the Labour administration. Similarly, the SMA opposed German rearmament despite a warning by Hastings, aware that this was an immensely divisive issue for the Labour Party, that it was not a matter for the Association.[22]

Even worse, from the Labour leadership's point of view, was the continuing presence in the SMA of Communist Party members, a situation which had existed since the mid-1930s and had led to a fierce internal debate over the organisation's attitude to the Second World War. After the resolution of this issue the Association resumed its 'popular front' approach, much to the annoyance of the NEC. It worked with the Labour Research Department, a body proscribed by both the Labour Party and the TUC. Both Honigsbaum and Earwicker point out that the SMA came close to expulsion from the party, probably saved only by the intervention of Morrison on the basis of their mutual involvement with the LCC and support for local authority control. This did not, however, stop the NEC from seeking the resignation of the communist Brian Kirman from the post of Association secretary, and requiring an assurance of its loyalty to the Labour Party from the SMA. The particular issue here was the participation of several leading activists – including Bourne and Hilliard – in the communist-front 'People's Convention' in January 1941. Similarly, Honigsbaum claims that important union leaders (he cites Bevin in particular) never forgot communist opposition to the war in the early 1940s, and that this too disposed them to a sceptical view of the Association.[23] It is therefore ironic that despite its growing influence on party health policy during the war, the organisation was already tainted by its communist associations.

In the post-war period the SMA continued to embrace Communist Party members and their activities. In September 1948, for example, a report was made to Council on a *Daily Worker* peace conference, and it was agreed that all Association branches should do all possible 'to cooperate with working class and all other organisations in their locality, in any joint campaign for preserving world peace'.[24] This was hardly the sort of behaviour designed to appease the dominant Cold Warrior element in the Labour Party. From the summer of 1949 to early 1951 the SMA's Liverpool branch suffered severe disruption through differences between Communist and Labour Party members. At various points not only the SMA, but also the Liverpool Trades Council and the Labour Party's national agent and national secretary were involved. The whole affair was reported in the national press, no doubt to the intense annoyance of the party leadership. The net result was a split in the branch caused by the departure of Labour supporters – including H.H. MacWilliam – unwilling to accept the behaviour of their communist colleagues. After numerous meetings and investigations, an uneasy resolution was reached which still involved the two groups working separately. Murray, who had done much of the investigating and negotiating, was congratulated by Hastings for carrying out 'this very difficult and unpleasant task'.[25]

The Liverpool branch's problems were about more than just parochial political differences, important as these undoubtedly were to the participants and to other labour movement bodies in the city. As Hastings's comments imply, the whole complex affair was both disruptive and immensely time-consuming. We noted that the Association was inclined to leave responsibilities to a few leading activists. The Liverpool situation can only have added to this burden at exactly the period when leading figures such as Gilliland were attempting to politically revitalise the organisation. It is further likely that the disruption in Liverpool not only saw the loss of Labour supporters such as MacWilliam, but that it also discouraged potential new members or caused other existing ones to leave. Communist activities had had this result on at least one previous occasion, during the debate in 1940 over the Association's approach to the war. As Murray noted in his report for the EC, the issue was being used throughout the Liverpool region 'to label the SMA as a Communist controlled organisation', a piece of publicity the Association could well have done without.[26]

The episode thus highlights a central weakness in the SMA, for what happened in Liverpool was not an isolated incident. On the contrary, it was the direct outcome of the decision to admit communists in the mid-1930s and to allow them to remain thereafter. As the Association itself attempted to argue, it was a body primarily concerned with health matters. But given that it also argued that health was bound up with wider political and socio-economic circumstances and its own engagement with overtly political issues, this was, at best, naive. The unremitting hostility of the Labour leadership to communism was well known and meant that it could not help but look upon the SMA as a compromised organisation. There can be little doubt that many in the Association genuinely believed in the need for all 'progressive' forces to unite to advance the cause of socialised medicine, and that this was a direct reflection of the lessons drawn from the experiences of the 1930s.

But purely from the point of view of political pragmatism, the admission and retention of Communist Party members was a tactical mistake which did little to endear the SMA to the most influential sections of the labour movement. More specifically, it can be argued that the Labour Party was prepared to use the Association and more or less tolerate its political radicalism during the 1930s and 1940s, when it had a valuable part to play in devising plans for medical reconstruction. But after the war, with the NHS in place and the world dividing into communist and non-communist blocs, the party was equally prepared to quietly marginalise the politically unreliable SMA. In any assessment of the Association, the negative impact of its left-wing stance and membership must be a factor of considerable weight.

Further obstacles in the Association's path

So far it has been argued that the problems the Association faced after 1945 contributed to its decline from a position of some influence over Labour health policy to one of increasing marginalisation; that these problems were inherent in the nature of the organisation itself; and that it was consequently in a difficult position when it argued for further progress towards what it considered a truly socialised service. This should, nonetheless, not obscure the fact that at the end of the Second World War Labour's health policy was largely that of the SMA. We have seen that this was in part overridden by Bevan, and sought to explain how this came about. However the creation of the National Health Service was an immensely complex process, and to have fully achieved the Association's programme would have involved the removal or circumvention of major structural and political obstacles as well as large-scale capital investment. Its only partial realisation is therefore attributable not only to the issues already discussed, but also to the following further, and related, factors.

First, Honigsbaum claims that one characteristic of the SMA was its misreading of the mood of its fellow professionals.[27] There is certainly a strong case to be made here. In the last chapter, for example, we found MacWilliam claiming rather optimistically that opposition to the NHS among medical practitioners would have been lessened had Bevan pursued a more vigorous line on health centres. Similarly, the Association argued that the BMA leadership was a reactionary clique and that many doctors, and especially the younger ones, were more disposed to a socialised service. This may have been partly true, but it is equally the case that the SMA had only limited success in one of its declared aims of converting medical practitioners to its view of how, and to what ends, health services should be organised. This might not have mattered had the Association been able to command broad popular support, or tap into general discontent with the NHS. Part of Gilliland's analysis in the late 1940s included, as we have seen, the assertion that the organisation was preoccupied with routine administration to the neglect of public demands for expansion of the service. Once again, this seems wildly optimistic. While there was certainly opposition to the introduction of charges, as witnessed by the heckling of Summerskill, the NHS as an institution was nonetheless highly popular. There was also a fair degree of scepticism among the British population about the apparent pace of change in the post-war period.[28] In short, at this stage there was no widespread desire for the further advances sought by some Association members. This appears to have been the case among medical practitioners, the public at large, and the majority of the Labour Party itself.

This problem was recognised by Hastings in two pieces in the early 1950s. In the first, discussing the recent general election defeat, he claimed that in his own constituency people had lost interest in politics, having gained their short-term desires without having absorbed the 'high ideals of the socialist movement'. This was, he continued, largely the fault of the movement itself, since 'we have insisted too much on immediate palliatives and too little on basic principles'. The second piece argued that the post-war governments had changed the 'whole outlook and conception of society' but that difficulties nonetheless remained. To get the best out of socialist legislation it was necessary that all who participate in it must have the 'Socialist outlook'. But it was hard even for those who 'had accepted the Socialist creed to practice what they preach'. Hastings attributed this to 'spending most of our lives as members of an acquisitive society'. The use of this Tawnyesque phrase reminds us of the basis of Hastings's political philosophy and it may also be significant that the piece was entitled 'Problems of the Welfare State', a perhaps unconscious echo of the recently published volume by Richard Titmuss. His remarks are also worth placing along-side the contemporary comments of G.D.H. Cole, who claimed that the Labour government had 'conceived socialisation as merely state busi-ness replacing private business, without any change of spirit'.[29]

In any event, Hastings was acknowledging not only that the bulk of the population had to be fully educated in socialist principles, but also that fellow-socialists too needed reminding of these fundamental ideas. This brings us to our second major point. We noted above that there were internal divisions within the SMA, and that these acquired par-ticular significance when confronted with the scheme Bevan put in place. As will have become evident in the course of this work, these differences extended to the wider labour movement. Important sections of the Fabian Society, for instance, were deeply sceptical about local authority control on the basis that a nationally uniform delivery of medical services, irrespective of where the patient/consumer happened to live, was required. Local government, in any case in dire need of reform, was seen as incapable of doing this.

Similarly the TUC, a body with considerable influence on the Labour Party, was much more sympathetic to the medical profession's sensibili-ties than the SMA. On the question of a salaried service, for example, in principle it desired such a scheme. But as Earwicker points out, the TUC was also careful to hedge its support 'against the overriding need to secure the co-operation of doctors'. It is also clear that it saw social welfare in the broader context of collective bargaining and of the social wage, and of its desire to cooperate on policy matters with the Labour government. In such circumstances there seems little doubt that, as Francis puts it, the trades unions 'frequently restricted the options open to Labour's socialist policy makers'.[30] Consequently the TUC, although strongly in favour of a state health service, was more concerned with the actual delivery of medical care than with the finer administrative details. It was also, of course, a nationally organised body, with deep roots in the organised working class, in marked contrast to the Associa-tion. Finally, a number of leading TUC figures were avowed anti-communists, and thereby deeply suspicious of the SMA's left-wing political stance. In any battle of ideas between the two organisations the Association was clearly at a considerable disadvantage.

Third, there is the nature of the Labour Party itself. We noted in the previous chapter that the sympathetic historian of the post-war Labour governments claims, rather curiously, that the SMA had 'forced' its policy on the party in 1934. But Morgan does make the useful point that this was achieved despite Labour's 'labyrinthine and cumbersome' structures, and perhaps what is most noticeable here is that this came about while the party was in opposition and still reeling from the debacle of 1931. However, being in government is clearly a vastly different matter and it was in this context that Bevan, as Brooke succinctly puts it, 'stood Labour Party policy on its head'.[31] The difficult nature of the structural relationship between organisations such as the SMA and the party as a whole is illuminated by a brief examination of another affiliated body, in this case concerned with education.

The National Association of Labour Teachers (NALT) was founded in 1927, and like the SMA in respect of health sought to convert both professional colleagues and the Labour Party to its vision of a socialist education system. It too had a strong base on the London County Council, while being weak in other parts of the country. The LCC experience, although as with the SMA rather frustrating in terms of outcomes, nonetheless convinced the organisation of the possibilities of 'multilateral' (that is, 'comprehensive') schools. Also like the SMA, the NALT had a significant presence on the party policy committee set up in 1937. By 1939, as Rodney Barker puts it, Labour was not publicly committed to multilateralism, but was nonetheless 'publicly associated' with the idea, with the war further increasing pressure for educational reform. However as in health policy, and despite the NALT's activities, there were different approaches inside the labour movement to education with bodies such as the TUC preferring a more gradualist strategy when compared with that of the professional organisation. Ultimately Labour accepted the socially-divisive 1944 Education Act. At 1945 conference the NEC made a commitment to multilateralism, but as Barker further points out the attitude of the parliamentary party in particular was one of 'whole-hearted support' for every aspect of the Act. Consequently the Labour government's policy was essentially a continuation of the system set up in 1944. While the Labour Teachers continued to press for a reconstruction of secondary education, in the immediate term at least, little real progress was made.[32]

The parallel experiences of the SMA and the NALT are striking. Both were professionally-based bodies which at certain points succeeded in having significant aspects of their radical and innovative policies accepted by the Labour Party. Their authority derived from professional knowledge allied to their socialist vision. However both were also small organisations, concentrated in London, and unable to put down deep roots in the broader labour movement. Their policies, because of (or despite) their very radicalism, could be accepted when the party was in opposition or in the wartime coalition. But their actual realisation became much more problematical when Labour was governing in its own right. Furthermore both had powerful critics within the movement, more inclined to a pragmatic or gradualist approach and able to call on support from throughout the country and across occupational boundaries, and not just from metropolitan professionals. In short, Labour's 'laby-rinthine and cumbersome' structures could be subverted or penetrated when policy alternatives were absent, or when there was no immediate prospect of political power. But when government became a reality, the very nature of the Labour Party could work against small, narrowly-based organisations such as the SMA.

Fourth, we have seen that many of the reservations about the practi-cality and desirability of parts of the SMA's programme were shared by Aneurin Bevan, a politician with a significant power base in the Labour Party nationally. Bevan's relationship with the Association, not close in the first place, was put under increasing strain by its post-war critique of his scheme. The advice proffered by SMA members may have been further unwelcome as coming from middle class socialists who were also members of an élite profession, two groups to whom the Health Minister was not over-sympathetic. For Bevan the Association was 'pure but impotent' – an organisation which had, implicitly, the luxury of coming up with radical, even utopian, ideas without the responsibil-ity of actually implementing them. Bevan, by contrast, held real political power and was thereby obliged to engage in complex negotiations with a range of interested parties.

The role of Bevan's personality in achieving his own version of a socialised service should not be neglected. Even the sceptical Murray, while making the usual proviso about no one individual being able to change the course of history, described him as a 'revolutionary force', albeit one which 'appeared to have expended itself in the great effort of placing the National Health Service Act on the statute book'. Webster has recently reinforced the idea of Bevan as central to the creation of the NHS, while Stephen Taylor shrewdly pointed out that Bevan's repu-tation as a left-winger made the Labour Party 'ready to accept much which, from other hands, would have led to revolts'. From a rather different angle, Earwicker observes that Bevan entered the Commons as 'a champion of local rights' but was then 'absorbed into its procedures and possibilities', ending up a firm believer in the doctrine of parlia-mentary responsibility. He quotes to effect Bevan's parliamentary private secretary, who later recalled that the Minister 'did not consider himself bound to accept advice or ideas on the basis of their origin or of their association with the Labour movement. He was, above all, a parliamen-tarian ... '. It was in this context that, as Earwicker further suggests, Bevan devised a hospital plan which 'contravened the letter and spirit of every Labour Party policy document on health', thus exchanging the 'traditional Labour view of accountability in social policy, where lo-cally-elected representatives took the decisions, for one which stressed ministerial responsibility to Parliament'.[33]

Finally on Bevan, it is clear that he was primarily concerned with the delivery of free and comprehensive medical services rather than with potentially irresolvable issues such as control and remuneration – hence his assertion that free health care was pure socialism. Related to this, Beach argues that Bevan's view of citizenship emphasised rights more than participation. One implication of these two different approaches was divergent ideas about how democracy and citizenship were expressed. In rejecting local accountability, Bevan was clearly coming down in favour of the imposition of national, uniform standards controlled through parliament. There were therefore fundamental philosophical differences between Bevan and the Association over the status of local and consumer rights. In passing it is worth noting here that, as Beach and Brooke both point out, by the late 1940s questions were being asked within the labour movement, for example by Cole and by Michael Young, as to whether more participation and local variation might be allowed in both the welfare services and society generally.[34] This was what the SMA had long argued but such criticisms had, at least in the short term, little impact on the newly-created structures of the 'welfare state'.

Fifth, the context in which the Association operated was not simply confined to the labour movement, nor was it isolated from broader structural factors. Civil servants at the Ministry of Health were certainly aware of the Association's activities, especially on the LCC. Important as this was as an indicator of the dissemination of SMA ideas these public officials were, both Webster and Rodney Lowe argue, ultimately neither especially proactive in formulating policy nor able to effectively resist the pressure exerted by, in particular, the BMA.[35] This suggests the need to examine the policy process more closely in the light of Association aspirations.

The BMA was hostile to key elements in the SMA programme, for example the proposal that medical practitioners become salaried state employees. Bevan was prepared to concede on precisely this sort of issue in order to realise what he considered the essential core of his plan. Of course this was not simply one-way traffic – the profession too was forced to compromise, for example over the sale of practices – and this process of negotiation has been analysed by a number of political scientists. Christopher Ham reminds us that creation of the NHS was characterised by the relative unimportance of parliament. By contrast, he continues, of central significance were extra-parliamentary forces, especially 'major pressure groups with an interest in health services'. Civil service records make clear that these included the BMA, but not the SMA. One implication of this, as a 1978 government report acknowledged, is that since the 1940s the profession's 'independence' has remained 'a central feature of the organisation and management of health services'.[36]

The consequences of this are further highlighted by those – and particularly R.A.W. Rhodes – concerned with 'policy networks'. Here the NHS is cited as the prime example of a 'professional network', characterised by the 'pre-eminence of one class of participants in policy making – the profession'. Expanding on this, Gerald Wistow concludes that the history of the NHS confirms that the 'values and interests' of the dominant medical practitioners have provided a powerful integrating mechanism within the health service, as well as 'insulating' it from outside forces. Effectively, therefore, there is a 'health service policy community rather than a health one'. Furthermore both political and managerial influences, and the demands of service users, have been subordinated to those of the medical profession.[37]

A number of points pertinent to the history of the SMA arise from these analyses. First, the Association's success in influencing Labour policy, winning votes at party conference, and even in having a group of representatives in parliament, has to be seen in the light of the ability of organisations such as the BMA to deal directly with ministers and civil servants and thereby to shape the policy agenda. Second, the 'vested interest' of the medical profession, of which the SMA had long warned, had indeed gained control of the NHS; and, moreover, once entrenched was able to dictate the terms of health policy with little outside interference. Hence even by the late 1940s it would have required a huge effort of political will, and certainly more influence than the Association was by itself able to command, to introduce into the service features actively opposed by the dominant professional group. Third, Wistow's distinction between a health service policy community and a health community, and the lack of importance attached to the wishes of health service consumers, vindicates the SMA's fears that in such a system curative medicine would triumph over preventive medicine, and that its version of the 'right to health' would not be fully realised.

Yet another political scientist, Douglas Ashford, sees in the development of the British 'welfare state' an inherent tendency towards 'subordinating ... localities'. This process, he argues, was furthered by local government's difficulties in imitating 'Whitehall methods', notably during the discussions of the later wartime period on social reconstruction. In the specific context of health policy, and when combined with the medical profession's antipathy to local government, 'traditional Westminster distrust of local governing capacities' resulted in the creation of 'fixed boundaries' between national and local responsibilities. This was despite the fact that a complex activity such as health care 'inescapably reaches across levels of government'. So while politically the NHS was an 'immense success', in terms of its capacity 'to adapt to new conditions, to redefine the aims of health and to accommodate a variety of political interests' it became an 'awkward and unwieldy instrument' – hence the various subsequent attempts at administrative reform. Finally, Ashford notes the 'irony' that one of the Labour government's 'great achievements' became, through the introduction of charges, the source of bitter party in-fighting, and thereby a prime example of the 'strange divorce of politics and policymaking in Britain'.[38]

While not all historians would agree with every aspect of Ashford's overall analysis, these particular points are illuminating in that, first, he places the fundamental disagreement between the SMA and Bevan over local control in the wider context of the evolution of British government. If, as he suggests, there was an overall trend away from devolved power, then the Association faced an even bigger task than it consciously realised. Second, Ashford's depiction of the inbuilt problems of the administrative structures created in 1946 would certainly have been agreed to by the SMA. Murray's remark that the service had to develop rather than stand still similarly gains credibility from such an analysis.

Third, Ashford's comment on the introduction of health service charges as exemplifying the 'divorce' between politics and policy making throws into sharp relief the radically different approaches to this issue taken by the government and by the SMA. For the former, Edith Summerskill saw no fundamental problem in imposing fees. This was simply a policy adjustment to take account of Treasury concerns over the level of public expenditure. The Association, by contrast, adopted the wholly political attitude that it was a betrayal of one of the most basic ideas on which a socialised service should be built. But, again from the government's point of view, this might be seen as a stance untainted by the responsibility of having to actually exercise power. The SMA was, by such a criterion, 'pure but impotent', and Bevan's dichotomy can be seen as a specific instance of Ashford's more general point. His analysis also should be seen in the context of Brooke's observation, noted in Chapter Eight, that after Beveridge the Labour Party shifted from making to evaluating policy.

In the light of all these considerations, it is tempting to see Bevan's jibe as cruel, but accurate. The SMA was a relatively small organisation which had significant problems in putting down roots in the broader labour movement and outside London. It had within it dissenting voices, both over the future direction of health policy and over loyalty to the Labour Party. In its attempts to achieve its radical vision of a socialised health service it faced powerful opponents, including others inside the labour movement as well as such predictable bodies as the BMA. Given these weaknesses, the Association was excluded from the most essential of the negotiations over the form and organisation of the health service. The nature of these negotiations also countered the SMA's ability to shape Labour health policy, since they took place without any significant reference to parliament or party conference.

It was, moreover, wildly optimistic about the mood of its fellow professionals, being over-inclined to see in the BMA position simply the rearguard action of a reactionary clique. The victory of the 'vested interest' of the medical profession, and the complex administrative structure over which it exerted so much influence, further ensured that matters close to the SMA's heart were unlikely to be realised in the now-established health service. Finally, the very nature of British politics appeared to operate against the type of devolved power promoted by the Association, and against its highly political view of the policy process. In short, political, professional, and structural factors conspired to ensure that the SMA's vision remained just that, rather than the comprehensive blueprint for a fully socialised health service.

The SMA's achievements

However we should not dismiss the SMA too lightly, for two broad reasons: it had a number of positive achievements in the period 1930 to 1951, and its analyses can be argued to have, in retrospect, a certain validity. One consequence of the latter point is that the Association's ideas continue to raise important questions about the nature of both social welfare and socialism. The positive achievements can be placed in three categories. First, the SMA's active support for medical refugees fleeing fascist persecution and for the democratic forces in the Spanish Civil War both merit considerable praise. Driven by an internationalist philosophy, medical and political, the SMA's humanitarianism was in marked contrast to the stance of bodies such as the BMA and the MPU.

Second, the Association played a significant role on the LCC in the 1930s, and was instrumental in shaping its health policy after 1934. This was closely scrutinised by the Ministry of Health, an indication of the influence which the country's largest single provider of medical care exerted on the wider community. Labour's victory was important to the broader labour movement and reinforced an existing component of left-wing thought favourable to devolved welfare services. The majority of SMA members involved with the council subscribed to this view, as well as gaining practical experience of administering health care. For Somerville Hastings in particular participation on the LCC was a defining moment in his own and his organisation's history. Of course, as he acknowledged, the Labour administration faced formidable obstacles to the full achievement of what he and his colleagues sought, and its health care record in the 1930s was mixed. But this should not obscure its successes, and the SMA's part in bringing them about. The LCC experience was therefore crucial not just for the people of London, but also for the Association in the refining of its plans for a socialised health service, these in turn feeding into Labour health policy.

And this brings us to the third point. It is easy to highlight the differences between, most obviously, Bevan and the SMA, and to suggest that the rejection of some of its more 'radical' proposals thereby constituted 'failure'. But it should also be borne in mind that when the Association was founded in 1930 Labour had little in the way of a detailed health programme. The organisation, by definition, focused on this issue. In so doing, it came up with new proposals as well as drawing on a tradition of socialist and reforming ideas stretching back to the Edwardian era. The SMA identified the Labour Party as the political vehicle most likely to bring about the kind of service it desired. The first fruits of this strategy were its successes at party conference in 1932 and in 1934, the latter marking a commitment on Labour's part to some form of state service. The Association also worked within the party's own policy-making structures and was thereby responsible for numerous policy documents and statements, culminating in *National Service for Health* in 1943. These various texts between them laid out in considerable detail plans for a universal and comprehensive service, free at the point of consumption and financed out of communal funds rather than some extended form of health insurance. Such a service was justified on the grounds that both the individual and society would benefit, in economic as well as health terms; of socialism, with its opposition to the anarchy, inequalities, and instabilities of capitalism; and of the full achievement of citizenship, health being as fundamental a right as, say, education. If not all features of its plan were realised through the NHS, nonetheless significant parts of it were.

None of this is to suggest that had the SMA not existed, then there would have been no National Health Service. But it did exist, and its part in articulating and shaping Labour's health policy through its writings and speeches; its committee work; its influence on the LCC; and its participation in party conferences should receive due acknowledgement. The attacks on the organisation by the BMA in the mid-1940s are in themselves evidence that the medical establishment took the Association 'threat' seriously. Stephen Taylor, in later life highly dismissive of the SMA, nonetheless acknowledged that at the end of the Second World War the 'Labour Party's preconceptions about the health service had been fostered by the Socialist Medical Association'.[39] We saw previously that the organisation was convinced that the NHS derived from the schemes it first laid out in the 1930s. There is certainly more to it than this, but on the other hand there is a significant measure of justification in the organisation's view that the service owed much to its own hard work, if not always in the fine detail then certainly in at least some of the general principles.

The Association therefore could feel justifiably proud of its activities in the 1930s and 1940s, its problems notwithstanding. With the benefit of historical hindsight it can also be argued that some of its analyses, dismissed or ignored at the time, have been vindicated. Its warnings over matters such as the implications of the tripartite structure of the NHS have been largely justified, as subsequent attempts at administrative reform attest. The SMA's predictions about the consequences of ceding power to the medical profession likewise have at least in part been realised, although the significance to be attached to this is rather more problematic, and is returned to briefly below.

Another area of concern to the SMA was, as we have repeatedly seen, local control of a socialised service. The argument used against this in the 1940s was that existing boundaries were unsuitable; that local authorities had shown themselves incapable of carrying out even existing health functions; that in consequence what was required was a national service; and that in any case the medical profession was adamant in its opposition. The SMA itself acknowledged that local government was in dire need of reform, and its inappropriateness to carry out the health functions of a socialised service has become received wisdom. As George Godber, in the 1940s a medical officer at the Ministry of Health, put it on the 25th anniversary of the NHS, areas that were 'quite appropriate for recruiting a Saxon fyrd a thousand years ago' were completely irrelevant when it came to the creation and administration of a modern health service. However, as Martin Powell has recently shown, close examination of municipal government's health care record in the 1930s shows it making significant advances throughout the country. The problems local authorities faced were as much to do with lack of resources, unsurprising during a decade of economic depression, than with any failure of political will on their own part.[40]

What all this suggests is that not only did the Association have tangible achievements during the 1930s and 1940s, but also that at least some of its radical and innovative policies need not necessarily be consigned to the dustbin of health service history. Indeed, a number of issues raised by the SMA pose serious questions about the nature of health service provision in advanced societies with characteristics such as political democracy and a high degree of division of labour. The first of these concerns the role of the consumer in a truly socialised health service. The Association promoted a participatory view of democracy, with power being both devolved and accountable, this in turn being an integral component of a socially responsible society. This was a version of socialism widely subscribed to by the democratic left in the 1930s and 1940s, and seen as a necessary safeguard against an over-central-ised and bureaucratic state. The SMA was therefore as concerned with means as with ends in the achievement of socialism, and as we noted in Chapter Four this places them in what Clarke describes as the 'moral' rather than the 'mechanical' reformist tradition.

If it is agreed that health service consumers should have a greater say in its administration, then this brings into serious question doctors' dominant role in shaping health policy. But it also raises a matter with which the Association grappled unsuccessfully throughout the 1930s and 1940s. For the SMA was concerned with both democratic account-ability and the preservation of professional autonomy and clinical judgement. As we saw in Chapter Three, its ideas were certainly social-ist in inspiration, but it also had a strong professional ethos. Both these issues are related to broader questions such as whether direct democ-racy and state welfare are, in the last resort, compatible; and whether professional power, autonomy, and judgement can, or indeed should, be reconciled with any form of democratic control.

On the latter point it is worth bearing in mind that Godber saw the decision in the 1940s to have Hospital Boards appointed rather than elected as 'the vital one for the future of the Health Service'. Appoint-ment allowed for, among other things, 'rational staffing' to be carried out by specialists able to guard against 'local favouritism on the one hand and favouritism from the academic centres on the other'.[41] From this medical dominance flows a number of other important points raised by the SMA, for example how should medical practitioners be remunerated; and, if it is accepted that the medical profession is more concerned with curative than with preventive medicine, how can a shift to the latter be effected? All these are matters of significance to both non-socialists and socialists. But for the latter they also raise issues of what is meant by a socialist health service, and of the role of welfare services in social transformation.

A socialist health service?

In late 1997, just prior to the 50th anniversary of the NHS, the journal *Health Care Analysis* took as its theme socialism and health. Address-ing the question 'Is a Socialist Health Service Possible?', its editorial concludes that the answer is 'yes', although not in the short term. Clear definitions of both 'health service' and 'socialist', it continued, are required. Similarly, the perceived tension between 'democracy' and 'socialism' has to be addressed, for example in areas such as private practice where it is often asserted that socialists wish to restrict individual 'freedom of choice'. Martin Powell, dealing specifically with the NHS, concludes that it was not in any real sense socialist when set up. He highlights, for example, the failure to introduce a salaried service, democratic control, and preventive medicine. Socialist medicine, Powell suggests, is not simply 'better distributed "capitalist medicine"' – qualitative change is also required. Calum Paton, analysing the 'necessary conditions' for a socialist health service, argues that this is 'more likely to flourish in a society which is more generally socialist'. Among his conditions for such a service are that it be 'integrated'. Dealing with administration he points out that while a socialist service would be democratically accountable, deciding at what level this would operate is 'not ... an easy choice'. Local government control, Paton suggests, can have negative as well as positive consequences, for instance through lack of adequately expert knowledge.[42]

As will be evident, these concerns are strikingly similar to a number of central SMA preoccupations. Powell's argument that a socialist health service involves not simply the allocation of resources but also qualitative change echoes Hastings's contrast between the Association's programme and the 'bulk purchase of the services of capitalist medicine'. The early introduction, by a Labour government, of prescription charges might be seen as highlighting the vulnerability of the latter approach. Paton, as well as drawing attention to the perennial problem of reconciling democracy with expert knowledge, implies problems in instituting a socialist health service in a predominantly capitalist society. Murray, 20 years previously, claimed that the failings of the NHS were at least in part due to the paradox of 'the idea behind the service (being) a socialist one although framed in a capitalist society'. This had led to an escalation of 'inevitable contradictions'.[43] If this was the case, however, does it mean that a truly socialist health service must await more widespread political and socio-economic change rather than, as the SMA's founders had hoped, playing a key role in the bringing about of a socialist society? This, for socialists, is a serious question, and harks back to the point noted above about the differences in the labour movement over the means and ends of socialism.

It is easy, of course, to stress the conceptual difficulties faced by Association members in their attempts to envisage a socialist medical service. Other examples might include the rather coercive nature of aspects of the 'right to health', noted in Chapter Seven, and Hastings's argument in the 1940s that the problem of 'reactionary' local authorities could be solved by obligatory rather than permissive legislation.[44]

This poses the obvious question: why have local autonomy in the first place, if its discretion is to be nationally circumscribed? However these contradictions do not necessarily undermine the validity of some key SMA ideas, especially for socialists. If it is the case that to achieve a socialist health service clear definitions of both 'socialism' and 'health service' are required, then for all their faults the Association's plans of the 1930s and 1940s bear re-examination and deserve applause. In particular the SMA's emphasis on a devolved and popularly accountable system which views health as more than simply the provision of medical services is worthy of reappraisal. This is particularly so at a time, such as the present, when the centralised, unaccountable institutions of the British welfare state are under increasing criticism, and when socialists themselves are having to review, reinvent, or rediscover central aspects of their ideology.

Notes

1. Donoughue and Jones, *Herbert Morrison*, p. 541.
2. See Murray, *Why a National Health Service?*, pp. 102–4 for a tribute to Hastings. Murray himself was the new president.
3. For a full account of the imposition of charges see Webster, *The Health Services since the War*, Ch. 5; Jim Tomlinson, 'Why So Austere? The British Welfare State of the 1940s', *Journal of Social Policy*, 27, January 1998; DSM 1/2, Minutes of Council, 30 November 1947; Parliamentary Debates, 5th series, vol. 470, cols 2241–9, 2251–4.
4. DSM (2) 4, cutting from *London News*, November 1949; DSM 1/3, EC Minutes, 2 November 1949.
5. DSM 6/25, 'Letter to Press from South London Doctors/SMA members to Press re Prescription charges', 3 February 1950.
6. DSM 5/4, cuttings from *The Daily Telegraph*, 2 May 1951, and from the *Fulham Gazette*, 11 May 1951.
7. DSM 1/3, EC Minutes, 2 May 1951; Parliamentary Debates, 5th series, vol. 470, cols 2275–6, 2283–6; DSM 1/3, EC Minutes, 4 January 1950.
8. DSM 1/25, Charles Brook, 'Health Centres', undated but 1946; *BMJ*, 1948, I, p. 272.
9. See the Labour Party annual reports for the relevant years; Anne Digby, *The Evolution of British General Practice, 1850–1948*, Oxford, Oxford University Press, forthcoming, Ch. 13 – I am grateful to Anne Digby for the opportunity to see an early draft of this chapter; DSM 1/2, EC Minutes, 20 October 1948; DSM 4/2, 'Report of a Meeting at the House of Commons on Wednesday 10 November, 1948'.
10. DSM 1/3, EC Minutes, 1 March 1950; SMA, *Bulletin*, 117, June–July 1950, p. 1.
11. DSM 1/3, EC Minutes, 17 July 1949; DSM 1/31. The Policy Committee prepared drafts for various Association publications.
12. DSM 1/2, Minutes of Council, 6 March 1949; Ian Gilliland, 'A Socialist Health Service', *MTT*, vol. 7, no. 1, Spring 1949, pp. 5–6.

13. *MTT*, vol. 8, no. 1, Spring 1951, p. 1.
14. Aneurin Bevan, *In Place of Fear*, Heinemann, 1952, p. 81; Francis, *Ideas and Policies under Labour*, p. 102; Webster, *The Health Services since the War*, pp. 148–9, 184.
15. Brooke, *Labour's War*, p. 330; DSH, File 22, 'NHS Miscellaneous', SMA, 'Conference at Battersea Town Hall, 29 October 1955: the Decline of the National Health Service'; Klein, *The New Politics of the NHS*, p. 29.
16. MH 133/63 and 64; Stewart, 'The "Back-Room Boys of State Medicine"', p. 229.
17. DSM 1/3, Minutes of Council, 23 October 1949.
18. DSM 1/3, Minutes of Council, 24 June 1951.
19. Honigsbaum, *Division in British Medicine*, p. 169.
20. MSS.79/MPU/1/2/2, Minutes of Council, 7 October 1948; DSM 1/3, EC Minutes, 21 September 1949; MSS.79/MPU/1/2/2, Minutes of Council, 11 December 1946.
21. MSS.79/MPU/1/1/1, Executive Committee Minutes, 10 November 1948; MSS.79/MPU/1/2/2, Minutes of Council, 8 December 1948; DSM 1/3, EC Minutes, 30 November 1949.
22. SMA, *Bulletin*, 117, June–July 1950, p. 2; DSM 1/3, EC Minutes, 10 January and 7 February 1951.
23. Honigsbaum, *Division in British Medicine*, pp. 272, 262; Earwicker, thesis, p. 208; DSH, File 49 'Socialist Medical Association, Miscellaneous Papers'; NEC Minutes, 26 February 1941.
24. DSM 1/2, Minutes of Council, 26 September 1948.
25. DSM 1/2, EC Minutes 1 June, 15 June, 29 June 1949; DSM 1/3, EC Minutes, 1 March 1950, Minutes of Special Meeting of the EC, 3 May 1950, EC Minutes, 11 October 1950 and 24 January 1951.
26. DSM (2) 18.
27. Honigsbaum, *Division in British Medicine*, pp. 284–6.
28. Fielding, Thompson, and Tiratsoo, *'England Arise!'*, p. 172.
29. DSH, file 15, 'Socialism', typescript by Somerville Hastings, 'Our Socialist Faith Restored', no date, but 1951; DSH, file 6, 'National Health Service', typescript by Somerville Hastings, 'Problems of the Welfare State', no date, but early 1950s (?); quoted in Brooke, *Labour's War*, p. 331. I am grateful to Stephen Brooke for pointing out Cole's critique of the post-war Labour governments, and its similarities with that of the SMA.
30. Earwicker, thesis, citing a joint TUC/BMA meeting in July 1944; Noel Whiteside, 'Creating the Welfare State in Britain, 1945–1960', *Journal of Social Policy*, 25, January 1996, pp. 89–93; Francis, *Ideas and Policies under Labour*, p. 7.
31. Morgan, *Labour in Power*, p. 16; Brooke, *Labour's War*, p. 337.
32. Rodney Barker, *Education and Politics 1900–1951: a Study of the Labour Party*, Oxford, Oxford University Press, 1972, Chs 4 and 5; Brooke, *Labour's War*, pp. 114–25, 198–200, 336–7.
33. *MTT*, vol. 8, no. 1, Spring 1951, p. 1; Charles Webster, 'Introduction', in Webster, Charles (ed.), *Aneurin Bevan on the National Health Service*, Oxford, University of Oxford Wellcome Unit for the History of Medicine, Research Publication Series, no. X, 1991; *idem, The National Health Service: A Political History*, Ch. 1; Taylor, *A Natural History of Everyday Life*, p. 296; Earwicker, thesis, pp. 350, 314; see also Francis, *Ideas and Policies under Labour*, p. 102ff.

34. Beach, thesis, pp. 241–2; Brooke, *Labour's War*, pp. 4, 285, 289–92.
35. Webster, 'Conflict and Consensus', pp. 143–7; Rodney Lowe, *The Welfare State in Britain since 1945*, Macmillan, 1993, pp. 42–5 – Chapter 3 of this work provides a useful introduction to, in its own words, 'The Nature of Policymaking'.
36. Christopher Ham, *Health Policy in Britain*, Macmillan, 3rd edn, 1992, p. 15, and citing the Normansfield Report p. 178.
37. R.A.W. Rhodes and David Marsh, 'Policy Networks in British Politics', in Marsh, David and Rhodes, R.A.W. (eds), *Policy Networks in British Government*, Oxford, Oxford University Press, 1992, pp. 13–14; Gerald Wistow, 'The Health Service Policy Community', in Marsh, David and Rhodes, R.A.W. (eds), *Policy Networks in British Government*, pp. 51–74.
38. Douglas Ashford, *The Emergence of the Welfare States*, Oxford, Blackwell, 1986, pp. 121–32, 275, 288–94.
39. Taylor, *A Natural History of Everyday Life*, p. 296.
40. Sir George Godber, *The Health Service: Past, Present and Future*, Athlone Press, 1975, pp. 18–19; Martin Powell, 'An Expanding Service: Municipal Acute Medicine in the 1930s', *Twentieth Century British History*, 8, 3, 1997.
41. Godber, *The Health Service*, pp. 16–17.
42. David Seedhouse, 'Is a Socialist Health Service Possible?', Martin Powell, 'Socialism and the British National Health Service'; and Calum Paton, 'Necessary Conditions for a Socialist Health Service', *Health Care Analysis*, 5, 3, 1997, pp. 183–5, 187–94 and 205–16 – cf. Francis, *Ideas and Policies under Labour*, p. 102 where he suggests that in the post-war era Labour supporters accepted that 'even after concessions had been made, the new service still successfully satisfied a number of socialist maxims', for example hospital nationalisation.
43. David Stark Murray and Joan Sohn-Rethel, *Health for 1000 Million People*, 1976, p. 1.
44. DSH, File 8, 'Social Medicine', typescript Somerville Hastings, 'An Attack on Democracy Through Health', n.d. but pre-NHS.

Bibliography

Primary sources

Archives

Socialist Medical Association Papers, Brynmor Jones Library, University of Hull. The following files have been used in the preparation of this study:

DSM 1/1, Minutes (Signed) of Annual General Meetings, with Reports of Executive Committee, 1931–39 – Reversed: SMA Bulletins (with Index) 1938–40.

DSM 1/2, Minutes (Signed) of Council and Executive Committee, 1946–49.

DSM 1/3, Minutes (Signed) of Council and Executive Committee, 1949–52.

DSM 1/6, File of Minutes of Executive Committee and Sub-Committees, 1941–46.

DSM 1/25, File of Policy (National Health Service) Committee Minutes (Signed) and Papers.

DSM 1/30, File of Policy Committee Memoranda, 1942–46.

DSM 1/31, File of Policy Committee Memoranda, 1948–51.

DSM 1/36, Sub-Committees.

DSM 4/1, Circulars 1930–39.

DSM 4/2, Circulars 1940–49.

DSM 5/1, Unbound Volume of Press Cuttings 1943–45.

DSM 5/4, Loose Press Cuttings 1938–65.

DSM 6/1, Notes on the History of the SMA.

DSM 6/10, Chadwick Lecture, Somerville Hastings, October 1944.

DSM 6/25, Letter to Press from South London Doctors/SMA members on Prescription Charges.

DSM 6/43, Cards for SMA Exhibition on Health Service.

DSM (2) 1, Minute Book of the State Medical Service Association, 1912–31.

DSM (2) 4, Press Cuttings – Articles and Reviews by David Stark Murray.

DSM (2) 5, General Correspondence, 1930–40.

DSM (2) 6, Bulletins, Circulars, Notices, Resolutions, Accounts etc., 1930–40.

DSM (2) 7, Various items, including Bevan correspondence.

DSM (2) 9, Circular and Posters.
DSM (3)/3, Honorary Secretary's correspondence.
DSM (3)/14, London Branch.

Somerville Hastings Papers, Brynmor Jones Library, University of Hull. This comes in two forms: first, 68 files of printed material, very loosely classified; second, three reels of microfilm of notes, and correspondence. Both of these are prefixed 'DSH'.

Fabian Society Papers, British Library of Political and Economic Science.

Arthur Greenwood Papers, Bodleian Library, Oxford.

Labour Party Papers, Museum of Labour History, Manchester. The material used in this study comes from both classified and unclassified material: see specific note references. Use has also been made of the microfilm/microfiche editions of the records of the Labour Party published by Research Publications.

Labour Spain Committee Papers, Churchill College, Cambridge.

London County Council Papers, London Metropolitan Archives, in the notes in the format LCC/MIN/XXXX.

London Labour Party Papers, London Metropolitan Archives, in the notes in the format Acc2417/X/X.

Medical Planning Commission Papers, British Medical Association Archive, BMA House, London.

Medical Practitioners' Union Papers, Modern Records Centre, University of Warwick, in the notes in the format MSS.79/MPU/X/X/X.

Ministry of Health Papers, Public Record Office, Kew, in the series MH 58, 71, 76, 77, 79, 80, 133. One of these, MH 77/63, is devoted entirely to the Socialist Medical Association.

Piercy Papers, British Library of Political and Economic Science.

Society for the Protection of Science and Learning Papers, Bodleian Library, Oxford.

Trades Union Congress Papers on Health Policy, Modern Records Centre, University of Warwick, in the notes in the format MSS/292/XXX/X.

Published material

Books and pamphlets

Attlee, Clement (1954), *As It Happened*, London: Heinemann.
Barker, Brian (1946), *Labour in London: a Study in Municipal Achievement*, London: Routledge and Sons.
Beckett-Overy, H., Hastings, Somerville and Freeman, Arnold (1910), *The Medical Proposals of the Minority Report: an Appeal to the Medical Profession*, London: H. and W. Brown.
Benjamin, Lawrence (1935), *The Position of the Middle-Class Worker in the Transition to Socialism*, The Labour Party.
Bevan, Aneurin (1952), *In Place of Fear*, London: Heinemann.
Bourne, Aleck (1942), *Health of the Future*, Harmondsworth: Penguin.
Brockway, Fenner (1949), *Bermondsey Story: the Life of Alfred Salter*, London: George Allen and Unwin.
Brook, Charles (1946), *Making Medical History*, London: Percy P. Buxton.
Brown, Irwin (David Stark Murray) (1948), *Back-Room Boys of State Medicine*, Socialist Medical Association.
Bunbury, Elizabeth (1941/42), *Health and the Medical Services*, Socialist Medical Association.
Hastings, Somerville (1923), *Labour, the Children's Champion*, TUC/Labour Party.
Hastings, Somerville (1926?), *Why this Poverty?*, Reading: Reading Labour Party.
Hastings, Somerville (1932), *Medicine in Soviet Russia*, n.p.
Hastings, Somerville (1932), *The People's Health*, The Labour Party.
Hastings, Somerville (1934), *A National Physiological Minimum: Fabian Tract 241*, The Fabian Society.
Hastings, Somerville (1941), *The Hospital Services: Research Series no. 59*, Fabian Society/Victor Gollancz.
Herbert, S.M. (1937), *Britain's Health*, Harmondsworth: Penguin.
Huxley, Julian et al. (1943), *When Hostilities Cease: Papers on Relief and Reconstruction prepared for the Fabian Society*, London: Victor Gollancz.
Labour Party (1921), *Memoranda Prepared by the Advisory Committee on Public Health: the Organisation of the Preventative and Curative Medical Services and Hospital and Laboratory Systems under a Ministry of Health; The Position of the General Medical Practitioner in a*

Reorganised System of Public Health; The Ministry of Health, Labour Party.

Labour Party (1924), *The Hospital Problem: the Report of a Special Conference of Labour, Hospital, Medical and Kindred Societies, held in the Caxton Hall, Westminster, on April 28th and 29th, 1924*, Labour Party.

Labour Party (1927), *Draft Report on the Nursing Profession*, Labour Party.

Labour Party Research Department (1931), *Reports Hospitals and the Patient; and a Domestic Workers Charter*, Labour Party.

Labour Party (1943), *National Service for Health*, Labour Party.

Labour Party (1943), *Notes for Discussion Groups on National Service for Health*, Labour Party.

London County Council (1946), *The Hospital Service*, London County Council.

London County Council (1949), *The LCC Hospitals: a Retrospect*, London County Council.

London Labour Party (1935), *Socialist Planning in London*, London Labour Party.

London Labour Party Health Research Group (1934), *The Public Health of London*, London Labour Publications.

London Trades Council and the Socialist Medical Association (1951), *TB: Report of Conference*, Socialist Medical Association.

Moore, Benjamin (1911), *The Dawn of the Health Age*, London: J. and A. Churchill.

Moore, Benjamin (1913), *First Steps Towards a State Medical Service*, State Medical Service Association.

Morrison, Herbert and Daines, D.H. (1935), *London under Socialist Rule*, Labour Party.

Murray, David Stark (1936), *Science Fights Death*, London: Watts and Co.

Murray, David Stark (1942), *The Future of Medicine*, Harmondsworth: Penguin.

Murray, David Stark (1948), *The Search for Health*, London: Watts and Co.

Murray, David Stark and Sohn-Rethel, Joan (1976), *Health for 1000 Million People*, Socialist Medical Association.

Murray, David Stark (1971), *Why a National Health Service?*, London: Pemberton Books.

Shirlaw, G.B. (1940), *Casualty: Training, Organisation and Administration of Civil Defence Casualty Services*, London: Secker and Warburg.

Shirlaw, G.B. and Troke, Clifford (1941), *Medicine Versus Invasion*, London: Secker and Warburg.

Sigerist, Henry E. (1937), *Socialised Medicine in the Soviet Union*, London: Victor Gollancz.

Socialist Medical Association (1933), *A Socialised Medical Service*, Socialist Medical Association.

Socialist Medical Association (1936), *Gas Attacks – Is there any Protection?*, Socialist Medical Association.

Socialist Medical Association (1941/42), *Medicine Tomorrow*, Socialist Medical Association, rev. edn.

Socialist Medical Association (1942), *The Socialist Programme for Health*, Socialist Medical Association.

Socialist Medical Association, *SMA Leaflet no. 1: the Beveridge Report and the Health Services*, Socialist Medical Association, n.d. but 1943?

Socialist Medical Association, *SMA Leaflet no. 2: Assumption B or the 'Panel'*, Socialist Medical Association, n.d. but 1943?

Socialist Medical Association (1943), *Health: What Needs to Be Done*, Socialist Medical Association.

Socialist Medical Association (1944), *A Socialised Health Service*, Socialist Medical Association.

Socialist Medical Association, *A National Health Service: the White Paper Examined: SMA Leaflet no.3*, Socialist Medical Association, n.d. but 1944?

Socialist Medical Association, *Child Health: a Survey and Proposals*, Today and Tomorrow Publications, n.d. but probably 1948.

Socialist Medical Association (1948), *A Socialised Dental Service: a Report produced by the Dental Group of the Socialist Medical Association*, Socialist Medical Association.

Socialist Medical Association (1949), *A Socialist Health Service*, Socialist Medical Association.

Socialist Medical Association (1951), *Get the Health Centres Going NOW*, Socialist Medical Association.

Socialist Medical Association, *The SMA and the Foundations of the National Health Service*, Socialist Medical Association, n.d. but 1980.

Spanish Medical Aid Committee (1937), *British Medical Aid in Spain*, Spanish Medical Aid Committee.

Taylor, Stephen (1944), *Battle for Health: a Primer of Social Medicine*, London: Nicholson and Watson.

Taylor, Stephen (1946), *National Health Service: Labour Party Discussion Series no.6*, Labour Party.

Taylor, Stephen (Lord Taylor of Harlow) (1988), *A Natural History of Everyday Life: a Biographical Guide for Would-Be Doctors of Society*, The Memoir Club.

Thomas, R.B. (1940), *The Health Services: Research Series no. 49*, Fabian Society.

Thompson, Brian (1942), *A Letter to a Doctor: Fabian Letter no. 6*, Fabian Society.

Trades Union Congress and the Labour Party (1922), *The Labour Movement and the Hospital Crisis*, Trades Union Congress and the Labour Party.

Trades Union Congress/Labour Party (1928), *Joint Committee on the Living Wage etc: Interim Report on Family Allowances and Child Welfare*, TUC/Labour Party.

Trades Union Congress (1930), *Family Allowances: Text of the Minority and Majority Reports issued by the TUC and Labour Party Joint Committee: Verbatim Report of the Debate at the Nottingham Conference*, TUC.

Webb, Sidney and Beatrice (1910), *The State and the Doctor*, London: Longmans, Green.

Major essays and chapters

Cole, Margaret (1948), 'Social Services and Personal Life', in Munro, Donald (ed.), *Socialism: the British Way*, London: Essential Books.

Hastings, Somerville (1948), 'Public Health', in Tracey, Herbert (ed.), *The British Labour Party – vol. II*, London: Caxton Publishing.

Murray, David Stark (1963), 'The National Health Service in Britain', in Evang, Karl, Murray, David S. and Lear, Walter J. (eds), *Medical Care and Family Security*, New Jersey: Prentice-Hall.

Periodicals and reports

British Medical Journal, *Bulletin* (of the Socialist Medical Association), *Fabian News*, *Fabian Quarterly*, *The Guardian*, *Labour Magazine*, *The Labour Woman*, *Lancet*, *London Labour Chronicle*, *London News*, *Medicine Today and Tomorrow*, *Socialist Doctor*; British Parliamentary Papers, Hansard (Parliamentary Debates, 5th series), Labour Party Annual Reports, Minutes of the London County Council.

Secondary sources

Books

Abel-Smith, Brian (1964), *The Hospitals 1800–1948*, London: Heinemann.

Ashford, Douglas (1986), *The Emergence of the Welfare States*, Oxford: Blackwell.

Barker, Rodney (1972), *Education and Politics 1900–1951: a Study of the Labour Party*, Oxford: Oxford University Press.

Bartrip, P.W.J. (1990), *Mirror of Medicine: a History of the BMJ*, London and Oxford: BMJ and Oxford University Press.

Bartrip, Peter (1996), *Themselves Writ Large: the British Medical Association 1832–1966*, London: BMJ Publishing Group.

Brooke, Stephen (1992), *Labour's War: the Labour Party during the Second World War*, Oxford: Oxford University Press.

Bryder, Linda (1988), *Below the Magic Mountain*, Oxford: Oxford University Press.

Buchanan, Tom (1991), *The Spanish Civil War and the British Labour Movement*, Cambridge: Cambridge University Press.

Campbell, John (1987), *Nye Bevan*, London: Hodder and Stoughton.

Clarke, Peter (1978), *Liberals and Social Democrats*, Cambridge: Cambridge University Press.

Collins, Kenneth (1988), *Go and Learn: the International Story of Jews and Medicine in Scotland*, Aberdeen: Aberdeen University Press.

Digby, Anne (forthcoming) *The Evolution of British General Practice, 1850–1948*, Oxford: Oxford University Press.

Donoughue, Bernard and Jones, G.W. (1973), *Herbert Morrison: Portrait of a Politician*, London: Weidenfeld and Nicolson.

Durbin, Elizabeth (1985), *New Jerusalems: the Labour Party and the Economics of Democratic Socialism*, London: Routledge and Kegan Paul.

Eckstein, Harry (1958), *The English Health Service*, Cambridge, Mass.: Harvard University Press.

Fielding, Steven, Thompson, Peter and Tiratsoo, Nick (1995), *'England Arise': the Labour Party and Popular Politics in 1940s Britain*, Manchester: Manchester University Press.

Foot, Michael (1975), *Aneurin Bevan 1945–1960*, London: Granada.

Foote, Geoffrey (1986), *The Labour Party's Political Thought*, 2nd edn, London: Croom Helm.

Fox, Daniel (1986), *Health Policies, Health Politics: the British and American Experience, 1911–1965*, Princeton, New Jersey: Princeton University Press.

Francis, Martin (1997), *Ideas and Policies under Labour, 1945–1951*, Manchester: Manchester University Press.

Fyrth, Jim (1986), *The Signal was Spain*, London: Lawrence and Wishart.

Gilbert, Bentley B. (1966), *The Evolution of National Insurance in Britain*, London: Michael Joseph.

Godber, Sir George (1975), *The Health Service: Past, Present and Future*, London: Athlone Press.

Graves, Pamela (1994), *Labour Women*, Cambridge: Cambridge University Press.

Ham, Christopher (1992), *Health Policy in Britain*, 3rd edn, London: Macmillan.

Hennessy, Peter (1992), *Never Again: Britain 1945–1951*, London: Jonathan Cape.

Hollis, Patricia (1997), *Jennie Lee: a Life*, Oxford: Oxford University Press.

Honigsbaum, Frank (1970), *The Struggle for the Ministry of Health*, Occasional Papers in Social Administration no. 37.

Honigsbaum, Frank (1979), *The Division in British Medicine*, London: Kogan Page.

Honigsbaum, Frank (1989), *Health, Happiness and Security: the Creation of the National Health Service*, London: Routledge.

Horne, John N. (1991), *Labour at War: France and Britain 1914–1918*, Oxford: Oxford University Press.

Howell, David (1976), *British Social Democracy*, London: Croom Helm.

Klein, Rudolf (1995), *The New Politics of the NHS*, 3rd edn, London: Longman.

Lee, Jennie (1980), *My Life with Nye*, London: Jonathan Cape.

Lindsey, Almont (1962), *Socialized Medicine in England and Wales*, Chapel Hill: University of North Carolina Press.

Lowe, Rodney (1993), *The Welfare State in Britain since 1945*, London: Macmillan.

McBriar, A.M. (1987), *An Edwardian Mixed Doubles*, Oxford: Oxford University Press.

McGucken, William (1984), *Scientists, Society and State: the Social Relations of Science Movement in Britain*, Columbus, Ohio: Ohio State University Press.

Mackenzie, Norman and Jeanne (1977), *The First Fabians*, London: Weidenfeld and Nicolson.

McKibbin, Ross (1974), *The Evolution of the Labour Party 1910–1924*, Oxford: Oxford University Press.

Marks, Lara (1996), *Metropolitan Mortality*, Amsterdam: Rodopi.

Morgan, Kenneth and Jane (1980), *Portrait of a Progressive*, Oxford: Oxford University Press.

Morgan, Kenneth (1984), *Labour in Power 1945–1951*, Oxford: Oxford University Press.

Navarro, Vicente (1978), *Class Struggle, the State and Medicine*, Oxford: Martin Robertson.

Pater, John (1981), *The Making of the National Health Service*, King's Fund Historical Series 1.

Perkin, Harold (1989), *The Rise of Professional Society*, London: Routledge.

Pimlott, Ben (1977), *Labour and the Left in the 1930s*, Cambridge: Cambridge University Press.

Prochaska, Frank (1992), *Philanthropy and the Hospitals of London*, Oxford: Oxford University Press.

Pugh, Martin (1993), *The Making of Modern British Politics*, 2nd edn, Oxford: Blackwell.

Rivett, Geoffrey (1986), *The Development of the London Hospital System 1832–1982*, King Edward's Hospital Fund for London.

Sherman, A.J. (1994), *Island Refuge: Britain and Refugees from the Third Reich*, 2nd edn, Ilford: Frank Cass.

Tanner, Duncan (1990), *Political Change and the Labour Party, 1900–1918*, Cambridge: Cambridge University Press.

Trueta-Raspall, Josep (1967), *Joseph Trueta: a List of his Appointments, Distinctions, and Publications*, Oxford, n.p.

Watkins, Steve (1987), *Medicine and Labour: the Politics of a Profession*, London: Lawrence and Wishart.

Webster, Charles (1988), *The Health Services since the War: vol. 1 Problems of Health Care – The National Health Service before 1957*, London: HMSO.

Webster, Charles (ed.) (1991), *Aneurin Bevan on the National Health Service*, Oxford: University of Oxford, Wellcome Unit for the History of Medicine, Research Publication Series no. X.

Webster, Charles (1998), *The National Health Service: A Political History*, Oxford: Oxford University Press.

Werskey, Gary (1988), *The Visible College*, London: Free Association Books.

Williams, A. Susan (1997), *Women and Childbirth in the Twentieth Century*, Stroud: Sutton.

Articles and chapters

Berghahn, Marion (1984), 'German Jews in England', in Hirschfeld, Gerhard (ed.), *Exile in Great Britain*, Leamington Spa: Berg.

Burleston, Louise (1993), 'The State, Internment and Public Criticism in the Second World War', in Cesarani, David and Kushner, Tony (eds), *The Internment of Aliens in Twentieth-Century Britain*, Ilford: Frank Cass.

Clarke, Peter (1983), 'The Social Democratic Theory of the Class Struggle', in Winter, Jay (ed.), *The Working Class in Modern British History*, Cambridge: Cambridge University Press.

Deakin, Nicholas and Wright, Anthony (1995), 'Tawney', in George,

Vic and Page, Robert (eds), *Modern Thinkers on Welfare*, Hemel Hempstead: Prentice Hall/Harvester Wheatsheaf.

Digby, Anne and Bosanquet, Nick (1988), 'Doctors and Patients in an Era of National Health Insurance and Private Practice, 1913–1938', *Economic History Review*, 2nd series, vol. 41, no. 1.

Earwicker, Ray (1979), 'A Study of the BMA-TUC Joint Committee on Medical Questions, 1935–1939', *Journal of Social Policy*, vol. 8.

Earwicker, Ray (1981), 'The Emergence of a Medical Strategy in the Labour Movement 1906–1919', *Bulletin of the Society for the Social History of Medicine*, no. 29, December.

Esping-Andersen, Gosta (1987), 'Citizenship and Socialism: De-Commodification and Solidarity in the Welfare State', in Rein, Martin, Esping-Andersen, Gosta and Rainwater, Lee (eds), *Stagnation and Renewal in Social Policy*, Armonk, New York: M.E. Sharpe Inc.

Fox, Daniel (1986), 'The National Health Service and the Second World War: the Elaboration of Consensus', in Smith, H.L. (ed.), *War and Social Change*, Manchester: Manchester University Press.

Hall, Phoebe (1975), 'The Development of Health Centres', in Hall, Phoebe et al., *Change, Choice and Conflict in Social Policy*, London: Heinemann.

Jefferys, Kevin (1987), 'British Politics and Social Policy During the Second World War', *Historical Journal*, vol. 30, no. 1.

Joicey, Nicholas (1993), 'A Paperback Guide to Progress: Penguin Books 1935–c. 1951', *Twentieth Century British History*, vol. 4, no. 1.

Kerr, David (1960), 'Politics and the National Health Service', in SMA (ed.), *Aneurin Bevan: an Appreciation of his Services to the Health of the People*, Socialist Medical Association.

Lee, Roger (1988), 'Uneven Zenith: towards a Geography of the High Period of Municipal Medicine in England and Wales', *Journal of Historical Geography*, vol. 14, no. 3.

Lewis, Jane and Brookes, Barbara (1983), 'The Peckham Health Centre, "PEP", and the concept of General Practice during the 1930s and 1940s', *Medical History*, vol. 27.

Lindsay, Kenneth (1981), 'PEP through the 1930s: Organisation, Structure, People', in Pinder, John (ed.), *Fifty Years of Political and Economic Planning*, London: Heinemann.

London, Louise (1990), 'Jewish Refugees and British Government Policy, 1930–1940', in Cesarani, David (ed.), *The Making of Modern Anglo-Jewry*, Oxford: Blackwell.

Loudon, Irvine (1986), 'Deaths in Childbed from the Eighteenth Century to 1935', *Medical History*, vol. 30.

Marwick, Arthur (1964), 'Middle Opinion in the Thirties: Planning,

Progress and Political Agreement', *English Historical Review*, vol. LXXIX.

Marwick, Arthur (1967), 'The Labour Party and the Welfare State in Britain', *American Historical Review*, December.

Meisel, Joseph S. (1994), 'Air Raid Shelter Policy and its Critics in Britain before the Second World War', *Twentieth Century British History*, vol. 5, no. 3.

Nicholson, Max (1981), 'PEP through the 1930s: Growth, Thinking, Performance', in Pinder, John (ed.), *Fifty Years of Political and Economic Planning*, London: Heinemann.

Paton, Calum (1997), 'Necessary Conditions for a Socialist Health Service', *Health Care Analysis*, vol. 5, no. 3.

Pelling, Henry (1986), 'The Impact of the War on the Labour Party', in Smith, H.L. (ed.) *War and Social Change*, Manchester: Manchester University Press.

Porter, Dorothy (1992), 'Changing Disciplines: John Ryle and the Making of Social Medicine in Britain in the 1940s', *History of Science*, vol. XXX.

Porter, Dorothy (1993), 'John Ryle: Doctor of Revolution?', in Porter, Dorothy and Porter, Roy (eds), *Doctors, Politics and Society: Historical Essays*, Amsterdam: Rodopi.

Powell, Martin (1994), 'The Forgotten Anniversary? An Examination of the 1944 White Paper, "A National Health Service"', *Social Policy and Administration*, vol. 28, no. 4.

Powell, Martin (1997), 'Socialism and the British National Health Service', *Health Care Analysis*, vol. 5, no. 3.

Powell, Martin (1997), 'An Expanding Service: Municipal Acute Medicine in the 1930s', *Twentieth Century British History*, vol. 8, no. 3.

Rhodes, R.A.W. and Marsh, David (1992), 'Policy Networks in Britain', in Marsh, David and Rhodes, R.A.W. (eds), *Policy Networks in British Government*, Oxford: Oxford University Press.

Ritschel, Daniel (1995), 'The Making of Consensus: the Nuffield College Conferences during the Second World War', *Twentieth Century British History*, vol. 6, no. 3.

Seedhouse, David (1997), 'Editorial: Is a Socialist Health Service Possible?', *Health Care Analysis*, vol. 5, no. 3.

Sheldrake, John (1989), 'The LCC Hospital Service', in Saint, Andrew (ed.) *Politics and the People of London: the London County Council 1889–1965*, London: Hambledon Press.

Stewart, John (1993), 'Ramsay MacDonald, the Labour Party, and Child Welfare, 1900–1914', *Twentieth Century British History*, vol. 4, no. 2.

Stewart, John (1995), 'Socialist Proposals for Health Care Reform in

Inter-War Britain: the Case of Somerville Hastings', *Medical History*, vol. 39, July.

Stewart, John (1996), '"The Children's Party, therefore the Women's Party": the Labour Party and Child Welfare in Inter-War Britain', in Digby, Anne and Stewart, John (eds), *Gender, Health and Welfare*, London: Routledge.

Stewart, John (1996), 'The "Back-Room Boys of State Medicine": David Stark Murray and Bevan's National Health Service', *Journal of Medical Biography*, November.

Stewart, John (1997), '"For a Healthy London": the Socialist Medical Association and the London County Council in the 1930s', *Medical History*, vol. 41, October.

Stewart, John (forthcoming) 'Somerville Hastings' and 'David Stark Murray', in the *New Dictionary of National Biography*, British Academy/Oxford University Press, forthcoming 2004.

Terris, Milton (1986), 'Epidemiology and the Public Health Movement', *Journal of Chronic Diseases*, vol. 39, no. 12.

Thane, Pat (1985), 'The Labour Party and State "Welfare"', in Brown, K.D. (ed.), *The First Labour Party*, London: Croom Helm.

Thane, Pat (1993), 'Women in the British Labour Party and the Construction of State Welfare, 1906–1939', in Koven, Seth and Michel, Sonya (eds), *Mothers of a New World*, London: Routledge.

Tomlinson, Jim (1992), 'Planning: Debate and Policy in the 1940s', *Twentieth Century British History*, vol. 3, no. 2.

Tomlinson, Jim (1998), 'Why So Austere? The British Welfare State of the 1940s', *Journal of Social Policy*, vol. 27, January.

Wasserstein, Bernard (1984), 'The British Government and the German Immigration 1933–1945', in Hirschfeld, Gerhard (ed.), *Exile in Great Britain*, Leamington Spa: Berg.

Webster, Charles (1988), 'Labour and the Origins of the National Health Service', in Rupke, Nicolaas (ed.), *Science, Politics and the Public Good*, London: Macmillan.

Webster, Charles (1990), 'Doctors, Public Service and Profit: General Practitioners and the National Health Service', *Transactions of the Royal Historical Society*, 5th series, vol. 40.

Webster, Charles (1990), 'Conflict and Consensus: Explaining the British Health Service', *Twentieth Century British History*, vol. 1, no. 2.

Webster, Charles (1993), 'The Metamorphosis of Dawson of Penn', in Porter, Dorothy and Porter, Roy (eds), *Doctors, Politics and Society: Historical Essays*, Amsterdam: Rodopi.

Weindling, Paul (1991), 'The Contribution of Central European Jews to Medical Science and Practice in Britain, the 1930s–1950s', in Mosse,

W.E. (ed.), *Second Chance: Two Centuries of German-speaking Jews in the United Kingdom*, Tübingen: J.C.B. Mohr.

Whiteside, Noel (1996), 'Creating the Welfare State in Britain, 1945–1960', *Journal of Social Policy*, vol. 25, January.

Wistow, Gerald (1992), 'The Health Service Policy Community', in Marsh, David and Rhodes, R.A.W. (eds), *Policy Networks in British Government*, Oxford: Oxford University Press.

Unpublished theses

Earwicker, Ray (1982), 'The Labour Movement and the Creation of the National Health Service 1906–1948', PhD, University of Birmingham.

Beach, Abigail (1996), 'The Labour Party and the Idea of Citizenship, *c.* 1931–1951', PhD, University of London.

Index

Printed and bound by CPI Group (UK) Ltd, Croydon, CR0 4YY

21/10/2024

01777087-0015